Physical Activity and Health Promotion:
...tice

Edited by

Lindsey Du

Diane Cror

and

Rebecca M

This book is due for return on or before the last date shown below.

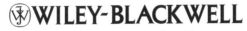

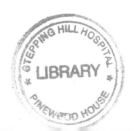

ⓦWILEY-BLACKWELL
A John Wiley & Sons, Ltd., Publication

This edition first published 2009
© 2009 Blackwell Publishing Ltd

Blackwell Publishing was acquired by John Wiley & Sons in February 2007.
Blackwell's publishing programme has been merged with Wiley's global Scientific,
Technical, and Medical business to form Wiley-Blackwell.

Registered office
John Wiley & Sons Ltd, The Atrium, Southern Gate, Chichester, West Sussex,
PO19 8SQ, United Kingdom

Editorial offices
9600 Garsington Road, Oxford, OX4 2DQ, United Kingdom
2121 State Avenue, Ames, Iowa 50014-8300, USA

For details of our global editorial offices, for customer services and for information
about how to apply for permission to reuse the copyright material in this book
please see our website at www.wiley.com/wiley-blackwell.

The right of the author to be identified as the author of this work has been asserted
in accordance with the Copyright, Designs and Patents Act 1988.

Library of Congress Cataloging-in-Publication Data
Physical activity and health promotion: evidence-based approaches to practice/edited
by Lindsey Dugdill, Diane Crone, Rebecca Murphy.
    p. ; cm.
  Includes bibliographical references and index.
  ISBN 978-1-4051-6925-7 (pbk. : alk. paper)
  1. Exercise. 2. Health promotion. 3. Evidence-based medicine. I. Dugdill, Lindsey.
  II. Crone, Diane. III. Murphy, Rebecca.
  [DNLM: 1. Exercise. 2. Evidence-Based Medicine. 3. Health Behavior.
  4. Health Promotion. QT 255 P57215 2008]

  RA781.P5615 2008
  613.7—dc22

                                                        2008030013

A catalogue record for this book is available from the British Library.

Set in 10/12.5 pt Palatino by Newgen Imaging Systems Pvt. Ltd, Chennai, India
Printed in Singapore by C.O.S Printers Pte Ltd

1   2009

Contents

Contributors

Colin Baker, BA (Hons), MSc, Dip FTST
Colin is a PhD research student at the Faculty of Sport, Health and Social Care at the University of Gloucestershire. His main research interests are in evaluating methods of delivery for community sport and physical activity initiatives and the role played by professionals in exercise provision.

Jeff David Breckon, BSc (Hons), MSc, PGCert HE, PhD, C Psychol
Jeff is senior lecturer in exercise psychology at Sheffield Hallam University. He is a member of BASES, the BPS and the Motivational Interviewing Network of Trainers. He has published internationally in physical activity counselling and has over 14 years experience of physical activity referral schemes across the UK.

Nick Cavill, BA (Hons), MPH
Nick is an independent health promotion consultant, a research associate of the University of Oxford BHF Health Promotion Research Group, an associate of the BHF National Centre for Physical Activity and Health at Loughborough University and honorary senior research fellow, University of Salford. He specialises in the development of policy and programmes on physical activity and sport and sustainable transport.

Margaret Coffey, BA (Hons), PhD
Margaret is a senior lecturer in Health at Liverpool Hope University. She is a member of the Institute of Health Promotion & Education and the UK Public Health Association. Her main research interests are on the impact of the work environment on stress, health and well-being.

Diane Crone, BSc (Hons), PhD
Diane is reader in exercise science at the Faculty of Sport, Health and Social Care at the University of Gloucestershire and is a BASES accredited exercise scientist (support and research). Her main research interests and activities are in the evaluation of exercise referral schemes and the holistic role of physical activity for people with mental health problems.

Lindsey Dugdill, BA (Hons), MA, MPhil, PhD
Lindsey is reader in exercise and health at the University of Salford. She worked (1993–2000) as research advisor on the Health Education Authority's Health at Work in the NHS programme and has been a consultant for the World Health Organization publishing work on health evaluation. Her current research focuses on physical activity promotion in all community settings.

Chris Gidlow, BSc (Hons), MSc, PhD
Chris is a researcher within the Centre for Sport and Exercise Research at Staffordshire University. His main research interests and activities are in exercise referral, children's physical activity, and more recently, the relationship between physical activity and the environment.

Linda Heaney, MBBS, LLM, MRCPsych
Linda Heaney is a consultant psychiatrist working in a Support and Recovery Team in Bristol. She is keen to promote physical activity as part of a holistic approach in working towards recovery in mental health problems.

Andrew John Hutchison, BSc (Hons), MSc
Andrew is a doctoral student at Sheffield Hallam University. His research interests are centred around physical activity behaviour change. His PhD is using a grounded theory methodology to investigate how people make long-term behavioural changes to their physical activity habits.

Lynne Halley Johnston, BA (Hons), MSc, PhD, CPsychol
Lynne is a chartered psychologist (BPS), an Accredited Sport and Exercise Psychologist (BASES), and a recognised trainer in Motivational Interviewing (MINT). She has supervised several PhD students and published internationally on physical activity promotion. Formerly a reader in exercise psychology, at Sheffield Hallam University, she is currently completing her second doctorate in Clinical Psychology at Newcastle University.

Jim McKenna, BHum (Hons), MPhil, PhD
Jim is professor of physical activity and health at Leeds Metropolitan University and is head of the Active Lifestyles research centre. He publishes extensively and was a scientific contributor to the Chief Medical Officer's Report (2004). He researches workplace and community interventions, currently focusing on ageing and health literacy.

Sara Moore
Sara Moore is the programme lead for Public Health and Physical Activity, Offender Health, Department of Health. This work involves her in policy development as well as operational implementation. Sara is a Fellow of the Royal Institute of Public Health.

Rebecca Murphy, BSc (Hons), PGCert, LTHE, PhD

Rebecca is lecturer in exercise and health at Liverpool John Moores University, on the BSc Physical Activity, Exercise and Health degree programme. Rebecca's doctoral work investigated the effectiveness of an exercise referral programme using key stakeholder perspectives (participants, exercise professionals and health professionals).

Christopher Stephen Owens, BSc (Hons), PGCert, MSc (Res)

Christopher is a PhD student in the Faculty of Sport, Health and Social Care at the University of Gloucestershire. His main research interests are around sport and physical activity participation in adolescents and the place and promotion of well-being for service users within mental health services.

Andy Smith, BA (Hons), PhD, FBASES

Andy is the director of Institutional Advancement at York St John University. He is a professor of exercise and sports science and was made an Honorary Fellow of BASES for his 'exceptional contribution'. Andy has written extensively on physical activity. His current interests are rehabilitation from neurosurgery and futurology.

Afroditi Stathi, BSc (Hons), MSc, PhD

Afroditi is a lecturer in exercise psychology in the School for Health at the University of Bath. Her research focuses on two inter-related themes: the relationship between physical activity and well-being, particularly in older adults, and the effectiveness of physical activity interventions.

Gareth Stratton, BHum (Hons), PGCE, MPhil, PhD

Gareth is professor in paediatric exercise science at Liverpool John Moores University. He chairs the Research into Exercise, Activity and Children's Health (REACH) Group and the National Institute for Health and Clinical Excellence group, currently writing national guidelines for physical activity in young people. His current reseach involves evaluating physical activity interventions in children and adolescents.

Paula Watson, BSc (Hons), MSc

Paula is principal researcher on the GOALS project at Liverpool John Moores University, working with agencies across the North-West of England to develop and evaluate a family-centred lifestyle intervention for obese children. Paula's research interests lie in the psychosocial process of adopting and adhering to a physically active lifestyle, particularly in the role played by the family in children's experiences of activity.

Foreword

This book must be placed in the context of contemporary lifestyles, the widely varying physical activities of people and the morbidities associated with long-term sedentary behaviour. Among the disorders due to an imbalance between daily energy intake and energy expenditure are the cardiovascular diseases, metabolic syndrome, overweight and obesity, mental health problems and certain forms of cancer – the list is long and the evidence for a link is well established. Yet denial is a commonplace reaction of individuals in the community at large, solutions are offered but the problems persist or are getting worse. The increased prevalence of obesity across developed countries, and through the lifespan from childhood, is on a scale that causes bewilderment with regard to how easily humans can activate a virtual self-destruct button. Defective genes, conspicuous consumption, fast-food facilities, and sloth have all been in the firing line but the causes and remedies are complex. We need to have a better understanding of these causal phenomena if this adverse trend is to be halted and reversed. The content of this book should go some way towards developing this understanding from individual to societal levels and to providing frameworks within which solutions may be implemented and evaluated.

It is clear that physical activity and exercise programmes have a role to play alongside nutrition and habitual activity patterns in both disease prevention and health promotion. The gains are manifold, ranging from benefits of self-satisfaction and personal worth to the workplace benefits of enhanced mobility, fitness status and improved weight control. Yet for those who might gain most health-wise from activity programmes, compliance is a persistent and obdurate challenge. It is a truism that humans are reluctant to change, particularly from a passive lifestyle that encourages indulgence. In this text various theories of behaviour change are considered and placed in the context of exercise as a public health intervention.

The editors have done a remarkable job in pulling together the expert contributions from different authors in order to draw out the many contemporary issues associated with promoting healthy lifestyles.

They accommodate a range of perspectives including medical and non-medical models of health and place a number of current policies and initiatives in context. The interdisciplinary nature of the text enhances its readability, with explanations of the social and political milieu for different schemes. The material is supported by a comprehensive evidence base and augmented by illustrations where appropriate.

The book should be a valuable learning resource for a range of health professionals and students with an interest in physical activity and exercise. The former includes personnel employed in various guises as health promotion specialists. The latter includes those working towards academic qualifications in health studies, exercise and health, sport and exercise sciences, physiotherapy and related disciplines. It should be an essential reference for those engaged in health-related projects and for healthcare professionals and their peers in community schemes. All of these readers should benefit from the information provided in this text as well as gain inspiration from the enthusiasm and commitment of the contributors to this book. It is a landmark volume which is authoritative and informative.

Thomas Reilly, BA, Dip PE, M Sc, PhD, DSc,
DHC, F Erg S, FI Biol, FRSM

Director, Research Institute for Sport and Exercise Sciences,
Liverpool John Moores University

Dedication

To our parents with dearest love and thanks to Tom Reilly, a much valued friend, colleague and mentor

Acknowledgements

The editors would like to thank everyone who has supported the production of this book. Firstly, the contributors – for their wide-ranging expertise, enthusiasm and engagement with the material for this book. It would not have been possible without their dedication to the task and for that we are very grateful.

Secondly, the publishing team at Wiley-Blackwell, including Amy Brown, who have made the process both enjoyable and enlightening.

To colleagues and in particular, Linzi Mackie at University of Salford, for technical support.

To our families who have, as always, supported us throughout the process of writing this book. It is their love and support that makes all things possible.

Finally, very sincere thanks to all the practitioners, professionals, general public and students whom we have worked with. The contribution of each individual has helped to shape our interest and understanding of physical activity and its promotion in the community.

Part I Concepts for the development of physical activity practice

Part I consists of four chapters: Chapter 1 provides an introduction to physical activity promotion by presenting definitions, explanations and health promotion approaches to improving health. Chapter 2 presents a critical appraisal of health behaviour theory and provides a contemporary perspective for practice. In Chapter 3 the importance of policy and the political context of physical activity promotion is analysed. Chapter 4 concludes the section with an explanation of the process of evaluation to guide the reader through key principles of intervention evaluation.

1 Physical activity, health and health promotion

Rebecca Murphy, Lindsey Dugdill and Diane Crone

Introduction

Physical activity research has clearly established the link between inactivity and poor health status in populations (United States Department of Health and Human Services, 1996; Department of Health, 2004 a,b,c; Department of Health, 2005). In addition, it is widely accepted that population physical activity levels in the UK are lower than that recommended for ensuring optimal health. Physical inactivity is becoming an issue of extreme public health importance to all health professionals and agencies within the UK, across Europe and in other Western industrialised countries. A range of global and international health policies outline the significance to public health of promoting healthy lifestyles in the twenty first century (Department of Health, 2004a, 2008; World Health Organisation [WHO], 2004; Wanless, 2004; Hillsdon *et al.*, 2004). In the UK, physical activity is cited as a key intervention to tackle many health problems (Department of Health 2004a). The Department of Health has a joint public service agreement with the Treasury, the Department for Education and Skills and the Department for Culture Media and Sport (DCMS, 2002) to halt the year-on-year rise in obesity among children under 11 by 2010, in the context of a broader strategy to tackle obesity in the population as a whole (Dugdill and Stratton, 2007; Department of Health, 2008). In addition, the importance of physical activity as a risk factor for coronary heart disease is increasingly being recognised throughout Europe (Health Enhancing Physical Activity Guidelines [HEPA], 2000) and beyond (WHO, 2004).

Physical activity is a key component to maintaining a healthy lifestyle for all individuals. To assist in contextualising the significance of physical activity promotion to public health, this chapter outlines and considers definitions of health and health promotion, health trends, and current recommendations for physical activity within health promotion.

> **Learning outcomes**
>
> The aims of this chapter are to:
>
> 1. define concepts of physical activity, exercise, health and health promotion
> 2. introduce relevant policy drivers
> 3. describe current trends in physical activity participation
> 4. introduce concepts and determinants of health and health promotion
> 5. explain the public health importance of physical activity promotion
> 6. outline approaches to physical activity promotion in the UK

Defining exercise and physical activity

Physical activity is defined as any bodily movement produced by skeletal muscles that results in energy expenditure (Caspersen *et al.*, 1985). It has dimensions of 'volume (how much), duration (how long), frequency (how often), intensity (how hard) and mode (what type)' (Cale and Harris, 2005, p. 7). It is, therefore, a multi-faceted, complex and broad-ranging behaviour that may encompass activities of daily living (housework, gardening, stair climbing), occupation-related activity completed as part of one's job (walking, hauling, lifting and packing), transportation physical activity [walking, biking or wheeling (for wheelchair users), to and from places)] also known as active travel or transport, leisure time activity (exercise, sports recreation or hobbies), or engagement in specific prescribed interventions (Dugdill and Stratton, 2007). Exercise is considered a subset of physical activity which includes planned, structured, and repetitive bodily movement which is undertaken to improve or maintain one or more components of physical fitness (Casperson *et al.*, 1985).

Understanding the political climate

In recent years, the Chief Medical Officer has collated and summarised the scientific evidence on the contribution of active living to promoting health and well-being across the lifespan (Department of Health, 2004b). Evidence suggests that increasing physical activity participation could significantly contribute to the prevention and management of over 20 diseases and conditions. In addition it is estimated that the cost of inactivity in England could be £8.2 billon annually (DCMS, 2002). In recent years various targets for increasing participation levels in sport and physical activity have been proposed. These include a target to increase participation levels to 70% of individuals undertaking 30 minutes of physical activity 5 days a week by 2020 (DCMS, 2002), and a less ambitious target of an increase in participation to 50% by 2020

(Wanless, 2004) (see also Chapters 3 and 6). Physical activity promotion was a key target of the Public Health White Paper Choosing Health: Making Healthier Choices Easier (Department of Health, 2004a). Furthermore, Choosing Activity: A Physical Activity Action Plan (Department of Health, 2005) outlined the action that needs to be taken in order to promote physical activity in the UK, and documents Government priorities for physical activity promotion in the form of cross-departmental Public Service Agreement Targets, which are:

'To halt the year-on-year increase in obesity among children under 11 by 2010, in the context of a broader strategy to tackle obesity in the population as a whole.

By 2008, increase the uptake of cultural and sporting opportunities by adults and young people aged 16 and above from priority groups by increasing the number of people who participate in active sports, at least 12 times a year by 3% and increasing the number who engage in at least 30 minutes of moderate intensity level sport, at least 3 times a week by 3%.

Enhance the take-up of sporting opportunities by 5–16 year olds so that the percentage of school children in England who spend a minimum of two hours each week on high quality PE and school sport, within and beyond the curriculum, increases from 25% in 2002 to 75% by 2006 and 85% by 2008 in England, and at least 75% in each school sport partnership by 2008'.

(Department of Health, 2005, p. 7)

Physical activity prevalence and trends

Worldwide, 60% of the population are insufficiently active to benefit their health (WHO, 2004) and physical activity levels in the UK are exceptionally low (Department of Health, 2004b); e.g. only 21% of the adult population are regularly participating in sport or recreational activity (defined as taking part, on at least 3 days a week, in moderate intensity sport and active recreation, for at least 30 minutes continuously in any one session) (Sport England, 2006). Variation in participation exists according to demographic variables. More males (37%) than females (25%), residing within the UK, attain current recommended activity guidelines (Department of Health, 2004c), participation declines with age for both men and women and, compared with the general population, men from certain ethnic groups (Indian, Pakistani, Bangladeshi and Chinese) are less likely to meet physical activity recommendations (Department of Health, 2004c). According to the National Travel Survey (Department for Transport, 2001) between 1975–1976 and

1999–2001 average miles travelled by foot and bicycle had decreased by approximately 26%. In contrast, participation levels in selected leisure time physical activity such as walking, swimming and keep-fit/yoga were reported to have increased or at least remained the same between 1987 and 1996 (Department for Transport, 2001). In conclusion, therefore, over the past 20–30 years it seems that there has been a significant decrease in physical activity as part of daily routines and a small increase in activity during leisure time.

Health and health promotion

Health is a multidisciplinary concept, which encompasses states of both positive and negative well-being. Definitions of health arise from different perspectives, and as such, broad variations exist (Lucas and Lloyd, 2005). Historically, definitions have evolved with social change:

> 'The rising expectations of the past 150 years have led to a shift away from viewing health in terms of survival, through a phase of defining it in terms of freedom from disease, onward to an emphasis on an individuals ability to perform daily activities, and more recently to an emphasis on positive themes of happiness, social and emotional well-being, and quality of life'. (Lindau et al., 2003, p. 3)

In 1948 the World Health Organisation defined health as 'a complete state of physical, mental and social well-being, and not merely the absence of disease or infirmity' (cited in Nutbeam, 1998, p. 351). This definition encapsulates health as both a positive and holistic concept emphasising physical, mental and social elements. In contrast, biomedical models of health propose a negative definition, through which health is defined as freedom from disease, dysfunction or injury (Naidoo and Wills, 2000). In historical terms biomedical definitions of health were commonly adopted during the nineteenth and twentieth centuries, during which time the predominant focus of public health was to control disease and infection. Despite more recent acceptance of the holistic concept of health, arguably, the biomedical perspective remains the favoured definition adopted by health care professionals in the UK (Ewles and Simnett, 1999). In addition to biomedical and holistic approaches to defining health, Keleher and Murphy (2004) also outline sociological, socio-ecological, lay and health promotion approaches to understanding health.

The complexity of the concept of health is further evident when considering the various dimensions of health. Viewed from a holistic perspective, health can be experienced from a range of inter-related and interdependent dimensions, including physical, mental, emotional, social and spiritual (Ewles and Simnett, 1999), as such complex states of health can co-exist. Physical and mental health, arguably the most commonly described dimensions of health, are concerned with the mechanistic function of the body and the ability to think clearly and coherently, respectively. Emotional and social health are closely related to mental health and refer to the ability to recognise emotions and the ability to make and maintain relationships. Spiritual health is concerned with feeling at peace with oneself and the quality of 'innermost' feelings.

Determinants of health

Health is shaped by multiple factors including personal lifestyle and the social, cultural and physical environment within which a person exists. The multi-layered model of factors determining health status (Dahlgren and Whitehead, 1991) represents the inter-related nature of the determinants of health (Figure 1.1). At the centre of the model are non-modifiable (fixed determinants) factors such as age, gender and genetics. Extending from the centre of the model are layers of influence that are potentially modifiable (variable determinants) by manipulation of either the environment or individual behaviour. The inner most layer represents individual lifestyle factors such as physical activity or dietary behaviour. Elements of the social environment include family structure and social networks and the final outer layer represents physical environmental conditions that have been linked to health,

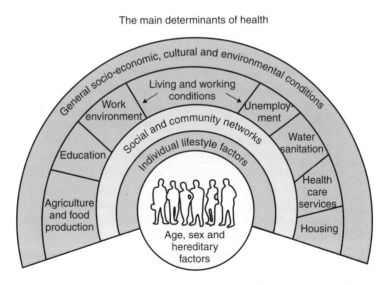

Figure 1.1 The social determinants of health as illustrated by Dahlgren and Whitehead (1991a,b). Reproduced with permission.

which include the provision of public services such as education, housing and healthcare. This model recognises the importance of the broader social, cultural and environmental determinants of health, and their inter-relationship with lifestyle choices of individuals.

Health and health promotion – an historical perspective

Expressed in terms of measurable biological outcomes, i.e. morbidity (disease) or mortality (death) rates, significant improvements in population health and well-being have been experienced. Such improvements have been attributed to rising standards of living (Department of Health, 2004a), advances in science, medicine and technology, and suppression of the incidences of infectious diseases, in developed countries (Naidoo and Wills, 2000). Over the last 50 years, global life expectancy at birth has increased by approximately 20 years, from 46.5 years in 1950 to 65.2 years in 2002 (WHO, 2003). In the UK, in 2004, female life expectancy was 81.1 years, for males 76.7 years (ONS, 2006). Increased life expectancy is not, however, synonymous with healthy life expectancy. Primarily as a consequence of non-communicable diseases individuals experience a significant number of unhealthy years at the end of life. Healthy life expectancy in the UK is currently 69.9 years and 67.1 years for females and males, respectively (ONS, 2006). In both developed and developing countries, non-communicable diseases represent 60% of the global disease burden (WHO, 2006). For example, circulatory diseases and cancer are the two most common causes of death and disability in the UK. Furthermore, coronary heart disease, diabetes and stroke are the most common illness to impair quality of life (ONS, 2006). In developed countries, therefore, a large proportion of illness and deaths can be attributed to a small number of lifestyle-behavioural risk factors, unhealthy diet, tobacco usage, physical inactivity and alcohol abuse (Wanless, 2004).

Health promotion has emerged as an increasingly important academic and professional multi-discipline (Ewles and Simnett, 1999). Measures designed to enhance health include health education (lifestyle and preventative) approaches alongside environmental (policy and fiscal) measures (Tones, 2001). The foundations of health promotion have emerged from the specialist areas of public health and health education (Edmonson and Kelleher, 2000). Public health is defined as 'the science and art of preventing disease, prolonging life and promoting health through the organised efforts of society' (Nutbeam, 1998, p. 352). In the nineteenth century, public health action was primarily concerned with the improvement of living conditions and infectious disease control with a focus upon better housing, education and sanitation. In contrast health education, when introduced in the 1960s, was primarily concerned with individual responsibility for health and illness and arose as a result of increasing lifestyle related diseases and the subsequent requirement to convey information regarding personal health behaviours (Egger *et al.*, 1999).

Health promotion emerged in an attempt to overcome the limited focus of both public health and health education on individual health behaviour, and recognised the importance of addressing environmental as well as individual (behavioural) determinants of health (Tones and Green, 2004). A wide range of actions constitutes the multi-disciplinary nature of health promotion practice (Rootman *et al.*, 2001); and since its inception, broad ranges of health promotion definitions have emerged (Rootman *et al.*, 2001). Explanations of health promotion action are underpinned by the different meanings attached to the concept of health, including considerations of the determinants of health (Naidoo and Wills, 2000). For example, WHO define health promotion as 'the process of enabling people to increase control over, and to improve, their health' (Ottawa Charter, 1986, p. 2).

Health promotion therefore includes the strengthening of individual capabilities to influence economic, societal and political actions in order to impact on public health (Naidoo and Wills, 2000). This is reflected in the Ottawa Charter (1986), a seminal document in the emergence and development of health promotion, which outlined five inter-related action areas for health promotion interventions, including: (1) building healthy public policy, (2) creating supportive environments, (3) strengthening community action, (4) developing personal skills and (5) reorienting health services.

The principles of, and strategies for health promotion can be applied to a variety of population groups (e.g. older people), risk factors (e.g. hyperlipidaemia), diseases (e.g. coronary heart disease) and settings (e.g. inner city areas) (O'Byrne, 2000). Over the past 10 years physical activity has become increasingly recognised as an activity that has positive health benefits in both treatment and prevention of ill health. As a consequence, physical activity exists within the context of health promotion and it is not unusual, for example for a primary care trust (PCT) to have a lead health professional, who has a remit for the strategic promotion of physical activity.

The role of physical activity in promoting health

The benefits of physical activity in health promotion and disease prevention are widely established and extensively documented (United States Department of Health and Human Services, 1996; Department of Health, 2004 a,b). Increasing levels of chronic, lifestyle-related diseases are causing concern for healthcare and other professionals in the UK

(National Institute of Health and Clinical Excellence [NICE], 2006). Furthermore, physical activity has a known positive relationship with these chronic conditions for prevention, treatment or in the management of diseases (Biddle *et al.*, 2000; Department of Health, 2004a). There is considerable evidence to indicate that individuals who are more physically active suffer from reduced morbidity and mortality from a wide range of diseases. Adults who are physically active have a 20–30% reduced risk of premature death and up to 50% less chance of developing major chronic diseases (Department of Health, 2004a). The benefits of physical activity are also experienced across the life course. In children, engagement in physical activity results in amelioration of risk factors for disease (Department of Health, 2004a); and in adults, it provides protection against the diseases themselves. For both adults and children, participation in physical activity can result in improvements in musculoskeletal health and can have a significant impact upon mental well-being. Evidence (Department of Health, 2004a) outlines the beneficial effect of exercise in relation to approximately 20 specific diseases. In particular, physical activity has a key role to play in the prevention of coronary heart disease, type II diabetes, and various cancers, for example colon cancer, Furthermore, there is evidence of a dose–response relationship for such diseases (Department of Health, 2004a).

Recommendations for physical activity

Public health recommendations for health-related physical activity, in adults, is 30 minutes of at least moderate intensity physical activity a day, on 5 or more days per week (Department of Health, 2004a,b). This advice is outlined for general health benefits across a wide range of diseases (Department of Health, 2004a,b), and may be achieved through structured bouts of exercise, or alternatively through physical activity that is integrated into daily life. In addition, 30 minutes may be achieved in one complete session or alternatively through several shorter bouts of 10 minutes or more (Murphy *et al.*, 2000). The aforementioned guidelines supplement the more vigorous exercise training–physical fitness (Haskell, 1994) guidelines of continuous aerobic activity, on 3–5 days per week at a vigorous intensity for 15–60 minutes per session (American College of Sports Medicine [ACSM], 1990).

ACSM (2007) have recently reviewed their guidelines for physical activity and public health and they currently recommend that healthy adults (under age 65) should participate in moderately intense cardio (aerobic) activity for at least 30 minutes a day, 5 days a week, or do vigorously intense cardio activity for 20 minutes a day, 3 days a week. In addition 8–10 strength training exercises should be performed, with 8–12 repetitions of each exercise, twice a week. The 30-minute recommendation is for the average healthy adult to maintain health and reduce the risk for chronic disease; however, in order to lose weight or maintain weight loss, 60–90 minutes of physical activity may be necessary. ACSM explicitly state that 'The new recommendation emphasizes the important fact that physical activity above the recommended minimum amount provides even greater health benefits. The point of maximum benefit for most health benefits has not been established but likely varies with genetic endowment, age, sex, health status, body composition and other factors. Exceeding the minimum recommendation further reduces the risk of inactivity-related chronic disease' (2007).

ACSM (2007) physical activity guidelines for adults aged over 65 (or adults aged 50–64 with chronic conditions, such as arthritis) state that they should participate in moderately intense aerobic activity for at least 30 minutes a day, 5 days a week or do vigorously intense aerobic activity for 20 minutes a day, 3 days a week. In addition 8–10 strength training exercises should be performed, with 10–15 repetitions of each exercise, twice or thrice a week. Adults at risk of falling are recommended to perform balance exercises and develop a physical activity plan with the advice of a health professional. Strength training is recognised as being 'important for all adults, but especially so for older adults, as it prevents loss of muscle mass and bone, and is beneficial for functional health' (ACSM, 2007).

The decision to recommend moderate as opposed to vigorous intensity physical activity at a population level is twofold. Firstly, unacquainted vigorous physical activity is potentially hazardous for previously sedentary individuals, and secondly, from a behavioural perspective, it may be difficult to encourage a previously sedentary individual to engage in vigorous physical activity (Hardman and Stensel, 2003).

Although these broad recommendations are helpful, the recommended frequency, intensity and duration can be varied according to specifically desired health outcomes. Adult recommendations for health enhancing physical activities are appropriate for elderly individuals, with additional activities encouraged to promote strength, co-ordination and balance. Children are recommended to accumulate 60–90 minutes of daily moderate to vigorous physical activity and, in addition, participate in activities, twice weekly, that improve and maintain muscular strength, flexibility and bone health (Anderson et al., 2006). However, despite this there is limited evidence regarding the dose–response relationship and specific health outcomes (Hardman and Stensel, 2003). For example, it is widely accepted that the aforementioned health-enhancing guidelines are insufficient in the prevention of weight gain or maintenance, and therefore, for obesity prevention it is recommended that adults participate in 45–60 minutes of at least moderate physical activity each day (Saris et al., 2003).

Health promotion approaches to improving health and physical activity

In acknowledgment of the clearly established link between inactivity and poor health status in populations, physical activity promotion has been the target of health promotion interventions, strategies and actions. In order to effectively promote physical activity, it is necessary to have an appreciation of the factors that influence participation. Physical activity behaviour has been linked to an extensive range of correlates (Sallis and Owen, 1999; Sallis et al., 2000). A review conducted by Sallis and Owen (1999) summarised approximately 300 studies of physical activity determinants, within which the following categories of determinants were proposed demographic and biological factors (e.g. age, education, gender, marital status, income); psychological, cognitive and emotional factors (e.g. attitudes, intention to exercise, self-efficacy, perceived health or fitness); behavioural attributes and skills (e.g. activity history during adulthood, type A behaviour pattern); social and cultural factors (e.g. group cohesion, physician influence, social support); physical environment factors (e.g. access to facilities) and physical activity characteristics (intensity, perceived effort). Correlates can, therefore, exist at the level of the individual or the environment (social or physical). Correlates associated with physical activity have been identified within all categories, the most consistent of which include enjoyment of exercise, self-efficacy, social support and perceived access to facilities. However, most research on the correlates of physical activity has focused upon individual level psychological and social variables (Gorely, 2005).

Knowledge of physical activity correlates is important since methods of physical activity promotion must be linked to explanations and understandings of factors that influence exercise behaviour. In this sense, unmodifiable correlates can be used to identify target populations who are least likely to engage in physical activity. Similarly, modifiable correlates can be used to identify specific strategies and actions that are used to intervene with such populations. Correlates can vary in strength in different population sub-groups and for different modes of physical activity, and therefore different intervention strategies must be used for different populations.

A broad range of approaches have been utilised to increase activity amongst different populations and in different settings. These include informational, behavioural/social and environmental/policy approaches (Kahn et al., 2002). Interventions to promote physical activity have been variously described, in health promotion terms, such approaches can be broadly categorised as individualist or structuralist in nature (MacDonald and Bunton, 1992). The approach utilised will be dependent upon assumptions regarding the factors that influence physical activity behaviour (i.e. individual or environmental).

Individual approaches to physical activity promotion emphasise the importance of cognitive antecedents of behaviour change, and consequently focus upon understanding and modifying the psychology of the individual. Intervention strategies that are synonymous with such an approach focus upon individual behaviour change. Interventions are delivered in a structured format and typically involve face-to-face training or counselling by a health or fitness professional. Techniques to change behaviour may involve fitness testing, health risk assessments, health education and cognitive behavioural-change techniques such as self-monitoring, goal setting or decisional balance. Cognitive behavioural interventions are derived from theories that reflect psychology and social psychology. The most dominant theories that have been applied to the promotion of physical activity include Social Cognitive Theory (Bandura, 1986); Theory of Reasoned Action/Planned Behaviour (Fishbein and Azjen, 1975; Azjen, 1991); the Transtheoretical Model (Prochaska and DiClemente, 1983) and the Health Belief Model (Rosenstock, 1966). The aforementioned theories focus upon understanding cognitions as mediators of behaviour and behaviour change. Social Cognitive Theory and the Transtheoretical Model demonstrate the importance of self-efficacy to predicting behaviour change. The Theory of Reasoned Action proposes that exercise behaviour is predicted by intention to engage in such behaviour which is in turn is influenced by attitudes and social norms. The key components of such models are located at the level of the individual. This approach consequently leads to an individual approach to health promotion (Becker, 1992).

It has been suggested that behaviour change needs to take place at a societal level, as well as an individual level, and long-term patterns of healthy behaviour established if real health gains are to be experienced at a population level. Radical changes to the environment, both cultural and structural, may be required if significant shifts in population physical activity levels are to be achieved (Sallis and Owen, 1999). Socio-ecological models of health purport that health behaviours and health outcomes represent the result of the reciprocal relationship between individuals and their environments (Cohen *et al.*, 2000; McLaren and Hawe, 2005). The general argument therefore is that environments restrict behaviour by promoting and demanding certain actions and discouraging or prohibiting other actions (Sallis *et al.*, 1998). Such models are holistic and multi-level, that endeavour to understand behaviour at a variety of levels. Five levels of behavioural determinants are specified; these include intrapersonal factors, interpersonal processes, institutional factors, community factors, and public policy (McLeroy *et al.*, 1988). In contrast to the individually orientated, structured approach of social cognitive models, ecological models of behaviour change endorse the use of environmental or policy approaches to behaviour change (see also Chapter 2). Indeed, environmental approaches to public health promotion have proven successful in legislation for seat belt use and, more recently, tobacco control. However, such approaches have rarely been applied in chronic disease control and, in particular, the promotion of physical activity (Sallis *et al.*, 1998).

Sallis and Owen (1999) have previously discussed the importance of the concept of socio-ecological models in understanding and promoting physical activity behaviour. Environmental interventions to promote physical activity must consider the influence of natural and constructed environments upon behavioural choice. In addition, policy interventions to promote physical activity may be related to incentives for activity (such as subsidised health club membership for employees) or resources and infrastructure for physical activity (such as provision of greater funding for walking and biking routes). Ecological models provide a general framework for explaining behaviour, and therefore this approach embraces models and theories that have focused upon individual level correlates of behaviour. Such models have moved the agenda for physical activity promotion away from a focus on individual behaviour change alone (which has had limited success) to a broader focus on the environmental structures and policies to promote physical activity. Socio-ecological approaches focus on the importance of the inter-connections between individuals, their environment and the subsequent impact on behaviour.

Physical activity promotion requires understanding of the scientific theory of exercise and health promotion from a multi-disciplinary (i.e. psychological, behavioural, social and physiological) perspective. Traditionally, health and physical activity research and practice have focused upon the natural science paradigm (e.g. physiological change of individuals) rather than social science paradigm (e.g. psychosocial factors such as social support) (Crone *et al.*, 2004). This is reflected in the predominance of individualistic approaches to physical activity promotion that advocate the philosophy of individual responsibility for, and personal control over, health (King, 1991).

Despite the advantages of such approaches, (e.g. they provide a convenient method of physical activity promotion with a range of strategies available to health and exercise professionals), there is increasing recognition of the limitations, and large resource implications, of using such interventions alone in order to improve population physical activity levels. Individual approaches have been further criticised from a behavioural change perspective. Despite recognition of the value of regular physical activity amongst population groups, there is evidence to suggest that such positive beliefs do not translate into actual behaviour (Kearney *et al.*, 1999). In response, multilevel (or socio-ecological) approaches, for example King (1991) and Figure 1.2, are increasingly being recognised as more appropriate in

Level of intervention	Channel (delivery mode)	Target group	Strategy
Personal	Face-to-face: physician's office; health clinic; health spas and clubs	Patients, clients	Information on health risk and benefits, counsellor support, personal monitoring and feedback, problem solving (relapse prevention)
	Mediated: telephone, mail etc.	As above	As above
Interpersonal	Classes, telephone/mail, health spas and clubs, peer-led groups	Patients, healthy individuals, families, peers	Information; peer, family and counsellor support; group affiliation; personal or public monitoring and feedback; group problem solving.
Organisational/environmental	Schools, worksites, neighbourhoods, community facilities (walk/bike paths), churches, community organisations, sites for activities of daily living (public stairs, shopping malls, car parks)	Students populations, employees, local residents, social norms	Curricula, point-of-choice education and prompts, organisational support, public feedback, incentives
Institutional/legislative	Policies, laws, regulation	Broad spectrum of the community or population	Standardisation of exercise-related curricula, insurance incentives for regular exercisers, flexible work time to permit exercise, monetary incentives for the development of exercise facilities

Figure 1.2 King's socio-ecological model showing levels of intervention (taken from King, 1991, p. 247).

understanding behaviour change. Figure 1.2 considers four levels of intervention that may be considered when designing and implementing a physical activity programme ranging from those that focus at the level of the individual to those that focus at an environmental and legislative level. Action at all levels within the model is more likely to result in population-level behavioural change.

To date, research concerning the effectiveness of health promotion programmes has focused predominantly upon individual approaches (Hillsdon *et al.*, 2004) (see also Chapter 4). However, despite the popularity of individual approaches, in both research and applied terms, they appear to have been unsuccessful in halting trends towards sedentary behaviour in the UK. The reasons for this are unclear; however, this may be as much to with the nature and transferability of research evidence as it is to do with the limitations of individual behaviour change techniques. For example, research evidence has tested the predictable power of cognitive variables upon physical activity behaviour; however, despite a strong relationship in terms of efficacy, there are problems when translating into practice (i.e. effectiveness). In future, the evaluation of physical activity will require an eclectic, portfolio approach to outcome measurement where wider aspects of health benefit, e.g. mental health, are recorded. The challenge for both researchers and practitioners is to measure real world physical activity behaviour and then appropriately translate research evidence into practice (Blamey and Mutrie, 2004).

Summary

Physical activity promotion has been identified as a public health priority for the twenty-first century (Department of Health, 2004a; WHO, 2004). Traditionally, biomedical models have predominated medical research, education and discourse in the UK (Suls and Rothman, 2004). This book aims to critically discuss physical activity promotion within a health promotion framework, in particular focusing on a socio-ecological approach. Because physical activity is a behavioural intervention or lifestyle choice, promoting it is a complex activity that requires input of many professional groups to achieve success (Hopman-Rock, 2000; McKenna and Riddoch, 2003; James and Johnston, 2004; Smith, 2004). Currently, there is a need to develop both theoretical and practitioner perspectives in order to improve the design, development, implementation and evaluation of physical activity interventions that are effective in sustaining behaviour change (McKay *et al.*, 2003) within a variety of population groups. The following chapters will address many contemporary issues relevant to this debate.

References

American College of Sports Medicine (1990) Position stand: The recommended quantity and quality of exercise for developing and maintaining cardio-respiratory and muscular fitness in healthy adults. *Medicine and Science in Sports and Exercise*, 22: 265–274.

American College of Sports Medicine (2007) *Physical Activity and Public Health Guidelines*. http://www.acsm.org/AM/Template.cfm?Section=Home_Page&TEMPLATE=/CM/HTMLDisplay.cfm&CONTENTID=7764 (accessed 08/01/08).

Anderson, L.B., Harro, M., Sardinha, L.B., Froberg, K., Ekeland, U., Bradge, S. and Andreson, S.A. (2006) Physical activity and clustered factor in children: A cross sectional study. The European Heart Study. *The Lancet*, 368: 299–304.

Azjen, I. (1991) The theory of planned behaviour. *Organisational Behaviour and Human Decision Processes*, 50: 179–211.

Bandura, A. (1986) *Social Foundations of Thought and Action*. Prentice-Hall, Englewood Cliffs, NJ.

Becker, M.H. (1992) A medical sociologist looks at health promotion. *Journal of Health and Social Behaviour*, 33: 1–6.

Blamey, A. and Mutrie, N. (2004) Changing the individual to promote health-enhancing physical activity: The difficulties of producing evidence and translating it into practice. *Journal of Sports Sciences*, 22: 741–754.

Biddle, S., Fox, K. and Boutcher, S. (2000) *Physical Activity and Psychological Well-being*. Routledge, London.

Cale, L. and Harris, J. (2005) Young people and exercise: Introduction and overview. In: *Exercise and Young People: Issues, Implications and Initiatives* (Eds L. Cale and J. Harris), pp. 1–8. Palgrave Macmillan, London.

Caspersen, C.J., Powell, K.E. and Christenson, G.M. (1985) Physical activity, exercise and physical fitness: Definition and distinctions for health related research. *Public Health Reports*, 100: 126–131.

Cohen, D.A., Scribner, R.A. and Farley, T.A. (2000) A structural model of health behaviour: A pragmatic approach to explain and influence health behaviours at the population level. *Preventive Medicine*, 30: 146–154.

Crone, D., Johnston, L. and Grant, T. (2004) Maintaining quality in exercise referral schemes: A case study of professional practice. *Primary Health Care Research and Development*, 5: 96–103.

Dahlgren, G. and Whitehead M. (1991a) *European Strategies for Tackling Social Inequities in Health: Levelling up Part 1. Copenhagen: World Health Organization Regional Office for Europe*. http://www.euro.who.int/document/e89384.pdf

Dahlgren, G. and Whitehead, M. (1991b) *Policies and Strategies to Promote Social Equity in Health*. Institute of Future Studies, Stockholm.

Dugdill, L. and Stratton, G. (2007) *Evaluating Sport and Physical Activity Interventions. A Guide for Practitioners*. University of Salford, Manchester.

Department of Culture Media and Sport (2002) *Game Plan: A Strategy for Delivering Government's Sport and Physical Activity Targets*. Cabinet Office, London.

Department of Health (2004a) *Choosing Health: Making Healthy Choices Easier*. HMSO, London.

Department of Health (2004b) *At Least Five a Week. Evidence of the impact of physical activity and its relationship to health*. A report from the Chief Medical Officer. HMSO, London.

Department of Health (2004c) *Health Survey for England 2003*. Vol. 2: *The Risk Factors or Cardiovascular Disease*. The Stationery Office, London.

Department of Health (2005) *Choosing Activity: A Physical Activity Action Plan.* HM Government, The Stationery Office.

Department of Health (2008) *Health Weight, Healthy Lives: A Cross-government Strategy for England.* http://www.dh.gov.uk/en/Publicationsandstatistics/Publications/PublicationsPolicyAndGuidance/DH_082378 (accessed 29/01/08).

Department for Transport (2001) *National Travel Survey 1999–2001: Update.* Department for Transport, London.

Edmonson, R. and Kelleher, C. (2000) *Health Promotion. New Discipline or Multi-Discipline.* Irish Academic Press, London.

Egger, G., Spark, R., Lawson, J. and Donovan, R. (1999) *Health Promotion Strategies and Methods.* McGraw-Hill, Sydney.

Ewles, L. and Simnett, I. (1999) *Promoting Health: A Practical Guide to Health Education.* Harcourt Publishers Limited, Edinburgh.

Fishbein, M. and Azjen, I. (1975) *Belief, Attitude, Intention and Behaviour: An Introduction to Theory and Research.* Addison-Wesley, Reading, MA.

Gorely, T. (2005) The determinants of physical activity and inactivity in young people. In: *Exercise and Young People Issues, Implication and Initiatives* (Eds L. Cale and J. Harris), pp. 81–102. Palgrave MacMillan, London.

Hardman, A.E. and Stensel, D.J. (2003) *Physical Activity and Health. The Evidence Explained.* Routledge, London.

Haskell, W.L. (1994) Health consequences of physical activity: Understanding and challenges regarding dose–response. *Medicine and Science in Sport and Exercise,* 26: 649–660.

HEPA Guidelines (2000) *European Network for Health Enhancing Physical Activity.* British Heart Foundation, European Commission, Oxford University, Oxford.

Hillsdon, M., Foster, C., Naidoo, B. and Crombie, H. (2004) *The Effectiveness of Public Health Interventions for Increasing Physical Activity Amongst Adults: A Review of Reviews.* Health Development Agency, London.

Hopman-Rock, M. (2000) Towards implementing physical activity programmes: The health promotion approach. *Science and Sports,* 15: 180–186.

James, A.D. and Johnston, L.H. (2004) The emerging role of the physical activity promoter within health promotion. *Health Education,* 104(2): 77–89.

Kahn, E.B., Ramsey, L.T., Brownson, R.C., Heath, G.W., Howze, E.H., Powell, K.E., Stone, E.J., Rajab, M.W. and Corso, P. (2002) The effectiveness of interventions to increase physical activity. *American Journal of Preventive Medicine,* 22(4): 73–107.

Kearney, J.M., Graaf, C.D., Damkjaer, S. and Engstrom, L.M. (1999) Stages of change towards physical activity in a nationally representative sample in the European Union. *Public Health Nutrition,* 2: 115–124.

Keleher, H. and Murphy, B. (2004) Understanding health: An introduction. In: *Understanding Health: A Determinants Approach* (Eds H. Keleher and B. Murphy), pp. 3–8. Oxford University Press, New York.

King, A.C. (1991) Community intervention for the promotion of physical activity and fitness. *Exercise and Sport Science Reviews*, 19: 211–259.

Lindau, S.T., Laumann, E.O., Levinson, W. and Waite, L.J. (2003) Synthesis of scientific disciplines in pursuit of health: The interactive biopsychosocial model. *Perspectives in Biological Medicine*, 46(3): 74–86.

Lucas, K. and Lloyd, B. (2005) *Health Promotion: Evidence and Experience*. Sage, London.

MacDonald, G. and Bunton, R. (1992) Health promotion. Discipline or disciplines? In: *Health Promotion. Discipline and Diversity* (Eds R. Bunton and G. Macdonald), pp. 6–41. Routledge, London.

McKay, H.A., Macdonald, H., Reed, K.E. and Khan, K.M. (2003) Exercise interventions for health: Time to focus on dimensions, delivery, and dollars. *British Journal of Sports Medicine*, 37: 98–99.

McKenna, J. and Riddoch, C. (2003) *Perspectives on Health and Exercise*. Palgrave Macmillan, Hampshire.

McLaren, L. and Hawe, P. (2005) Ecological perspectives in health research. *Journal of Epidemiology and Community Health*, 59: 6–14.

McLeroy, K.R., Bibeau, D., Steckler, A. and Glanz, K. (1988) An ecological perspective on health promotion programmes. *Health Education Quarterly*, 15: 351–378.

Murphy, M.H., Nevill, A.M. and Hardman, A.E. (2000) Different patterns of brisk walking are equally effective in decreasing postprandial lipaemia. *International Journal of Obesity and Related Metabolic Disorders*, 24: 1303–1309.

Naidoo, J. and Wills, J. (2000) *Health Promotion: Foundations for Practice*. Harcourt Publishers, Edinburgh.

National Institute of Health and Clinical Excellence (2006) *Obesity: The Prevention, Identification, Assessment and Management of Overweight and Obesity in Adults and Children*. National Institute of Health and Clinical Excellence, London.

Nutbeam, D. (1998) Health promotion glossary. *Health Promotion International*, 13(4): 349–364.

O'Byrne, D. (2000) The future of health promotion: Jakarta conference. In: *Health Promotion. New Discipline or Multi-discipline* (Eds R. Edmondson and C. Kelleher), pp. 46–54. Irish Academic Press, Dublin.

Office for National Statistics (1998) *Living in Britain: Results from the 1996 General Household Survey*. The Stationery Office, London.

Office of National Statistics (2006) http://www.statistics.gov.uk/cci/nugget.asp?id=1657 (accessed 01/08/07).

Ottawa Charter (1986) http://www.who.int/hpr/NPH/docs/ottawa_charter_hp.pdf (accessed 08/01/08).

Prochaska, J.O and DiClemente, C.C. (1983) Stages and processes of self-change in smoking. Toward and integrative model of change. *Journal of Consulting and Clinical Psychology*, 51: 520–580.

Rootman, I., Goodstadt, M., Potvin, L. and Springett, J. (2001) A framework for health promotion evaluation. In: *Evaluation in Health Promotion. Principles and Perspectives* (Eds I. Rootman, M. Goodstadt, B. Hyndman, D. McQueen, L. Potvin, J. Springett and E. Ziglio), pp. 7–38. WHO Regional Publications, Denmark.

Rosenstock, I.M. (1966) Why people use health services. *Millbank Memorial Fund Quarterly*, 44: 94–124.

Sallis, J.F., Bauman, A. and Pratt, M. (1998) Environmental and policy interventions to promote physical activity. *American Journal of Health Promotion*, 15(4): 379–397.

Sallis, J.F. and Owen, N. (1999) *Physical Activity and Behavioural Medicine*. Sage, London.

Sallis, J., Prochaska, J. and Taylor, W. (2000) A review of correlates of physical activity in children and adolescents. *Medicine and Science in Sports and Exercise*, 32: 963–975.

Saris, W.H.M., Blair, S.N., Van Baak, M.A., Eaton, S.B., Davies, P.S.W., Di Pietro, L., Fogelholm, M., Rissanen, A., Schoeller, D., Tremblay, A., Westerp, K.R. and Wyatt, H. (2003) How much physical activity is enough to prevent unhealthy weight gain? Outcome of the IASO 1st stock conference concencus statement. *Obesity Reviews*, 4: 101–114.

Smith, A. (2004) What is exercise science? *Journal of Hospitality, Leisure, Sport and Tourism*, 3(2): 5–14.

Suls, J. and Rothman, A. (2004) Evolution of the biopsychosocial model: Prospects and challenges for health psychology. *Health Psychology*, 23(2): 119–125.

Sport England (2006) *Active People Survey*. http://www.sportengland.org/index/get_resources/research/tracking/active_people_survey.htm (accessed 01/08/07).

Tones, K. (2001) Health promotion: The empowerment imperative. In: *Health Promotion: Professional Perspectives* (Eds A. Scriven and J. Orme), pp. 3–18. Palgrave, Hampshire.

Tones, K. and Green, J. (2004) *Health Promotion: Planning and Strategies*. Sage, London.

United States Department of Health and Human Services (1996) *Physical Activity and Health: A Report of the Surgeon General*. USDHHS, Centres for Disease Control and Prevention, National Centre for Chronic Disease Prevention and Health Promotion, Atlanta, GA.

Wanless, D. (2004) *Securing Good Health for the Whole Population*. HMSO, London.

World Health Organisation (2004) *Global Strategy on Diet, Physical Activity and Health. World Health Organisation*. http://www.who.int/dietphysicalactivity/strategy/eb11344/strategy_english_web (accessed 14/12/05).

World Health Organisation (2003) *World Health Report*. World Health Organisation, Geneva. http://www.who.int/bookorders/anglais/detart1.jsp?sesslan=1&codlan=1&codcol=24&codcch=2003 (accessed 08/01/08).

World Health Organisation (2006) *Engaging for Health. 11th General Programme of Work, 2006–2015. A Global Health Agenda*. http://whqlibdoc.who.int/publications/2006/GPW_eng.pdf (accessed 08/01/08).

2 Influencing health behaviour: applying theory to practice

Lynne Halley Johnston, Jeff David Breckon and Andrew John Hutchison

Introduction

For more than a decade researchers in exercise psychology have recognised that much of the work in behaviour change lacked a sound conceptual or theoretical basis (e.g. Sonstroem, 1988; Rejeski, 1992). In 2001, Biddle and Mutrie (2001) reported that theoretical foundations had emerged within exercise psychology borrowing from well-known educational, motivational and social psychology theories. By providing insights into how people change, these health behaviour models have suggested more effective methods for achieving behaviour change than a traditional reliance on subjective interventions. Despite the obvious benefits of these models, there are a number of considerations that need to be addressed when applying theory to practice.

Learning outcomes

The aims of this chapter are to:

1. provide an outline of the dominant health behaviour change models in the context of exercise and physical activity
2. present contemporary research evidence to highlight and critique the application of the dominant model (i.e. the transtheoretical model, TTM) and its role in the development of physical activity behaviour change interventions
3. emphasise the need for researchers and practitioners to apply more stringent measures in order to protect the validity of applications of theory to practice
4. critically discuss and summarise the implications for practice and research

---

Models of behaviour change

There are a plethora of models and theories available to guide both researchers and practitioners towards the development and imple-mentation of physical activity and other health behaviour change interventions. These models attempt to explain the mechanisms behind how and why people change. As might be expected, there is no single theory or model that explains how best to assist individuals in adopting habitual physical activity behaviours (Marcus and Forsyth, 2003). As a result the physical activity behaviour change research literature incorporates a range of different models and theories to assist with the development of interventions.

Social cognition models

Health behaviour change models have been classified within categories determined by their social, cognitive or environmental foundations (Foster et al., 2005). Among these categories are social cognition models, which include Social Cognitive Theory (SCT; Bandura, 1986), the Health Belief Model (HBM; Becker and Maiman, 1975), Theory of Reasoned Action (TRA; Fishbein and Ajzen, 1975) and Theory of Planned Behaviour (TPB; Ajzen, 1985). Social cognition is concerned with how individuals make sense of social situations (Connor and Norman, 2005) and models are designed to better understand the correlates and determinants of health behaviours. Fiske and Taylor (1991) explain that these approaches focus on individual cognitions or thoughts as processes that intervene between observable stimuli and responses in real-world situations. However, it has been suggested that health behaviour change research has focussed too much on social cognition models and their practical utility has been questioned (e.g. Jeffery, 2005). This may suggest a reason for the shift toward other theories and more applied 'stage' models. For a more detailed explanation of social cognitive models, see Connor and Norman (2005).

Self-determination theory

An alternative approach to the prediction of health behaviour that is receiving increasing attention is Self-Determination Theory (SDT; Deci and Ryan, 1985; Ryan and Deci, 2000). SDT has been described as a theory of personality development and self-motivated behaviour change (Markland et al., 2005). SDT posits that people have an innate organizational tendency toward growth, integration of the self, and the resolution of psychological inconsistency (Ryan and Deci, 2000). The theory (as illustrated in Figure 2.1) suggests that individuals pursue self-determined (intrinsically motivated) goals to satisfy their basic psychological needs to independently solve problems, interact socially and master tasks (Hagger and Chatzisarantis, 2007). While there is

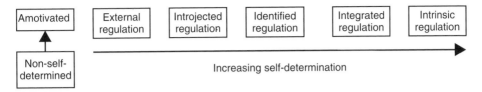

Figure 2.1 The continuum of autonomy: self-determination theory (adapted from Ryan and Deci, 2002, p. 16).

support for SDT as a tool for understanding motivation for physical activity behaviour change (e.g. Ntoumanis, 2001; Standage *et al.*, 2003), its applied implications are yet to be fully explored. Therefore, future research needs to consider exploring the efficacy of physical activity interventions developed using the principles of SDT. For a more detailed overview of SDT, see Ryan and Deci (2002; see Figure 2.1).

Stage models

Another set of models frequently cited in health behaviour change research are stage-based approaches. These focus on the idea that behaviour change occurs through a series of qualitatively different stages. The most dominant of these is the Transtheoretical Model (TTM: Prochaska, 1979; Prochaska and DiClemente, 1983), an integrative model of behaviour change (Velicer *et al.*, 1998) originally developed by Prochaska (1979) in response to the increasing theoretical diversity within psychotherapy. Since its conception, the model has been applied to a variety of behaviour change contexts such as HIV prevention (Prochaska *et al.*, 1994), substance abuse (Brown *et al.*, 2000), diet (Steptoe *et al.*, 1996) and physical activity (Kim *et al.*, 2004) [for a detailed overview of the TTM, see Prochaska *et al.* (1992) and Velicer *et al.* (1998)]. Other stage-based approaches include the precaution adoption process (Weinstein, 1988) and the health action process approach (Schwarzer and Fuchs, 1995).

The Transtheoretical Model: the dominant theoretical framework for physical activity behaviour change

Within physical activity, meta-analytical and systematic review-based research evidence (Marshall and Biddle, 2001; Marcus and Forsyth, 2003) and governmental reports on physical activity and behaviour change (United States Department of Health and Human Services [USDHHS], 1996; Foster *et al.*, 2005) suggest that the TTM is the most commonly adopted theoretical framework. The TTM is a multi-dimensional theoretical model commonly adopted by researchers to explain how people change various problem behaviours. The model is made up of four dimensions, which all contribute to explain not only the processes involved in behaviour change but when they are used and how they affect different types of outcomes. The four dimensions of the TTM are: the stages of change, the processes of change, self-efficacy/temptation and decisional balance. See Table 2.1 for an overview of each dimension. For a more detailed description of all the dimensions of TTM and their relationship to physical activity, see Biddle and Mutrie (2008).

Applying the TTM

If used appropriately, the four dimensions of the TTM potentially provide a valuable tool for the development of effective health behaviour change interventions. For example, the TTM construes change as a process that involves progress through a series of five stages. In order to explain how this change occurs the model describes 10 cognitive and behavioural processes that people use to progress through the stages. To accurately monitor a person's progress through the stages of change the model also incorporates decisional balance and self-efficacy dimensions which have been shown to change in a predictable pattern across the stages of change.

Using all dimensions of the model, Prochaska and Norcross (2001) explain that both the therapy relationship and treatment intervention can be tailored to meet an individual's specific needs based on their stage of change. For example, if a person is classified as a pre-contemplator, research has highlighted that processes such as 'consciousness raising' and 'dramatic relief' need to be emphasised in order to encourage stage progression (Prochaska and Velicer, 1997). Therefore, an appropriate intervention strategy might be to provide information about the risks associated with an individual's current health behaviour in order to increase their awareness (consciousness raising) and arouse negative emotions (dramatic relief) towards their current behaviour. In order to monitor any resultant changes and adapt the intervention accordingly, ongoing assessments of decisional balance and/or self efficacy might also be conducted (Figure 2.3).

Criticisms of the TTM

Despite the model's popularity, previous reviews have questioned the effectiveness of TTM based health promotion and physical activity

Table 2.1 The four dimensions of the transtheoretical model of behaviour change (adapted from Prochaska *et al.*, 1992; Velicer *et al.*, 1998; Prochaska and Norcross, 2001 and Hutchison *et al.*, 2008).

Dimension	Description	Role in TTM-based physical activity interventions

Stages of change	■ The stages of change represent ordered categories along a continuum of motivational readiness. The five stages are:
	  Pre-contemplation
	  Contemplation
	  Preparation
	  Action
	  Maintenance
	(See Figure 2.2 for a overview of the stages and how movement through them occurs.)
		Commonly referred to in the physical activity literature

Processes of change	■ The processes of change explain how individuals move through the stages of change ■ They are 10 strategies that describe the techniques that individuals use to modify their thoughts feelings and behaviour ■ Five of the processes are labelled as experiential and five are labelled behavioural ■ Experiential processes have been shown to be used primarily during the earlier stages of and behavioural during later stage transitions	Despite being the original dimension of the TTM, the processes of change are not acknowledged as frequently as the stages of change
Self-efficacy/ temptation	■ Self-efficacy represents the situation specific self-confidence that people have that they can cope with behaviour change without relapsing ■ It is an intermediate/outcome measure that is hypothesised to vary depending on stage of change (See Figure 2.3 for a overview of how self-efficacy and temptation relate to the stages of change.)	Rarely linked to TTM in the physical activity literature
Decisional balance	■ The decisional balance construct refers to the relative weighting of the pros and cons of change ■ It is an intermediate/outcome measure that is hypothesised to vary across the stages of change and with the type of behaviour being considered	Often not acknowledged as a dimension of TTM in the physical activity literature

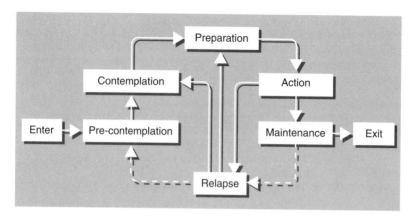

Figure 2.2   Movement through the stages of change (taken from Scales and Miller, 2003, p. 168).

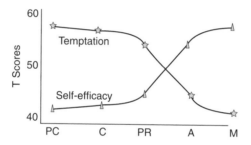

Figure 2.3   The relationship between the stages of change and both self-efficacy and temptation (taken from Velicer *et al.* 1998, p. 221).

interventions (e.g. Bunton *et al.*, 2000; Adams and White, 2003; Bridle *et al.*, 2005). For example, Adams and White (2003) produced evidence to suggest that TTM-based physical activity promotion interventions are reasonably effective in promoting physical activity adoption but have little influence on long-term maintenance of increased activity levels.

A number of arguments have been presented to explain the lack of support for TTM-based interventions. Firstly, it has been suggested that physical activity behaviour is more complex than single behaviours such as smoking and that individuals could be in a number of different stages of change depending on the type of activity being considered (Adams and White, 2005). Secondly, the importance of accurately determining current stage of change is necessary and yet many intervention studies lack validated algorithms to assess this (Bunton *et al.*, 2000). Thirdly, exercise behaviour may be influenced by a number of factors not considered by the TTM. For example, Adams and

White (2005) argue that the TTM focuses on personal motivation for behaviour change and does not take into account external and social factors such as age, gender and socio-economic position (e.g. Gidlow et al., 2006, 2007; James et al., 2008). Finally, it has been suggested that many of the previously reviewed interventions may not have been complex enough to do justice to the multidimensional nature of the TTM (Adams and White, 2005). Bridle et al. (2005) explained that many of the studies reported in their review of TTM-based health behaviour interventions were tailored only to stage of change and neglected the other dimensions of the model. Therefore, some TTM-based interventions may be conceptually flawed because they fail to fully represent the model.

While Adams and White (2005) questioned whether the physical activity interventions in their review were complex enough to do justice to the TTM, a limitation with their 2003 review is that they failed to conduct any assessment of the quality of each intervention and more importantly, the extent to which each intervention was based accurately on the TTM. A systematic review should identify the effectiveness of interventions based on a particular theoretical model, and within such a review, it is crucial to examine how accurately the intervention represents the theoretical model in question. Bridle et al.'s (2005) review of health behaviour change interventions based on the TTM did suggest that some of the components of the TTM may have been neglected, resulting in partial rather than full intervention tailoring. However, their review failed to present details regarding how many interventions neglected dimensions of the model and the impact that this might have on their efficacy. Therefore, the next section of this chapter reports on a systematic review, designed to assess the effectiveness and design of TTM-based physical activity interventions (Hutchison et al., 2008).

A systematic review of TTM-based physical activity interventions

The aims of the review were: to critically examine how the TTM is being applied to develop physical activity behaviour change interventions and to determine whether these TTM-based interventions are effective in promoting physical activity behaviour change. The review identified 24 physical activity behaviour change interventions based on the studies inclusion criteria (see Hutchison et al., 2008, for study design characteristics). Regarding the first aim, results revealed that only seven of the interventions (29%) were developed using all four dimensions of TTM (see Table 2.2 for full details). Therefore, very few studies are reporting to have applied all facets of the model and subsequently have

Table 2.2 TTM dimensions used in the development of physical activity interventions (Hutchison *et al.*, 2008).

Characteristic	No. of studies (%)
TTM dimensions	
Stages of change	24 (100)
Processes of change	17 (70.8)
Decisional balance	15 (62.5)
Self-efficacy	8 (33)
Number of TTM dimensions Included	
1	2 (8.3)
2	112 (45.8)
3	42 (16.7)
4	7 (29)

not acknowledged its multidimensional nature. As a result, it could be argued that only seven of the reviewed interventions can accurately claim to be based on the TTM.

In addition to the fact that researchers are clearly neglecting a number of the dimensions of the TTM, the review also identified some additional pitfalls associated with misrepresenting the model when applying it to the development of physical activity interventions.

TTM or the stages of change

Consistent with Bridle *et al.*'s (2005) findings, the stages of change was the dominant dimension of the model, as it was cited in the development of all the reviewed interventions. When describing the TTM, Velicer *et al.* (1998) clearly explain that the stages of change is just one of four key dimensions of the model. Despite this the TTM is often referred to as the 'stages of change model' (Bunton *et al.*, 2000; Adams and White, 2005) irrespective of the fact that the processes of change (cited in 71% of the reviewed interventions) was the original dimension. Bridle *et al.* (2005) explain that the stages of change construct is a variable, not a theory, and state that it is unclear why researchers would assume that a variable could facilitate consistent intervention effects. As a result, Bridle *et al.* suggested that many TTM-based interventions may be conceptually flawed because they are variable rather than theory driven. Therefore, it is crucial for researchers and practitioners to recognise that the stages of change are just one of the dimensions of the TTM.

The relationship between the processes and stages of physical activity behaviour change

Given that 71% of the reviewed interventions were developed with reference to both the stages and processes of change dimensions of TTM, it is important for researchers to demonstrate a good understanding of how these two variables interact with one another. There is evidence to suggest that the relationship between the stages and processes of change differs depending on the behaviour change context that they are applied to (Marcus *et al.*, 1992; Velicer *et al.*, 1998). Originally, the TTM was refined and tested based on a number of studies which investigated behaviour change within smoking cessation (e.g. DiClemente and Prochaska, 1982; Prochaska and DiClemente, 1983).

For physical activity adoption and maintenance, Marcus *et al.* (1992) found that the use of behavioural processes has been shown not to decline as individuals progress from action through to maintenance (as for smoking cessation) and the use of experiential processes peaks in the action stage for physical activity adoption compared to the preparation stage for smoking cessation. Therefore, any interventions based on these findings are likely to differ with regards to the timing of specific process related strategies. The results revealed that some of the interventions were developed with reference to the findings observed within smoking cessation and others were developed based on Marcus *et al.*'s (1992) physical-activity-based findings. Therefore, while all these interventions claim to be developed using the TTM, some of them have clearly failed to recognise the observed differences between physical activity behaviour change and smoking cessation with regards to stage and process interactions. As a result, the model is often applied without proper consideration regarding its application to physical activity.

Does a poorly applied theoretical framework influence the efficacy of interventions?

So far this chapter has presented research evidence which suggests that, in order to protect the validity of physical activity and other health behaviour change interventions, it is a crucial for those developing the interventions to demonstrate a good understanding of the theoretical models they choose to use. However, when this is not achieved and interventions fail to accurately represent the theoretical model in question, are they any less effective? While the findings of the review seem to reflect favourably on interventions that are accurately based on all four facets of the TTM (i.e. of the seven studies that demonstrated a complete understanding of the TTM six reported significant findings), a number of interventions that failed to consider every dimension of the TTM also reported significant findings.

Specifically, 17 of the interventions were not tailored to all four dimensions of the TTM, and of those, 12 (71%) reported significant short-term results in favour of the intervention group. One intervention (Hilton *et al.*, 1999; Steptoe *et al.*, 1999, 2001), which was tailored to only one dimension of the TTM (the stages of change), was shown to be effective in both the short and long term. Therefore, the extent to which interventions are accurately based on the TTM does not seem to be the only factor influencing their efficacy. As a result it is important for those developing interventions to consider the impact of other factors relating to the design and delivery of the intervention.

In order to explore the role of one such factor and provide a comprehensive picture of intervention integrity, the reviewed interventions were categorised into brief, medium or intensive. Results revealed that TTM based physical activity behaviour change interventions vary in their intensity from very brief interventions, involving only one delivery of intervention material, to intensive interventions which last for up to 6 months and involve multiple modes of delivery. Both intensive and medium intensity interventions were effective in the short term in 86% and 89% of studies respectively compared to 57% of brief intervention studies. Of the two interventions that reported significant long-term findings one was categorised as medium intensity and the other intensive. Therefore, consistent with findings presented by Marcus *et al.* (2006), the intensity of physical activity interventions does seem to influence their effectiveness. Thus, the application of theory to practice is not simply a case of accurately applying the principles of a theoretical model such as TTM because the role of other design related factors and their relationship with the theoretical model in question must be considered. For example, the TTM posits that behaviour change is a process that involves progression through a series of stages. Therefore, TTM-based interventions should arguably involve multiple patient contacts and follow ups in order to adapt the intervention to the changes that individuals are going through.

Implications for practitioners: TTM

While the TTM continues to provide a popular framework for the development of physical activity interventions, numerous inconsistencies regarding the development and implementation of interventions based on the model have been observed. As a result, it is difficult to determine whether findings are simply due to factors relating to intervention implementation or to a poorly conceptualised intervention. In order to draw more concrete conclusions about the efficacy of TTM and other theoretical model-based approaches, it is crucial for those developing interventions to fully articulate the nature of the interventions within the study protocol. To achieve this, future studies need to apply treatment fidelity measures to encourage researchers to fully describe the exact nature of their interventions. Applying such measures to accurately describe the nature of interventions is a crucial part of applying theory to practice.

Treatment fidelity and the Behaviour Change Consortium (BCC) framework

This chapter has highlighted the increase in research into physical activity behaviour change; there are, however, concerns over the lack of detail of physical activity interventions. For example, there is little discernable reporting of the content and type of intervention, the theoretical underpinning, or competence of the physical activity professional (or researcher) in delivering the intervention. Treatment fidelity refers to the methodological strategies used to monitor and enhance the reliability and validity of behavioural interventions (Bellg et al., 2004). The following section will consider treatment fidelity measures and provide recommendations for practitioners and researchers.

In comparison to physical activity interventions, 'health' behaviour change research has for some time embedded fidelity tests into interventions and research (Hahn et al., 2002; Dusenbury et al., 2003; Fiander et al., 2003) in order to preserve the internal validity and enhance the external validity of studies (Bellg et al., 2004). In order to address the issue of treatment fidelity for behaviour change settings, a consortium of health behaviour change studies was gathered in the US under the auspice of the National Institute of Health Behavior Change Consortium (BCC). The BCC group recommended five areas for implementing fidelity treatment measures in behavioural trials. The five components are summarised as a need to encourage fidelity at the design, training, delivery, receipt and enactment stages.

It is important to examine the potential efficacy of health behaviour change fidelity measures in order to ensure reliable, valid and robust interventions based on sound theoretical and scientific principles. Intervention fidelity testing is therefore a key methodological requirement for research into physical activity behaviour change. It provides a systematic process for the intervention design and when applied correctly, should ensure consistent and reliable results (Resnick et al., 2005). Treatment fidelity therefore plays a central role in ensuring that an intervention has been accurately evaluated. A recent synopsis of research projects into behaviour change fidelity has suggested that treatment fidelity requirements are only met if: (a) the treatment provided was given consistently to all participants randomised to treatment, (b) there was no evidence of non-treatment-related effects, and (c) the intervention was true to the goals and theory underpinning the research (Bellg *et al.*, 2004). For a more in-depth description of each fidelity goal, description and strategy the reader is referred to the BCC guidelines (Bellg *et al.*, 2004).

Physical activity counselling interventions and treatment fidelity

Within physical activity behaviour change settings, counselling based interventions are becoming increasingly popular in a variety of primary, secondary and community health care settings (Kennedy and Meeuwisse, 2003; Kirk *et al.*, 2003; McKenna and Vernon, 2004; Melanson *et al.*, 2004) to the point that physical activity counselling is becoming part of normal healthcare in the prevention, treatment and management of chronic diseases (Foster *et al.*, 2005). In the UK, the first guidelines for conducting an exercise (or physical activity) consultation were produced in 1995 by Loughlan and Mutrie. While these early guidelines filled a void, subsequent interventions applying these principles have compromised and confused the original guidelines (Kirk *et al.*, 2001, 2003; Hughes *et al.*, 2002).

Accurate descriptions of physical activity interventions are often lacking with little or no detail as to the fidelity, and therefore quality, of the intervention. Moreover, there is often no standardised measurement of physical activity outcome, physical activity counselling content, technique or patient readiness and receptiveness to the intervention (Kennedy and Meeuwisse, 2003). Table 2.3 represents an application of the five treatment fidelity components to the physical activity counselling setting along with the strategies for achieving each criterion (adapted from Breckon *et al.*, 2008).

In order to highlight the extent to which treatment fidelity measures are being adopted within physical activity counselling, the next section of this chapter reports on a systematic review of physical activity counselling interventions in clinical and community settings.

A review of physical activity counselling interventions

The review (Breckon *et al.*, 2008) identified 26 articles that examined the efficacy of physical activity/exercise counselling or consultations. Although the search criteria were for studies between 1995 and 2006, only one of the included studies was published before 2000 (Harland *et al.*, 1999) and 15 of the 26 studies (63%) were published after 2003, highlighting the increasing popularity of counselling-based physical

Table 2.3 Treatment fidelity components and physical activity counselling applications.

Component of treatment fidelity	Definition and description	Application to an physical activity counselling intervention
Design	Treatment fidelity applied at the design stage to ensure that the intervention can adequately test the proposed hypotheses. This in relation to underlying theory and clinical processes	Intervention consistent with behaviour change theory such as TTM, self-determination or social learning theory. Clear physical activity counselling protocol developed
Training	To ensure that those delivering the intervention have been satisfactorily trained, assessment is carried out of their skills and competencies in relation to the study	A combination of supervised role-playing, clinical supervision and reviews of audiotapes applied as an adjunct to a training manual
Delivery	Treatment fidelity processes are applied to monitor that the intervention is delivered in line with the proposed design	Physical activity counselling interventions audio taped and reviewed using a behavioural checklist based on the study protocol. Correction of observed intervention deviations
Receipt	The focus is toward the recipient of the intervention. The fidelity facet here aims to ensure that the intervention or treatment received is understood by the individual and that they can apply the intervention at a cognitive and behavioural level	Evaluation of the effects of the physical activity counselling intervention using post-session questionnaires or interviews (cognitive) and checklist of participant strategies employed (behavioural)
Enactment	An analysis is taken of the application of the treatment by the individual. This monitoring ensures that behavioural and cognitive strategies are applied in real-life settings	Completion of intervention strategy goals specific to the study outcomes. Clients encouraged to record accurately completed and missed sessions and to report occurrences of relapse

activity interventions. The results revealed that very few physical activity counselling interventions address treatment fidelity issues. At best, the physical activity counselling interventions reviewed indicated a theoretical underpinning but did not fully articulate the application of theory to practice by specifically detailing how components of the theoretical model (e.g. TTM) had been applied.

Table 2.4 Physical activity counselling studies and treatment fidelity (adapted from Breckon *et al.*, 2008).

Characteristic	No. of studies (%)
Experimental design	
Randomised control trial (RCT)	24 (92%)
Quasi-experimental	2 (8%)
Interventionist	
Research assistant	7 (27%)
Physical activity/Exercise professional	3 (12%)
Health professional[a]	12 (46%)
Unknown	4 (15%)
Assessment of interventionist competence?	
Yes	5 (19%)
No	21 (81%)
Outcome measure	
Behavioural	6 (23%)
Cognitive	0 (0%)
Epidemiological/Physiological	2 (7%)
Combination (with cognitive component)	9 (35%)
Combination (without cognitive component)	9 (35%)

[a] including GP/physician, practice nurse, dietitian, physiotherapist and health visitor.

Results also highlighted the vast array of health professionals that are currently being used to deliver physical activity counselling which in itself may help to explain the range of skills and level of competency. Indeed, the review emphasised the dearth of competence testing for those delivering the physical activity counselling component (only 19% of studies) and the variety of outcomes that are taken as a measure of intervention success. Table 2.4 summarises the main findings from the review.

For more details of the methods and inclusion criteria of this review see Breckon *et al.* (2008). The next section of this chapter discusses the findings of the review in more detail and presents recommendations regarding how treatment fidelity measures can be incorporated into the development of physical activity interventions.

Applying treatment fidelity measures to physical activity interventions

The BCC framework raises awareness of the need for a greater integration of theory to practice. It highlights the importance of a clear design and the processes involved, not just the outcomes that result. Many of the interventions highlighted in the review did provide some outline of the underlying theoretical construct upon which the intervention was based, the dominant model being the TTM (see Stage Models section). Several studies cited Loughlan and Mutrie's (1995) guidelines and an approach based on the stages of change and the TTM (Kirk *et al.*, 2001, 2003, 2004; Hughes *et al.*, 2002; Kim *et al.*, 2004). However, while this provides evidence of a theoretically grounded approach it does not inform practitioners how to interact with the client, elicit their perceptions of the need and desire for change and how to deal with issues such as ambivalence and resistance.

The dominance of randomised controlled trial (RCT) designs is clearly illustrated in the current review (92% of the studies) and emphasises the research preference for control of variables and extraneous factors. However, the lack of ecological validity in RCT designs is a major concern as this does not reflect the diverse nature (and reality) of community settings where the majority of physical activity interventions are delivered (Estabrooks and Gyureski, 2003; Dugdill *et al.*, 2005; Gidlow *et al.*, 2008 – see also Chapter 4). Further, RCT's do not necessarily ensure high-quality delivery of interventions, yet there is an implicit assumption that because the intervention is part of an RCT design that it is somehow standardised. Practitioners may be better advised to ensure a sound theoretical framework and competence in delivering a robust and reliable intervention. Further, qualitative studies are clearly required to systematically examine the process factors associated with physical activity counselling interventions (Gidlow *et al.*, 2008).

Applying treatment fidelity measures to training and delivery

Ensuring internal and external validity of behaviour change interventions is fundamental for methodological rigour. However, scant attention is paid to these in research-training curricula and there is a perceived lack of importance in published research (Bellg *et al.*, 2004). Indeed, it has been suggested that without understanding these issues researchers and clinicians 'application of behavior change technologies is likely to be slow, with wheels being re-invented rather than re-applied' (Michie and Abraham, 2004, p. 30). However, in-service training of GP's in the US and UK has shown that a systematic patient-centred protocol for physical activity promotion is efficacious (McKenna and Vernon, 2004).

Seven of the studies reviewed described the intensity, frequency or duration of training in physical activity counselling delivered to those providing the intervention. While these suggested that the interventionists had acquired the appropriate skills, or a level of competence in the application of these skills, it is not clear how robust the assessment actually was. When compared to vague guidelines or recommendations that are not underpinned with provision or training into the how and what to deliver, clear protocols may remove ambiguity inherent in physical activity counselling (Leventhal and Friedman, 2004). There are a limited number of strategies (in-health behaviour change) which do embed treatment fidelity by applying treatment manuals (Resnick *et al.*, 2002), mentored support (Williams *et al.*, 2002) and videotape monitoring (Sher *et al.*, 2002). The current systematic review indicated that to date there is no application of such comprehensive fidelity checks within physical activity behaviour change research. Thus, when developing interventions researchers must ensure that those delivering the intervention have received satisfactory training and an assessment should be carried out of their skills and competencies in relation to the study.

Applying treatment fidelity measures to ensure receipt and enactment

The BCC framework highlights the importance of ensuring the acquisition of behaviour change skills and techniques of the recipient (e.g. client or patient). This would ensure that the counselling recipient (or client) understands, and is able to enact, the techniques discussed in an action planning phase of, in this case, physical activity counselling. While this is paramount to creating an autonomous and independent individual, no studies reported how well the recipient understood the intervention delivered and their ability to apply it both cognitively and behaviourally.

The most common outcome measures were behavioral and epidemiological (17 studies) with only 9 (35%) of the reviewed studies including a cognitive outcome measure which may enable an assessment of the cognitive receipt and/or enactment. Other aspects such as physical activity and health information recall could have been applied within follow-ups considering the relatively high number of studies that applied this design (Harland *et al.*, 1999; Aittasalo *et al.*, 2004; Melanson *et al.*, 2004). Practitioners should then consider using regular contact with clients not just to re-assess their physical and behavioural adaptations but also their motivational and emotional state (and changes) as a result of the physical activity intervention.

Implications for practitioners: treatment fidelity

Equivocal results (both behaviourally and physiologically) have resulted from physical activity counselling interventions. It appears that studies have not fully analysed (or reported) the design, training of interventionists, quality of delivery of the intervention, receipt of the intervention by the patient and their ability to enact the new strategy. It is imperative that studies fully report not just what they have done but also how it was done. This need to include monitoring and evaluation of intervention processes at all stages. Only when this is common-place can practitioners have confidence in physical activity counselling techniques.

However, while there appears to be an unequivocal argument for increased treatment fidelity and consistency across health behaviour change interventions, a note of caution has been sounded by some authors, suggesting the demand for fidelity testing may be inappropriate for all steps (Leventhal and Friedman, 2004). They purport that the approach suggested by the BCC group ignores two things; firstly, that there are few theoretically grounded empirical studies of the processes involved in the successful attainment of this sequence. Secondly, trials with perfect fidelity may produce evidence that lacks a conceptual basis for adaptation across different diseases, treatments, patients, practitioners, institutions and cultures and may therefore lack applicability in clinical practice. In light of this it is important for behaviour change interventions to identify the core principles of treatment fidelity that are fundamental to achieving high quality interventions through research design, interventionist training and delivery, to client receipt and enactment. However, while the BCC strategies may appear exhaustive and potentially restrictive (Leventhal and Friedman, 2004), the BCC approach is based on validity and reliability checks from other settings and offers a framework which has never been applied within the context of physical activity counselling.

Conclusion

This chapter has illustrated that when applying theory to practice in health behaviour change settings, a number of considerations need to be taken into account to maintain the validity of behaviour change interventions. For example, for many TTM-based approaches, limited evidence is being presented to suggest that an adequate understanding of TTM is being demonstrated. Therefore, while some interventions may claim to be based on a particular theoretical model, in reality they may only reflect part of the model in question. With the wide range of theoretical approaches available, and in order to draw more concrete conclusions about their efficacy, it is crucial for those developing interventions to fully articulate the nature of the interventions within the study protocol. This can be achieved by applying treatment fidelity measures to physical activity behaviour change in order to preserve the internal validity and enhance the external validity of studies (Bellg *et al.*, 2004). This chapter has presented evidence to suggest that within physical activity behaviour change there is a lack of intervention quality control. Therefore, if treatment fidelity measures are not applied to such settings then it appears reasonable to request that authors justify why they have not been applied and to report alternative safeguards for quality assurance.

References

Adams, J. and White, M. (2003) Are activity promotion interventions based on the transtheoretical model effective? A critical review. *British Journal of Sports Medicine*, 37: 106–114.

Adams, J. and White, M. (2005) Why don't stage-based activity promotion interventions work? *Health Education Research*, 20: 237–243.

Aittasalo, M., Miilunpalo, S. and Suni, J. (2004) The effectiveness of physical activity counseling in a work-site setting: A randomized controlled trial. *Patient Education and Counseling*, 55: 193–202.

Ajzen, I.M. (1985) From intentions to actions: A theory of planned behaviour. In: *Action-control: From Cognition to Behaviour* (Eds J. Kuhl and J. Beckman), pp. 11–39. Springer, New York.

Bandura, A. (1986) *Social Foundations of Thought and Action: A Social Cognitive Theory*. Prentice-Hall, Englewood Cliffs, NJ.

Becker, M.H. and Maiman, L.A. (1975) Sociobehavioral determinants of compliance with health care and medical care recommendations. *Medical Care*, 13: 10–24.

Bellg, A.J., Borrelli, B., Resnick, B., Hecht, J., Minicucci, D.S., Ory, M., Ogedegbe, G., Orwig, D., Ernst, D. and Czajkowski, S. (2004) Enhancing treatment fidelity in health behavior change studies: Best practices and recommendations from the NIH behavior change consortium. *Health Psychology*, 23: 443–451.

Biddle, S.J.H and Mutrie, N. (2001) *Psychology of Physical Activity: Determinants, Well-being and Interventions*. Routledge, London.

Biddle, S.J.H. and Mutrie, N. (2008) *Psychology of Physical Activity: Determinants, Well-being and Interventions* (2nd edn). Routledge, London.

Breckon, J.D., Johnston, L.H. and Hutchison, A. (2008) Physical activity counseling content and competency: A systematic review. *Journal of Physical Activity and Health*, 5: 398–417.

Bridle, C., Riemsma, R.P., Pattenden, J., Sowden, A.J., Mather, L., Watt, I.S. and Walker, A. (2005) Systematic review of the effectiveness of health behaviour interventions based on the transtheoretical model. *Psychology and Health*, 20: 283–301.

Brown, V.B., Melchior, L.A., Panter, A.T., Slaughter, R. and Huba, G.J. (2000) Women's steps of change and entry into drug abuse treatment: A multidimensional stages of change model. *Journal of Substance Abuse Treatment*, 18: 231–240.

Bunton, R., Baldwin, S., Flynn, D. and Whitelaw, S. (2000) The 'stages of change' model in health promotion: Science and ideology. *Critical Public Health*, 10: 55–69.

Connor, M. and Norman, P. (2005) *Predicting Health Behaviour*. Open University Press, Berkshire.

Deci, E.L. and Ryan, R.M. (1985) *Intrinsic Motivation and Self-determination in Human Behaviour*. Plenum Press, New York.

DiClemente, C.C. and Prochaska, J.O. (1982) Self-change and therapy change of smoking behaviour: A comparison of processes of change in cessation and maintenance. *Addictive Behaviours*, 7: 133–142.

Dugdill, L., Graham, R. and McNair, F. (2005) Exercise referral: The public health panacea for physical activity promotion? A critical perspective of exercise referral schemes; their development and evaluation. *Ergonomics*, 48: 1390–1410.

Dusenbury, L., Brannigan, R., Falco, M. and Hansen, W.B. (2003) A review of research on fidelity of implementations for drug abuse prevention in school settings. *Health Education Research*, 18: 237–256.

Estabrooks, P.A. and Gyureski, N.C. (2003) Evaluating the impact of behavioral interventions that target physical activity: Issues of generalizability and public health. *Psychology of Sport and Exercise*, 4: 41–45.

Fiander, M., Burns, T., McHugo, G.J., Drake, R.E. (2003) Assertive community treatment across the Atlantic: Comparison of model fidelity in the UK and USA. *British Journal of Psychiatry*, 182: 248–254.

Fishbein, M. and Ajzen, I. (1975) *Belief, Attitude, Intention and Behaviour: An Introduction to Theory and Research*. Addison-Wesley, Reading.

Fiske, S.T. and Taylor, S.E. (1991) *Social Cognition* (2nd edn). McGraw-Hill, New York.

Foster, C., Hillsdon, M., Cavill, N., Allender, S. and Cowburn, G. (2005) *Understanding Physical Activity in Sport – A Systematic Review*. Sport England and University of Oxford British Heart Foundation Health Promotion Research Group, Oxford.

Gidlow, C., Johnston, L., Crone, D., Ellis, N. and James, D. (2006) A systematic review of evidence of the relationship between socio-economic position and physical activity. *Health Education Journal*, 65(4): 366–395.

Gidlow, C., Johnston, L., Crone, D., Morris, C., Smith, A., Foster, C. and James, D. (2007) Sociodemographic patterning of referral, uptake and attendance in Physical Activity Referral Schemes. *Journal of Public Health Medicine*, 29: 107–113.

Gidlow, C., Johnston, L.H., Crone, D. and James, D.V.B. (2008) Methods of evaluation: Issues and implications for physical activity referral schemes. *American Journal of Lifestyle Medicine*, 2(1): 46–50.

Hagger, M.S. and Chatzisarantis, N.L.D. (2007) *Intrinsic Motivation and Self-determination in Exercise and Sport*. Human Kinetics, Champaign, IL.

Hahn, E.J., Noland, M.P., Rayens, M.K. and Christie, D.M. (2002) Efficacy of training and fidelity of implementation of the life skills training program. *Journal of School of Health*, 72: 282–287.

Harland, J., White, M., Drinkwater, C., Chinn, D., Farr, L. and Howel, D. (1999) The Newcastle exercise project: A randomised controlled trial of methods to promote physical activity in primary care. *British Medical Journal*, 319: 828–832.

Hilton, S., Doherty S., Kendrick, T., Kerry, S., Rink, E. and Steptoe, A. (1999) A promotion of healthy behaviour among adults at increased risk of coronary heart disease in general practice: Methodology and baseline data from the change of heart study. *Health Education Journal*, 58: 3–16.

Hughes, A.R., Gillies, F., Kirk, A.F., Mutrie, N., Hillis, W.S. and MacIntyre, P.D. (2002) Exercise consultation improves short-term adherence to exercise during phase IV cardiac rehabilitation. *Journal of Cardiopulmonary Rehabilitation*, 22: 421–425.

Hutchison, A.J., Breckon, J., and Johnston, L.H. (2008) Physical activity behaviour change interventions based on the transtheoretical model: A systematic review. *Health Education and Behavior*. First published online on July 7, 2008 as doi:10.1177/1090198108318491.

James, D., Johnston, L., Crone, D., Sidford, A., Gidlow, C., Morris, C. and Foster, C. (2008) Factors associated with physical activity referral uptake and participation. *Journal of Sports Sciences*, 26: 217–224.

Jeffery, R.W. (2005) How can health behaviour theory be made more useful for intervention research? *International Journal of Behavioral Nutrition and Physical Activity*, 2(2): 194–201.

Kennedy, M.F. and Meeuwisse, W.H. (2003) Exercise counselling by family physicians in Canada. *Preventive Medicine*, 37: 226–232.

Kim, C., Hwang, A. and Yoo, J. (2004) The impact of a stage matched intervention to promote exercise behavior in physical activity participants with type 2 diabetes. *International Journal of Nursing Studies*, 41: 833–841.

Kirk, A., MacIntyre, P., Mutrie, N. and Fisher, M. (2003) Increasing physical activity in people with type 2 diabetes. *Diabetes Care*, 26: 1186–1192.

Kirk, A.F., Higgins, L.A., Hughes, A.R., Fisher, B.M., Mutrie, N., Hills, S. and MacIntyre, P.D. (2001) A randomised, controlled trial to study the effect of exercise consultation on promotion of physical activity in people with type 2 diabetes: A pilot study. *Diabetic Medicine*, 18: 877–882.

Kirk, A.F., Mutrie, N., MacIntyre, P.D. and Fisher, M.B. (2004) Promoting and maintaining physical activity in people with type 2 diabetes. *American Journal of Preventive Medicine*, 27: 289–296.

Leventhal, H. and Friedman, M.A. (2004) Does establishing fidelity of treatment help in understanding treatment efficacy? Comment on Bellg *et al.* (2004). *Health Psychology*, 23: 452–456.

Loughlan, C. and Mutrie, N. (1995) Conducting an exercise consultation: Guidelines for health professionals. *Journal of the Institute of Health Education*, 33: 78–82.

Marcus, B.H. and Forsyth, L.H. (2003) *Motivating People to be Physically Active*. Human Kinetics, Champaign, IL.

Marcus, B.H., Rossi, J.S., Selby, V.C., Niaura, R.S. and Abrams, D.B. (1992) The stages and processes of exercise adoption and maintenance in a worksite sample. *Health Psychology*, 11: 386–395.

Marcus, B.H., Williams, D.M., Dubbert, P.M., Sallis, J.F., King, A.C., Yancey, A.K., Franklin, B.A., Buchner, D., Daniels, S.R. and Claytor, R.P. (2006) Physical activity intervention studies: What we know and what we need to know. *Circulation*, 114: 2739–2752.

Markland, D., Ryan, R.M., Tobin, V.J. and Rollnick, S. (2005) Motivational interviewing and self-determination theory. *Journal of Social and Clinical Psychology*, 24: 811–831.

Marshall, S.J. and Biddle, S.J.H. (2001) The transtheoretical model of behavior change: A meta-analysis of applications to physical activity and exercise. *Annals of Behavioral Medicine*, 23: 229–246.

McKenna, J. and Vernon, M. (2004) How general practitioners promote 'lifestyle' physical activity. *Patient Education and Counselling*, 4: 101–106.

Melanson, K.J., Dell'Olio, J., Carpenter, M.R. and Angelopoulos, T.J. (2004) Changes in multiple health outcomes at 12 and 24 weeks resulting from 12 weeks of exercise counseling with or without dietary counseling in obese adults. *Nutrition*, 20: 849–856.

Michie, S. and Abraham, C. (2004) Interventions to change health behaviours: Evidence-based or evidence-inspired? *Psychology and Health*, 19: 29–49.

Ntoumanis, N. (2001) A self-determination approach to the understanding of motivation in physical education. *British Journal of Educational Psychology*, 71: 225–242.

Prochaska, J. (1979) *Systems of Psychotherapy: A Transtheoretical Analysis*. Dorsey Press, Homewood.

Prochaska, J.O. and DiClemente, C.C. (1983) Stages and processes of self-change in smoking: Toward an integrative model of change. *Journal of Consulting and Clinical Psychology*, 5: 390–395.

Prochaska, J.O., DiClemente, C.C. and Norcross, J.C. (1992) In search of how people change: Applications to addictive behaviors. *American Psychologist*, 47: 1102–1114.

Prochaska, J.O. and Norcross, J.C. (2001) Stages of change. *Psychotherapy*, 38: 443–448.

Prochaska, J.O., Redding, C.A., Harlow, L.L., Rossi, J.S. and Velicer, W.F. (1994) The transtheoretical model of change and HIV prevention: A review. *Health Education Quarterly*, 21: 471–486.

Prochaska, J.O. and Velicer, W.F. (1997) The transtheoretical model of health behavior change. *American Journal of Health Promotion*, 12: 38–48.

Rejeski, W.J. (1992) Motivation for exercise behaviour: A critique of theoretical decisions. In: *Motivation in Sport and Exercise* (Ed G.C. Roberts), pp. 129–157. Human Kinetics, Champaign, IL.

Resnick, B., Bellg, A.J., Borrelli, B., DeFrancesco, C., Breger, R., Hecht, J., Sharp, D.L., Levesque, C., Orwig, D., Ernst, D., Ogedegbe, G. and Czajkowski, S. (2005) Examples of implementation and evaluation of treatment fidelity in the BCC studies: Where we are and where we need to go. *Annals of Behavioural Medicine*, 29: 46–54.

Resnick, B., Magaziner, J., Orwig, D. and Zimmerman, S. (2002) Testing the effectiveness of the Exercise Plus Program. *Health Education Research*, 17: 648–659.

Ryan, R.M. and Deci, E.L. (2000) Self-determination theory and the facilitation of intrinsic motivation, social development, and well-being. *American Psychologist*, 55: 68–78.

Ryan, R.M. and Deci, E.L. (2002) *Handbook of Self-determination Research*. University of Rochester Press, Rochester, NY.

Scales, R. and Miller, J.H. (2003) Motivational techniques for improving compliance with an exercise programme: Skills for primary care clinicians. *Current Sports Medicine Reports*, 2: 166–172.

Schwarzer, R. and Fuchs, R. (1995) Changing risk behaviors and adopting health behaviors: The role of self-efficacy beliefs. In: *Self-efficacy in Changing Societies* (Ed A. Bandura), pp. 259–288. Cambridge University Press, New York.

Sher, T.G., Bellg, A.J., Braun, L., Domas, A., Rosenson, R. and Canar, W.J. (2002) Partners for life: A theoretical approach to developing an intervention for cardiac risk reduction. *Health Education Research*, 17: 597–605.

Sonstroem, R.J. (1988) Psychological models. In: *Advances in Exercise Adherence: Its Impact on Public Health* (Ed R.K. Dishman), pp. 125–153. Human Kinetics, Champaign, IL.

Standage, M., Duda, J.L. and Ntoumanis, N. (2003) A model of contextual motivation in physical education: Using constructs from self-determination and achievement goal theories to predict physical activity intentions. *Journal of Educational Psychology*, 95: 97–110.

Steptoe, A., Doherty, S., Rink, E., Kerry, S., Kendrick, T. and Hilton, S. (1999) A randomised control trial of behavioural counselling in general practice for the promotion of healthy behaviour among adults at increased risk of coronary heart disease. *British Medical Journal*, 319: 943–948.

Steptoe, A., Kerry, S., Rink, E. and Hilton, S. (2001) The impact of behavioural counseling on stage of change in fat intake, physical activity, and cigarette smoking in adults at increased risk of coronary heart disease. *American Journal of Public Health*, 91: 265–269.

Steptoe, A., Wijetunge, S., Doherty, S. and Wardle, J. (1996) Stages of change for fat reduction: Associations with food intake, decisional balance and motives for food choice. *Health Education Journal*, 55: 108–122.

United States Department of Health and Human Services (1996) Physical activity and health: A report of the Surgeon General. U.S. Department of Health and Human Services, Centers for Disease Control and Prevention, National Centre for Chronic Disease Prevention and Health Promotion, Atlanta, GA.

Velicer, W.F., Prochaska, J.O., Fava, J.L., Norman, G.J. and Redding, C.A. (1998) Smoking cessation and stress management: Applications of the transtheoretical model of behavior change. *Homeostasis*, 38: 216–233.

Weinstein, N.D. (1988) The precaution adoption process. *Health Psychology*, 7: 355–386.

Williams, G.C., Minicucci, D.S., Kouides, R.W., Levesque, C.S., Chrikov, V.I., Ryan, R.M. and Deci, E.L. (2002) Self-determination, smoking, diet, and health. *Health Education Research*, 15: 512–521.

3 Promoting physical activity through policy change: art, science or politics?

Nick Cavill

Introduction

> '... almost all government policy is wrong, but ... frightfully well carried out'.   (Sir Humphrey Appleby in BBC's *Yes Minister*)

Previous chapters of this book have demonstrated that effective health promotion activity takes place at multiple levels, attempting to influence the social and political environment as well as changing individuals' behaviour. Of increasing importance in recent years have been attempts to influence the policies of public and private organisations to create better conditions for health (World Health Organisation, 1986; Cavill and Foster, 2006).

Learning outcomes

The aims of this chapter are to:

1. explain the meaning of the terms policy and strategy
2. discuss the potential importance of influencing public policy
3. critically analyse some of the limitations and challenges inherent in working to influence public policy

---

The term policy refers to a statement of intent, or a plan of action, usually issued by an organisation. Policies set out what an organisation plans to do, or how it intends to react to certain situations. For example employers are now required by law to implement equal opportunities policies, which require that they treat people fairly regardless of factors such as ethnic background or sexuality. In the physical activity domain, obvious examples might be a local authority's sport and activity policy, or a primary care trust's obesity policy, which might refer overweight or obese patients to exercise and healthy eating interventions.

Sallis *et al.* (1998) defined policy for physical activity as 'Legislative, regulatory or policy-making actions that have the potential to affect physical activity' (p. 380). Examples of legislation can be found in support of many areas of public health policy, such as speed limits, safety belt laws or health and safety legislation. Laws such as these are the most visible and tangible manifestations of government policy, however, it is important to understand that policy and legislation are separate issues. Primary legislation is influenced by policy and will often simply be an expression of the policy of the government. However, in many cases public policy leads only to guidance such as planning policy statements issued to local authorities.

It is also important to differentiate between policy and strategy, two terms often mistakenly used interchangeably. A strategy (usually a written document) sets out how the policies of an organisation will be carried out. So, for example, a government department may have a policy to increase cycling to work among its staff. This would have been agreed by the management team and may be published on the department's website, or noticeboard for example. However, it will be relatively meaningless without a strategy, which shows how the department will increase cycling: for example through improving bike parking, paying generous mileage rates for cycles used at work; or promotional activity. So it can be seen that an evaluation of the success of a policy will involve checking the extent to which the strategy has been implemented; who it has reached; who has taken action and so on.

The importance of working to influence policy is due to the great potential to influence large numbers of people. Interventions at the individual or group level such as exercise referral by a health practitioner, or led walks by a trained walk leader, have the potential to make significant improvements to the physical activity patterns and health of the people concerned. However, often these are small numbers of people, and the effects may be short-lived (Ogilvie *et al.*, 2007). In contrast, making changes to a policy, especially an aspect of government policy, has the potential to influence far more people, and potentially for a longer time. Consider the following two hypothetical examples:

Scenario one

Jan is a school crossing warden (otherwise known as a lollipop lady). She became concerned at the number of cars on the school run in her area, and when she chatted to some of the children she found that one of the issues was that while the children would like to walk to school, their parents are often in a rush to get to work so find it more convenient to drive them to school. So she set up a 'walking bus' and she walks with a group of children to school twice a week, picking them up from their homes as the 'bus' passes through the area. This has increased the number of children walking to school and many of them say that they try to walk on days when the bus does not run.

Scenario two

Jean is a councillor and mother and was distressed to find that the head teacher at her daughter's school had banned cycling to school as he felt it was too dangerous. Jean looked into this further and found that while not all schools in the local area had taken such a severe approach, many were not supportive of cycling and some had low rates of walking to school. She raised it at a council meeting and passed a resolution to improve policy on school travel in the area. Working with the local authority school travel plan coordinator she achieved the implementation of travel plans in all local schools, which set out targets for walking and cycling, along with strategies for achieving the targets. Schools have now committed to a 'car free day' every year and aim to review their policy annually to monitor achievements and check they are on track. Across the local authority, levels of walking and cycling have increased and in some schools, car drivers are in the minority.

Both scenarios described here are valid health promotion activities; both had an influence on public health, however, it can be seen that by influencing policy, scenario two had a greater level of influence, which had the potential to last longer. This is the appeal of policy interventions: making a difference at a population level. A true eco-logical approach however will include interventions at all levels, from interpersonal and community-level approaches through to policy and environmental change.

UK health policy on physical activity

In the UK, government policy on physical activity has mainly been the responsibility of the Department of Health. The first main impetus for this came with the publication of the National Fitness Survey (Health Education Authority and Sports Council, 1992), which showed low levels of physical activity and fitness in the population. This led the Department of Health to set up a physical activity task force of experts to consider the issue. They released a strategy statement on physical activity (Department of Health, 1996), which was only eight pages long and not published by HM Stationery Office (as was the norm for official government documents) and not given any sort of press launch. The reason would seem to be that ministers at the time were nervous about being seen to be the 'nanny state' – telling people that they had to exer-cise. This presents an important learning point about physical activity: that although promoting physical activity is generally about a positive change in behaviour (compared to legislation banning smoking in pub-lic places) it is still a political issue, bound up in debates about how far the state should intervene.

From 1996 to 2000, responsibility for physical activity largely passed to the Health Education Authority, which was given the mandate to promote the new message about moderate intensity physical activity through an integrated mass media campaign. This campaign was successful in raising awareness and knowledge about the physical activity recommendations, and supported professionals in their local work promoting activity, but this did not translate into measurable population level behaviour change (Hillsdon *et al.*, 2001).

It was not until 2005 that the Department of Health finally launched a strategy and action plan for physical activity: Choosing Activity: a Physical Activity Action Plan (Department of Health, 2005). This set out a range of proposals including a focus on the environment for physical activity. Choosing Activity set out the contribution of the environment as (i) creating and maintaining a wide range of opportunities for activity through sport, (ii) ensuring high-quality, well targeted and attractive facilities for walking and cycling, (iii) continuing to make our public spaces and the countryside more accessible and attractive.

In Choosing Activity, the environment was placed in a supportive role to helping people build more active lifestyles – similar to one of the five principles of the 1986 Ottawa Charter for Health Promotion (World Health Organisation, 1986). The environment can be seen to play a role through creating opportunities for physical activity by 'the delivery of cleaner, safer and greener public spaces and improvement of the quality of the built environment in deprived areas', as outlined in the Public Service Agreement of the Office of the Deputy Prime Minister (ODPM, 2002, PSA Target 8). The environment could also promote walking and cycling for travel, a central policy of the Department for Transport's walking and cycling action plan (Department for Transport, 2004). The policy describes the contribution of the environment to promoting walking and cycling via 'access to well-maintained, safe walking and cycling routes, attractive and affordable leisure and sports facilities, playgrounds, parks and the countryside' (Department of Health, 2005, p. 20).

Physical activity policy: everything or nothing?

Physical activity is a term that has come to have a broad meaning. This means that the development of public policy to support physical activity involves a large and diverse range of sectors, including sport; public health; transport; education; environment; countryside; green space and many others. Coordinating these efforts therefore requires a thorough understanding of these broad sectors, and the existing and potential links to physical activity.

Usually this broad approach is seen as an advantage, as physical activity can incorporate a wider range of views, and include a greater number of potential players. However, this can also be a weakness, as no-one takes overall ownership of the issue, and instead sees it as the

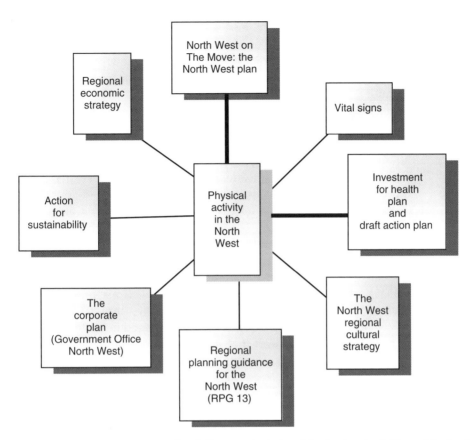

Figure 3.1 Strategic documents that influence physical activity in the North West of England (taken from Cavill *et al.*, 2005). Key: thin line = direct link; dark line = indirect link.

other's business. Figure 3.1 shows a policy map developed for an audit of physical activity policy in the North West of England (Cavill *et al.*, 2005). This audit was designed to have a strong focus on any strategy, policy or plan which was to be developed by a regional or sub-regional agency within three years that had the potential to impact on physical activity in its broadest terms. It therefore is forward looking, with the intention of developing an understanding of the best ways that the region's physical activity task force might work to influence public policy in support of physical activity.

Figure 3.1 shows the complexity of the physical activity policy environment, with a vast variety of public policy documents covering issues that have an influence on physical activity. For example, the regional spatial strategy influences where physical development occurs in the region, which can make a difference to creating environments for people to walk, cycle, and take part in other forms of physical activity. The cultural strategy sets out a plan for culture in the region, which includes provision of major sporting events. The Investment for Health plan sets out the health sector's response to issues such as childhood obesity and coronary heart disease. All of these have a relationship to physical activity, and all overlap in some way. Beneath this framework is a myriad of local strategies, plans, and targets (see Figure 3.1).

This policy complexity is also illustrated well by the Building Health Project (Cavill, 2006). This was a partnership between the National Heart Forum, Living Streets and the Commission for Architecture and the Built Environment. The project set out to increase awareness of the public health role of organisations concerned with urban design and improving the public realm, in particular in relation to population levels of physical activity, and to facilitate implementation of good health-promoting practice. The project brought together experts to discuss the issue of the built environment and to make recommendations about aspects of public policy that should be changed to help to create places that are more supportive of physical activity. The final report contains an extraordinarily complex mix of seventy-five recommendations spanning strategic planning, transport planning, architecture and building design. This is illustrated in Table 3.1.

These complexities mean that for progress to be made in physical activity policy, there needs to be leadership, with responsibility being taken by a lead agency, to coordinate actions by the various partners. This leadership can come from different sectors, according to local conditions and there are contrasting examples from around the world (Cavill, 2004). Historically, in Switzerland, most of the development work for physical activity policy was led by the sport sector, whilst in Finland and the UK it was mainly led by public health (Cavill *et al.*, 2006). At a local level this may be very different however, much of the development for the promotion of physical activity in the UK has been by local authorities' leisure services departments, which only relatively recently have forged links with health professionals, often as a result of exercise referral schemes (see Chapter 5).

Key issues for physical activity policy

The conflation of environment and policy in physical activity literature

There is an interesting issue relating to the literature on physical activity policy and the environment. The last ten years or so has seen a growing interest in the influence of the environment on physical activity among physical activity researchers. This has led to an increase in articles studying what have been termed environment and policy interventions (Sallis *et al.*, 1998). However, much of the literature tends to conflate the two issues of an environmental change (such as the

Table 3.1 Summary of key recommendations from Building Health (Cavill, 2006).

Topic	Issue	Examples of recommended policy changes
Strategic planning	Physical activity is not considered a priority within strategic planning	All government departments to apply a 'health check' to investment programmes with a focus on the impact on opportunities for physical activity
Urban planning	Motorised transport is given priority within urban planning	Local authorities should prioritise walking and cycling and produce an annual assessment of achievements
Streets and the public realm	Many public spaces are unattractive and do not encourage walking or outdoor activity	Local authorities should publish public realm strategies encouraging the informal and unconstrained use of streets and public spaces
Walking and cycling	Motorised transport is often prioritised by invisible subsidies	Government departments should identify and remove all subsidies to motorised transport such as free parking or car mileage allowances
Urban green space	Urban green space is not seen as a health resource	The Department of Health should provide funding for the development and maintenance of green infrastructure
Outdoor playing space	Planning policy allows for the loss of outdoor play space as long as there is judged to be 'a benefit to sport'	Policy should be reviewed so that outdoor play space can be retained
Building design	Architects and building designers appear to favour lifts over stairs	Stairs should be seen as an essential element within buildings (not just as a fire escape)

building of a new bike path) with the policy change that preceded it (such as a cycle strategy or similar statement setting out the intention to promote cycling through building more bike paths). The vast majority of these studies do not specifically isolate the policy component of these interventions, but focus on the actual change to the physical environment. This makes it difficult to tease out the specific effect of any policy change. It seems important to separate the two issues and ensure that the focus is on the components of public policy that might support effective interventions to promote physical activity through environmental change, or will provide a favourable background to the promotion of physical activity.

This is illustrated in Figure 3.2, which shows a conceptual model of how policy on the environment might be seen to influence levels of physical activity. Much of the policy and environment literature

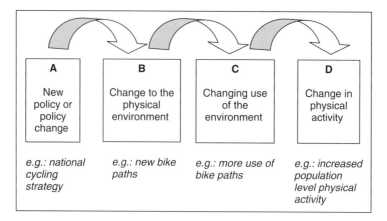

Figure 3.2 Conceptual model of physical activity promoting policy and the environment.

identifies changes in physical activity (box D) or use of a specific aspect of the environment (box C) that have arisen due to a change in the physical environment (box B), but studies rarely look at the policies that led to these changes in the first place (box A). So while our knowledge is improving of the specific interventions that can help to increase physical activity, we know little about how to make these interventions work, and how to integrate them into existing practice through policy change (National Institute of Health and Clinical Excellence [NICE], 2006).

The paucity of policy evaluations in the literature

This situation is exacerbated by the small number of policy evaluations in the literature. The author and colleagues conducted a search of the international literature on policy initiatives that had changed the environment to promote physical activity (NICE, 2006). We searched for studies that had assessed the impact of a stated policy (from any public body including the government, or a private body such as employers) on an aspect of the physical environment, and related this either to a direct measure of physical activity, or an outcome closely related to physical activity, such as footpath use. This was thought to be more appropriate for a review of public policies where an acceptable outcome might be an intermediate variable, and where physical activity might not be reported. The search strategy resulted in over 12000 potential studies, but after detailed screening and examination of papers, only three studies were found that actually met the criteria (see policy evaluation examples). This makes it very difficult to assess the effectiveness of policy interventions, and means that it is less likely that new policy will be based on studies of what has gone before.

There may be many reasons for the apparent lack of published evaluations of policy initiatives. Firstly, there are significant methodological challenges inherent in evaluating policy. How can the effects of the policy effectively be separated from all the potential confounding factors that may have influenced the eventual outcome? For example, it is generally thought that the high modal share of cycling in the Netherlands is a reflection of that country's strong commitment to cycling expressed in national policies such as the Dutch Bicycle Master Plan (Welleman, 1999), but how can we effectively separate the impact of these policies from other factors that may have more of an influence? Maybe Dutch people cycle more because of culture; because the country is flat; because bicycles are cheap; or all of these reasons. Evaluations of health promotion initiatives rarely lend themselves to controlled study designs, but this is even more the case with policy evaluations where it is particularly hard to control for all the potential confounding factors and demonstrate a causal link between the change in policy and the physical activity outcome.

Secondly, the physical activity intervention literature is relatively young, compared to other public health issues such as smoking or nutrition. This might lead researchers to focus initially on evaluating interventions that are more tangible and easier to focus on, like the effectiveness of GP exercise counselling or the use of pedometers in primary care, before exploring the more distal influences on health such as social or physical environment or policy. This leads to what is described as the 'inverse evidence law' where we seem to have the most evidence about factors that have the least importance, and know the least about the factors with the greatest potential to influence health (Ogilvie et al., 2007).

Finally, the paradigm from which researchers operate may have an important influence on their ability or inclination to publish studies of policy evaluations in the academic literature. For example, many professionals who have a significant influence on the built or natural environment, such as town planners or architects, do not normally conduct evaluations of their work, and if they do, do not tend to collect data on outcome measures such as physical activity. There is a significant literature on approaches to modifying the built environment, but it is rarely conducted to standards expected by the public health community, and tends to be restricted to case studies (NICE, 2006). This means that reviews such as the one mentioned above frequently find very few studies on which to draw conclusions.

Some of these issues can be explored through three contrasting examples taken from the systematic review referred to above (NICE, 2006).

Policy evaluation example: National policy on health and physical activity in Finland

Vuori *et al.* (2004) assessed the influence of sports and physical activity policies (including policies relating to the environment) on national physical activity trends in Finland. The study identified supportive policy change across a broad range of sectors, including education and sport; the health sector; transport sector; and multisectoral policies. Many of these policy changes included a focus on the environment. Significant examples included:

▪ The Sports Act 1999, which led to the Ministry of Education directing a major proportion of state support for the construction and maintenance of sites for the promotion of physical activity for people in their daily environments (e.g. small parks; playgrounds; and cycle paths).
▪ The national health program Health for All by the Year 2000 (1986), which recommended an increase in the availability of recreational areas and walking and cycling paths, and to develop land use and community planning to provide opportunities for all population groups to participate in physical activity in their own environments.
▪ The 1992 Ministry of Transport Finnish Cycling Policy, which set a goal to double the number of cycle trips made by Finns in seven years, by improving the conditions for cycling.
▪ Renewed efforts by the Ministry of Transport in 2001 to focus on cycling with a new cycling policy; and a walking policy.
▪ Multisectoral policies, notably the 2003 Government Resolution on Health Enhancing Physical Activity by the State Cabinet. This set out the obligation for municipalities to promote the well-being of all residents, including through physical activity. The resolution includes principles that emphasise collaboration among government sectors, increased consideration of physical activity in land use and environmental planning.

The authors reported annual trend data for adult population levels of self-reported physical activity between 1978 and 2002, and found a year on year increase in the proportions of adults (aged 15–64 years) reporting two or more occasions of at least 30 minutes leisure time physical activity in both women and men (62% of men, 66% of women in 2002 from 44% of men, 40% of women in 1978). Physical activity was also assessed in children and young people. The proportion of children and young people (3–18 years) reporting occasions of vigorous physical activity at least 4 times per week increased between 1995 and 2002, from 76% to 92%. The trend was similar for males and females within this age group. A slight increase (+4%) in the proportion of elderly adults (65–84 years) reporting their participation in physical activities (excluding walking) was reported between 1993 and 2001. However, the authors also reported a decrease in the proportion of adults (15–64 years) taking at least 15 minutes per day to travel and at least 30 minutes per day to travel to and from work walking or cycling between 1978 and 2002.

Supportive evidence for the impact of these policies on the Finnish population comes from a number of evaluation studies reported in the paper. For example, a survey showed that the most popular venues for physical activity were outdoor sites especially walking and cycling trails, used by at least nine out of ten Finns; and a study of perceptions among adults in Finnish regions showed that over 75% agreed with the statement that there are many possibilities in the vicinity of their residence to be physically active.

The authors concluded that policies promoting physical activity in Finland were perceived as at least satisfactory by the population. Other possible confounding factors or social changes may have influenced the self-reported levels of physical activity. One example could include an increase in the population's knowledge and awareness of the public health recommendations perhaps leading to over reporting of physical activity levels in the annual surveys.

In conclusion, Vuori *et al.* (2004) present balanced and cautious conclusions regarding the impact of physical activity promotion policies on population increases in physical activity, and recognised the limitations of studies of this type. However their conclusions are strengthened by the consistent use of the same population physical activity measure over twenty years.

Policy evaluation example: National transport policy on walking and cycling

Pucher and Dijkstra (2003) focused on the development of national transport policies to support increased levels of walking and cycling. They examined the national differences between active travel and traffic fatality rates in the USA, Germany and the Netherlands, and examined the relationship between population levels of travel related walking and cycling and the presence of supportive policies to promote these behaviours. They described the types of policies adopted by Germany and the Netherlands that may have contributed to higher levels of walking and cycling and lower levels of fatalities. These policies could be implemented at national, regional and local level. Examples of policies related to spatial planning, urban design including land use, traffic calming and cycling provision, restrictions on car use, traffic education, traffic regulations and enforcement. Of all policies identified, those including an environmental modification component included:

- Better facilities for walking and cycling. For pedestrians this has included 'auto-free' (car free) zones that cover many city centres. For cyclists the most notable policies have been heavy investment in cycle facilities. From 1976 to 1996 the Dutch more than doubled the extent of their 'already massive' network of bike paths and lanes from 9282 km to 18 948 km. From 1976 to 1995 the Germans almost tripled the extent of their bikeway network from 12 911 km to 31 236 km. Both countries also employ a number of engineering and planning measures to give bicycles priority over cars (e.g. changes to road infrastructure by building cycle lanes).
- Traffic calming of residential neighbourhoods. In both the Netherlands and Germany, 30 kph traffic calming is used on an area-wide basis, using physical barriers such as raised intersections or mid-block street closures.
- Urban design orientated to people and not cars. New suburban developments in both the Netherlands and Germany are designed to provide safe and convenient

pedestrian and bicycling access, and residential developments include facilities and services that can be reached easily on foot or by bike.

■ Restrictions on motor vehicle use. Dutch and German cities restrict auto use not only through traffic calming, auto-free zones and dedicated rights-of-way for pedestrians and cyclists, but also lower general speed limits, and restrictions on parking.

The study examined the effects of policies for transport-related walking and cycling on population rates of active travel and accidents. The authors assessed active travel behaviour using national travel survey data, and examined the variation of walking and cycling trips between countries. They compared the proportion of annual trips in urban areas made by walking and cycling in the USA, Canada and ten European countries (England and Wales, France, Italy, Switzerland, Germany, Austria, Sweden, Denmark and the Netherlands). The modal split for cycling and walking in the USA was 1% and 6% respectively, compared to 12% and 22% in Germany and 28% and 18% in the Netherlands. They reported the proportion of trips made in urban areas made by cycling and walking in the USA, Germany and the Netherlands, by age group, in 1995. They showed striking variations between the USA and other two European countries by age. For example in the USA for adults over 75 years the proportion of trips made in urban areas made by cycling and walking was 0.2% and 6%, 7% and 48% in Germany, and 24% and 24% in the Netherlands.

The study compared the pedestrian and cycling fatality and injury rates per trip and distance travelled between the three countries. Both fatality and injury rates were considerably higher in the USA compared to Germany and the Netherlands. Trends in pedestrian and cycling fatalities were reported as a proportion of a baseline level taken in 1975 to 2001. The rate of fatalities fell across all three countries however the rate of decline was far steeper and finally much lower in Germany and the Netherlands compared to the USA.

Six categories of traffic-related policy were identified based on their analysis of a range of publications, four of which included an environmental modification component:

■ Better facilities for walking and cycling
■ Traffic calming of residential neighbourhoods
■ Urban design orientated to people and not cars
■ Restrictions on motor vehicle use

The authors did not specify how these publications were selected or the methods to generate their categories. Furthermore, the impacts of policies were presented by listing the types of changes seen within each category but they did not outline which policies were relevant to which changes.

In conclusion, Pucher and Dijkstra (2003) present an argument that the presence of supportive policies for promotion of walking and cycling for transport is responsible for higher rates of these behaviours compared to the USA (presented as a country with unsupportive policy). Their approach makes this link overt and simplistic and unlike Vouri *et al.* (2004) they do not present any limitations to their study method or conclusions.

Policy evaluation example: National/regional planning policy

Schwanen *et al.* (2004) examined the impact that spatial policies and different urban forms in the Netherlands may have had on travel mode choice, and travel time and distance. Non-motorised transport behaviour was assessed using national travel survey data, sampled within populations living in areas of different urban density.

The policies identified in the paper included:

- Policies to counter urban sprawl, including the accommodation of urban growth outside the existing cities in a number of designated overspill or 'growth centres'.
- Investments in urban renewal, particularly in the old cores of the largest cities, focusing on the old private rental housing stock in the urban cores. This has led to the Big Cities Policy that includes the aim to renew and partially replace the social housing estates built in the 1950s and 1960s.
- A policy for the centralised location of firms that aimed to discourage the use of the private car and to promote the use of public transport together with cycling and walking.

The study examined the effects of these types of policies on active travel behaviour and travel time and distances at different level of urban density. Schwanen *et al.* (2004) described an evaluation of the possible impacts of the Netherlands' national physical planning policy on travel behaviour. They described four phases of planning between 1970 and 2000. They examined the possible impacts of these policies by comparing modal split by different areas of urbanisation. They examined modal split for commuting and shopping trips. Modal split by commuting and level of urbanisation for cycling was higher for adults living in more urbanised areas compared to less urbanised areas (32.1% vs. 22.6%). They reported a smaller difference between adults living in more urbanised areas for walking (5.2% and 4.0%). Modal split for shopping trips and level of urbanisation for cycling was slightly higher for adults living in more urbanised areas compared to less urbanised areas (33.8% vs. 30.0%). They reported a greater difference between adults living in more urbanised areas for walking as part of shopping trips (23.6% and 14.7%). They also compared the average daily travel distance (km) and time (minutes) per person for shopping activities, by cycling and walking. They reported that adults living in more urbanised areas travelled further and longer by cycling for shopping trips. They reported a difference between the average distances walked for shopping trips by adults living in more urbanised areas compared to less urban areas, but no difference in time travelled.

The authors then summarised these findings against the possible impacts of national spatial planning policies in terms of travel efficiency/mode. These impacts were summarised in one of three categories. They concluded that policies related to retail planning (supporting centralised retail development) and urban renewal, supported stimulation of cycling and walking. The authors argued that such policies also supported the development of integrated public transport systems within urban areas. Planning policies of the 1970s supported decentralised living, and shopping and employment development made a negative contribution to supporting cycling and walking trips.

In conclusion, Schwanen et al. (2004) highlight the relationship between national spatial planning policies and their impacts on walking and cycling in areas where they were adopted differently. They draw tentative conclusions that in the areas where the policies were adopted and implemented there are some positive effects on walking and cycling compared to non-adopting areas. Their conclusions are strengthened by using trend data for travel behaviour and a clear method to identify comparison areas using geographical information systems (GIS) and urban density data.

These three examples of studies from the systematic review referred to earlier (NICE, 2006) show just how difficult it is to conduct policy evaluations. In each case the links between the policy and the outcome appear to be intuitively right, but providing evidence for the association between them is very challenging. Perhaps this is what brings policy research closer to politics than science.

Evidence-based policy or policy-based evidence?

Finally, it is worth exploring the way that evidence is used in the policymaking process in order to understand the opportunities available for influencing policy. The concept of evidence-based public health has increased in importance in recent years, building on the strong tradition of evidence-based medicine (Cavill et al., 2006). The concept of evidence-based public health has been defined as '. . . the development, implementation, and evaluation of effective programs and policies in public health through application of principles of scientific reasoning, including systematic uses of data and information systems, and appropriate use of programme planning models' (Brownson, 1999, p. 87). This approach takes many of the principles of evidence-based medicine and applies them to public health. These include the initial quantification and assessment of the issue based on descriptive epidemiological data; developing and implementing intervention approaches based on the best available evidence on their effectiveness; and comprehensive evaluation to inform current and future practice. Although this may seem an obvious and logical approach to those schooled in scientific methods, it is not necessarily the preferred way of working for all professionals engaged in efforts to increase participation in health-enhancing physical activity (Cavill et al., 2006). In many ways it is even more of a leap of faith to expect these principles of application of evidence-based learning to apply to policymaking, which traditionally has been as much a political activity as a scientific one. But there are many examples of aspects of government policy being explicitly based on evidence of what works – the most striking recent example being the establishment of the National Institute of Health & Clinical Excellence (NICE) in the UK. NICE's role is to provide national guidance on promoting good health and preventing and treating ill health (www.nice.org.uk), with guidance based on tightly defined reviews of the scientific literature. In the NICE model, practitioners base their practice on guidance, which is in turn developed from the existing evidence of what works. However, this implies an over-rationalist model implicit in evidence-based health care (Gabbay and le May, 2004) and relies on the willingness of practitioners to override their own preferences for ways of working based on experience over many years. The reality however is often different. Gabbay and le May (2004) studied how primary care clinicians made decisions in two general practices in England. They found that the individual practitioners did not go through the steps that are traditionally associated with the linear-rational model of evidence-based health care. During their study period there was not a single occasion when they observed a doctor or nurse refer to a copy of the many clinical guidelines available. They concluded that most health professionals do not tend to refer directly to guidelines, but instead rely on 'mindlines': 'collectively reinforced, internalised tacit guidelines, which were informed by brief reading, but mainly by their interactions with each other' (p. 1013).

This seems even more likely to be the case with the development of public policy, which has the potential to be influenced strongly by many factors including politics, personal preferences, biases and previous experiences. So what is often seen instead, is a reversal of evidence-based policy to become what might be called policy-based evidence. Chapter 5 of this book critically discusses how the development of exercise referral schemes in the UK has been based on both limited government policy and evidence. The example of exercise referral schemes serves to show that the supposedly rational process of evidence-into-practice is often interrupted by real life concerns, opinions and practice of practitioners. This should perhaps be seen as a normal part of the policy development process, accepting that people all require different types of evidence or experience on which they can base their actions.

Conclusions

This chapter demonstrates how important policy initiatives can be in creating conditions and environments that make it easier for people to make healthier choices. By influencing policy there is potential to reach greater numbers of people, and also to change conditions that can have a longer-lasting impact. However, there are also significant challenges inherent in working in the policy domain. The most important challenge is to effectively demonstrate the impact of policy initiatives, and in particular to provide evidence that is acceptable to a public health audience. This challenge needs to be overcome if professionals are to work effectively at all levels in the socio-ecological model, influencing policy and the environment alongside more traditional inter-personal interventions.

References

Brownson, J. (1999) Evidence-based decision making in public health. *Public Health Management Practice*, 5: 6–97.

Cavill, N. (2004) *Promoting Physical Activity: International and UK Experiences*. Department of Health, London. http://www.dh.gov.uk/dr_consum_dh/idcplg?IdcService=GET_ FILE&dID=24876&Rendition=Web (accessed 28/01/08).

Cavill, N. (2006) *Building Health: Creating and Enhancing Places for Healthy Active Lives*. National Heart Forum, London.

Cavill, N., Dugdill, L. and Porcellato, L. (2005) *Physical Activity in the North West of England: A Policy Audit*. Commissioned by Sport England North West and Government Office North West (public health). http://www.nwph.net/regional%20documents/ nw%20physical%20activity%20policy%20audit.pdf (accessed 28/01/08).

Cavill, N. and Foster, C. (2006) How to promote health-enhancing physical activity? Community interventions. In *Health-Enhancing Physical Activity. Perspectives – The Multidisciplinary Series of Physical Education and Sports Science*, Vol. 6 (Eds O. Pekka and J. Borms), pp. 369–393. Meyer & Meyer Sport (UK) Ltd, Oxford.

Cavill, N., Foster, C., Oja, P. and Martin, B.W. (2006) An evidence-based approach to physical activity promotion and policy development in Europe: Contrasting case studies. *Promotion & Education*, XIII(2): 20–27.

Department of Health (1996) *Strategy Statement on Physical Activity*. Department of Health, London.

Department of Health (2005) *Choosing Activity: A Physical Activity Action Plan*. Department of Health, London.

Department for Transport. (2004) *Walking and Cycling: An Action Plan*. Department of Transport, London.

Gabbay, J. and Le May, A. (2004) Evidence based guidelines or collectively constructed "mindlines?" Ethnographic study of knowledge management in primary care. *British Medical Journal*, 329(7473): 1013.

Health Education Authority and Sports Council (1992) *Allied Dunbar National Fitness Survey*. Sports Council, London.

Hillsdon, M., Cavill, N., Nanchahal, K., Diamond, A. and White, I. (2001) National Level promotion of physical activity: Results from England's ACTIVE for LIFE campaign. *Journal of Epidemiology and Community Health*, 55: 1–6.

National Institute of Health and Clinical Excellence (NICE) (2006) *Physical Activity and the Environment, Review Four: POLICY*. NICE, London. http://www.nice.org.uk/ guidance/index.jsp?action=download&o=34744 (accessed 28/01/08).

Office of the Deputy Prime Minister. (2002) http://www.neighbourhood.statistics.gov.uk/dissemination/Info.do?page=archive.htm (accessed 28/01/08).

Ogilvie, D., Foster, C.E., Rothnie, H., Cavill, N., Hamilton, V., Fitzsimons, C.F., Mutrie, N. and Scottish Physical Activity Research Collaboration. (2007) Interventions to promote walking: Systematic review. *British Medical Journal*, 334(7605): 1204.

Pucher, J. and Dijkstra, L. (2003) Public health matters. Promoting safe walking and cycling to improve public health: Lessons from the Netherlands and Germany. *American Journal of Public Health*, 93: 1509–1516.

Sallis, J.F., Bauman, A. and Pratt, M. (1998) Environmental and policy interventions to promote physical activity. *American Journal of Preventive Medicine*, 15: 379–397.

Schwanen, T., Dijst, M. and Dieleman, F.M. (2004) Policies for urban form and their impact on travel: The Netherlands experience. *Urban Studies*, 41(3): 579–603.

Vuori, I., Lankenau, B. and Pratt, M. (2004) Physical activity policy and program development: The experience in Finland. *Public Health Reports*, 119: 331–345.

Welleman, A.G. (1999) *The Dutch Bicycle Masterplan: Description and Evaluation in a Historical Context (English Language Version)*. Directorate General for Passenger Transport, Ministry of Transport, Public Works and Water Management, The Netherlands.

World Health Organisation (1986) *Ottawa Charter for Health Promotion*. World Health Organisation, Geneva. http://www.opha.on.ca/resources/charter.pdf (accessed 28/01/08).

4 Developing the evidence base for physical activity interventions

Lindsey Dugdill, Gareth Stratton and Paula Watson

Introduction

This book has already identified that despite the unequivocal evidence for the benefits of physical activity on health (Department of Health, 2004), there is a dearth of evidence of effectiveness for physical activity interventions. The World Health Organisation recommend that between 10% and 20% of total intervention costs should be spent on evaluation. However, evaluation is sometimes seen as problematic and time consuming and takes lower priority compared to intervention delivery (Stratton *et al.*, 2005). Evaluation is essential to the effective management of any intervention programme and should inform practice. In general, evidence on the effectiveness of physical activity interventions across England is scarce and interventions with sound evaluations are required (National Institute of Health and Clinical Excellence [NICE], 2006a).

This chapter aims to address key issues that need to be considered when evaluating the impact of physical activity interventions and should inform practitioners who are working with Choosing Activity: a Physical Activity Action Plan (Department of Health, 2005) and attempting to evaluate strategies (Dugdill, 2001) developed within local area agreements, wider physical activity interventions or within health care or education settings. This chapter is an abridged version of a commissioned report produced for Sport England North West and the North West Public Health Group (Dugdill and Stratton, 2007, with permission).

> ## Learning outcomes
>
> This chapter aims to
>
> 1. introduce some methodological considerations for evaluation design
> 2. explain the key stages of the evaluation process and discuss principles of good practice when designing evaluations
> 3. critically discuss the range of tools available to evaluate physical activity in field settings
> 4. illustrate the complexity of evaluation design through the use of a developmental case study aimed at evaluating a family-based, community lifestyle intervention for overweight and obese children

Models of evaluation: methodological considerations

The previous chapter discussed the importance of applying appropriate evaluation designs to the intervention in question. The dominant naturalistic paradigm in this academic field has upheld the randomised controlled trial (RCT) as the gold-standard measurement for intervention effectiveness, and it has been difficult to move thinking beyond these approaches (see also Chapters 2, 5 and 8). An RCT approach requires very tight control over the intervention (in order to deliver a controlled, measured 'dose' of exercise), so much so that very often it becomes merely an artifact of the real-world intervention (Dugdill *et al.*, 2005; Gidlow *et al.*, 2008). The reality is that physical activity behaviour is often complex, erratic and variable on a daily basis and does not lend itself to a 'dose model'. Therefore, learning yielded from an RCT is limited because the model is probably not transferable back into a community setting; it may show if an intervention works but not why it works; it does not provide evidence of the complexity of physical activity as a social phenomenon; it does not report on the intervention processes that may lead to unintended yet positive health outcomes; and controversially, it may require potentially unethical assignation of participants to a control group when they may require (immediate) access to a necessary service (for further discussion, see Dugdill *et al.*, 2005). Guidelines from practice suggest that tailored interventions are more likely to be effective for participants and again this opposes the concept of a fixed-dose model.

Complex interventions may well require a mixed-method approach (qualitative and quantitative data, where a range (or portfolio) of data is collected (Patton, 1997; Goodstadt *et al.*, 2001; Dugdill *et al.*, 2005; Gidlow *et al.*, 2008). As South and Tilford state 'There is an emerging consensus that the complex nature of health promotion demands a pluralistic approach to evaluation and even relatively enthusiastic proponents of systematic reviews propose that these should integrate quantitative and qualitative research' (2000, p. 730). Participatory and action research orientated approaches to evaluation are often useful when trying to design an intervention where little is known about what works and practitioners are starting from scratch to achieve an intervention that meets the expressed health and social needs of stakeholders (Goodstadt *et al.*, 2001; Flores, 2008). The case study at the end of this chapter provides an example of participatory research in practice.

Evaluating interventions

Evaluation is made up of a number of progressive steps, the most important of which is the collection of appropriate data that is subsequently used to make a judgment about the value of an intervention. The evidence from an evaluation should enable practitioners to produce more effective interventions for participants. An evaluation should measure progress towards meeting the expressed aims and objectives of an intervention. Also, as the resources and skills available for evaluations are often limited, a choice of what to measure and why should be taken early on in the evaluation process. Thus, if an intervention aims to increase the number of people walking in a park, then counting the number of walkers around the park using an observational tool and a representative sampling period (morning, midday, afternoon and evening on week, and weekend days) would suffice.

Evaluation should always be seen as an integral part of the process of intervention design, especially new interventions; however, it is important to choose evaluation methods and types of data collection carefully. An appropriate evaluation should instigate improvements in intervention effectiveness or aid intervention sustainability (Boaz and Hayden, 2002). Furthermore, it is also useful to create a framework around evaluations.

An example of an evaluation framework: RE-AIM

The RE-AIM framework (for more detail see: www.re-aim.org) is perhaps a useful way for practitioners to think about structuring their evaluation.

- **Reach:** Whom did the intervention reach, e.g., through. monitoring of participant numbers through registers, post codes, questionnaires or facility usage?
- **Effectiveness:** How effective was the intervention at meeting its aims and objectives, e.g. physical activity increase, decrease in body mass index or increasing the contemplation to become physically active?

- **Adoption:** Have significant parts of the intervention been adopted elsewhere, e.g. exercise referral interventions have been adopted by most local authorities in the UK?
- **Implementation:** How was the intervention implemented and managed? How was the intervention funded? What skills did the staff have?
- **Monitoring:** What were the monitoring and evaluation strategies used to assess the quality of the intervention? Is the intervention sustainable?

This framework also allows a reporting structure to be used between partnerships. Thus, if 10 sport/physical activity interventions were in operation in one neighbourhood, each would report against the 5 RE-AIM sections allowing an overall report to be constructed using the RE-AIM headings. Many other such frameworks exist including a comprehensive evaluation framework for health promotion presented by Wimbush and Watson (2000) which covers all relevant stages of an intervention from the design and pilot stage (developmental evaluation) through implementation (monitoring, impact and outcome evaluation) to dissemination (see also Goodstadt *et al.*, 2001).

Stages of evaluation

Evaluation studies should assess process, impact and outcome of an intervention (Ovretveit, 1998; Dugdill, 2001). Outcome evaluation alone is not sufficient as it does not explore the reasons why an intervention has been successful. The researcher/practitioner should ask what, how and why a physical activity intervention is successful if the evaluation is to be meaningful. Well-designed evaluation studies should follow a series of principles of good practice outlined below (see also Wimbush and Watson, 2000). This evidence can be collected, collated and disseminated at various stages:

Stage one – planning

- Stakeholder involvement and participation – evaluation should be carried out by a team who represent all stakeholder views. A balance between insider (management) and outsider involvement (consultants, academics) in evaluation is the ideal and can help keep the balance between subjectivity/objectivity and rigorous practice.
- Needs analysis is useful for a range of reasons: for example it helps identify stakeholders priorities; it begins the evaluation cycle and provides baseline data; it identifies current good practice and/or gaps in provision; it helps to establish how and when to intervene and finally it helps to develop links with different groups.

- Clarifying aims of the intervention – stakeholders can use the needs analysis to decide on priorities for action, intervention aims and goals and implementation delivery.
- Setting evaluation objectives – this involves several stages:
  - Deciding the evaluation questions – once the aims and objectives of the evaluation are decided it should be reasonably straightforward to clarify the questions that the evaluation will address. Clarity at this stage can ensure that only relevant, rather than redundant information is collected.
  - Choosing appropriate indicators – indicators chosen to reflect stakeholder agendas will produce data of real interest and this is more likely to lead to action as a result.
  - A balance of process, impact and outcome indicators are required to avoid a focus on short-term impacts rather than longer-term outcomes. To be effective, evaluation should have a balanced range of all indicators. For instance, failure of an intervention may be due to the manner of implementation rather than the content of the intervention – only process indicators will detect this. Short-term impact measures are important to give participants and stakeholders a view as to the progress being made and can keep people engaged with the process. Outcome measures help to identify if an intervention is still on track at a later time and whether change has been maintained or lost. The boundaries between process, impact and outcome indicators can become blurred, particularly with ongoing interventions as the cyclical nature of action, evaluation and reflection can overlap.

A variety of other factors may influence evaluation design – target group, for example age, gender, disability; seasonality and climate; geographical location of intervention, for example rural and urban; resources and skills for evaluation; for example current policy supporting health practices; and environmental, cultural and socio-demographic issues.

Stage two – measurement

It is important to choose a measurement method appropriate to the evaluation question and type of intervention. A variety of research methods could be employed to gather layers of data on a topic which can be cross referenced to each other to add validity and rigour to the evaluation. Measuring process, impact and outcome will normally entail the collection of both quantitative and qualitative data.

Gaining ethical approval

There are a number of key principles that describe ethical protection when measuring physical activity (Stratton, 2006). The most important aspect of ethical evaluation is voluntary and informed consent by participants aged 16 years and over. For participants under the age of 16 (or vulnerable adults), assent from both the participant and parent/carer is required. Participants must receive an information sheet outlining the type(s) of evaluation methods to be used, the time required, alterations to normal routine and potential recompense for participation. All participants have the right to withdraw from the evaluation aspect of the intervention without penalty and without reason. Data should be treated in accordance with the data protection act (www.dh.gov.uk/en/PolicyAndGuidance/OrganisationPolicy/RecordsManagement/DH_4000489). Guidance on NHS research ethics can be found on the National Research Ethics Service (NRES; www.nres.npsa.nhs.uk).

Measuring physical activity in practice

There are a variety of methods available for measuring physical activity levels but there is no gold standard (Welk, 2002; see also Table 4.1). Key parameters for physical activity measurement include frequency (when/how often it occurs), intensity (how hard it is), time (the duration) and type of activity (walking, running, swimming, etc.). There are over 30 methods available for measuring physical activity and their practicality or feasibility of use is illustrated in Figure 4.1. The challenge is to choose the most valid, accurate and reliable tool (or portfolio of tools) with which to measure physical activity within the intervention in question. A valid instrument measures what it purports to measure, whereas a reliable instrument quantifies the degree to which a measure produces stable and repeatable results when used under the same conditions.

The choice of a measure depends on a balance between feasibility (ease and cost) against validity (complexity and expense). Diaries, self-reports (questionnaire), pedometers, heart rate monitors, accelerometers and systematic observation tools move from high feasibility to low validity and low feasibility to high validity. The key issue here is one of practicality and realism.

Self-report (questionnaire) tools

The development of an appropriate, valid and reliable questionnaire to measure physical activity is a challenging task. Physical activity for health benefit comprises several components (e.g. intensity, frequency, duration and type) that can be performed in different domains (e.g. occupational physical activity, transport physical activity, and/or physical activity during discretionary or leisure time).

Self-report tools are frequently used as they are affordable and have low participant burden. Self-report can be used in a number of formats such as diaries and questionnaires (interview, self administered or proxy-administered, for example where parents may report on the activity of their children). Self-report is influenced by the ability to comprehend a survey question and to recall activity patterns and hence, the most reliable

Table 4.1 Strengths and weaknesses of methods for measuring physical activity (Dugdill and Stratton, 2007).

Physical activity measure	Instruments available	Strengths	Limitations
Self-Report	IPAQ GPAQ GPPAQ 7DPAR Active People Survey PAQ-C/A (children/adolescents)	Captures qualitative and quantitative information. Inexpensive Low participant burden Possible to estimate energy expenditure from compendium of activities	Reliability and validity problems. Misinterpretation of questions, language problems. Problem for use in children <10 years. Potential recall bias
Accelerometer	MTI Actigraph RT3 triaxial	Objective indicator of body movement (acceleration). Provides a measure of frequency, intensity, duration. Non-invasive. Measuring frequency in seconds or minutes/ Large storage capacity (weeks). Easy data manipulation and analysis	Expensive. Less useful for detecting upper body movement, incline walking and cannot be used in water. Problems with the placements of the monitor during extended monitoring periods
Heart rate Monitoring	Polar team Polar	Indirect physiologic measure of activity. Provides a measure of frequency, intensity, duration. Non-invasive. Measuring frequency in seconds or minutes. Large storage capacity (weeks). Easy data manipulation and analysis. Useful for analyzing activity in structured sessions such as exercise classes/walking activities	Expensive. Occasional monitor discomfort. Heart rate affected by arousal, gender, fitness and temperature

Pedometers	Yamax Digiwalker	Inexpensive, non-invasive. Can be administered to large groups. Useful in a variety of settings. Useful for goal setting and promoting behaviour change. Good measure walking type programmes	Problems with between instrument variation. Can be tampered with. Lose accuracy during running activity or during intermittent activity such as exercise class or PE lesson
Systematic Direct Observation	SOPLAY SOPARK SOFIT	Can provide qualitative and quantitative information concurrently. Specific physical activity behaviours coded	Time to train observers. Time intensive data collection. Observer presence may alter behaviour
Geographic positioning Systems (GPS)	Garmin foretrak 201	Detects movement, speed of movement and distance travelled whilst outdoors. Download data and map activity patterns to geographical areas	Expensive. Does not work indoors. Can provide erroneous results (speed and distance whilst in a car). Some participant burdening. Signals can be poor in some built up areas or under cloud or tree cover

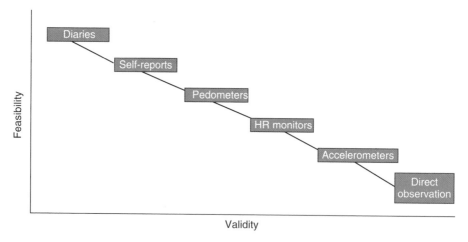

Figure 4.1 The feasibility and validity of a range of commonly used measures of physical activity (Dugdill and Stratton, 2007).

tools tend to be 3-day or 7-day recall (physical activity participation over past 3 or 7 days), as they have adequate reliability and validity in large populations (Welk, 2002). Some of the most widely used questionnaires are the International Physical Activity Questionnaire (IPAQ), and the Active People Survey. Population self-report of sport and physical activity has been inconsistent across the UK. Various tools have been used to gather data and all use slightly different measurement parameters (making trend analysis difficult) and methods (e.g. Health Survey for England, 2003; Active People Survey, 2006).

Self-report (questionnaire) tools: Active People Survey

The Active People Survey (2006) used a specially developed questionnaire (telephone interview survey) in order for Sport England to monitor sport and active recreation. Regular participation in sport and active recreation is defined by Sport England as taking part in moderate intensity sport and active recreation on at least three days a week (at least 12 days in the last 4 weeks) for at least 30 minutes continuously in any one session. Participation includes recreational walking and cycling (www.sportengland.org/active_people_results). Professionals can register to use the Active People Diagnostic (APD) tool to find information on sedentary levels, recreational cycling and walking, sport and recreation participation and volunteering (www.activepeoplesurvey.com). Whilst it is important to note that the APS only records sport and recreation activity that lasts for over 30 minutes, they provide the most up to date data on baseline participation rates in sport and active recreation in England. The APS does not assess occupational, household, gardening or transport-related physical activity (unless walking and cycling as a form of transport is a part of a healthy lifestyle choice).

Self-report (questionnaire) tools: International and Global Physical Activity Questionnaires (IPAQ: www.ipaq.ki.se/ipaq.htm) (GPAQ: www.who.int/chp/steps/GPAQ)

One of the most widely used self-report (telephone or self administered) tools is the International Physical Activity Questionnaire (IPAQ), of which there are short and long forms. Both forms include an assessment of walking, and moderate and vigorous physical activities (MVPA), and are recommended as a viable method of monitoring population levels of physical activity globally for populations aged 15–69. Some authors have found over reporting of physical activity by the IPAQ (Rzewnicki et al., 2003), whereas there is conflicting evidence on its reliability which has been reported as poor (Rutten et al., 2003) and acceptable (r = 0.8). Low criterion validity results were found between IPAQ and an accelerometer (Craig et al., 2003), whereas Ekelund et al. (2006) found similar criterion validity scores for the short IPAQ, suggesting that the specificity to correctly classify people achieving 30 minutes of physical activity per day was sound. In summary the IPAQ was not initially designed for research and evaluation purposes or in small scale interventions. However Ekelund et al.'s findings suggest that it is possible to use the long version of IPAQ to identify people who achieve activity guidelines (30 minutes per day). Therefore, it is our view that the long version IPAQ can be used for evaluation purposes and in representative samples. Technical expertise may be required with the cleaning and analysis phases of IPAQ use.

Comparing the IPAQ and GPAQ

The GPAQ (2nd version) is very similar to the long version of the IPAQ. Both assess frequency, duration and intensity of physical activity. The IPAQ includes Metabolic Equivalent (MET) values of 3.3, 4.0 and 8.0 for walking, moderate and vigorous activity respectively whereas the GPAQ only includes the 4.0 and 8.0 MET values. The IPAQ requires respondents to recall physical activity over the past 7 days compared to a 'typical week' in the GPAQ. The GPAQ has 15 questions in three domains (work, travel, recreation) and is validated for use in 16–84 year olds compared to 25 questions across 4 domains in the IPAQ (job, transport, domestic/gardening, recreation), which is validated for use in 15–69 year olds. The GPAQ data can also be cleaned and analysed using free public health analysis software (www.cdc.gov/epiinfo).

Self-report (questionnaire) tools: Physical Activity Questionnaire for Older Children and Adolescents (PAQ-C/A)

The Physical Activity Questionnaire for Older Children (PAQ-C) and Adolescents (PAQ-A) are validated (Crocker et al., 1997), self-administered,

7-day recall questionnaires, which assess general levels of physical activity in 9- to 15-year-old children. There are no valid questionnaires for children under the age of 9.

IPAQ and GPAQ and PAQ-C/A are examples of a number of forms of self-report or interview administered questionnaire. Many others can be found in a special edition of *Medicine and Science in Sports and Exercise: A Collection of Physical Activity Questionnaires* (Pereira *et al.*, 1997).

Accelerometry and heart rate monitoring

Accelerometers and heart rate telemeters are objective measures of physical activity and will be discussed together. It is unlikely that practitioners will use these because of the cost, technical expertise required for use and the complexity of data analysis. Nevertheless a brief explanation of these monitors will be described here.

Heart rate monitoring usually uses a telemetric system (http://www.polar.fi) with a transmitter which comes in the form of a belt and fits around the chest and detects electrical impulses from the heart and converts these to beats per minute. These data are either stored in the belt or transmitted to a receiver in the form of a wristwatch. Heart rate telemeters can be programmed to record heart rate second to second or minute to minute (recording interval is called an epoch) continuously for weeks.

Accelerometers (www.theactigraph.com) are small box devices usually placed on the waistband (on the wrist in wheelchair users) which record the vertical (uni-axial) or vertical, horizontal and diagonal (tri-axial) acceleration of the body. These accelerations are subsequently converted to gravitational counts per epoch duration. These instruments can record in second by second or minute-by-minute epochs. The main advantage of heart rate monitoring and accelerometry is the relatively low participant burden and the relative ease by which data can be collected and more importantly analysed. Both heart rate telemeters and accelerometers are first initialised in conjunction with their respective software programmes when names, monitor numbers and start and end recording dates and times are set up for each individual. On completion of data collection the instruments are interfaced with a PC and data downloaded. Data can then be analysed by frequency, intensity and time and patterns of activity assessed across each minute of the day.

Data produced by heart rate and movement methods is extremely valuable and is not beset by problems of recall, although most studies also use objective methods alongside a diary which requires participants to record getting up and going to bed times. For example, high heart rates at unusual times may be recorded in a diary and allow the evaluator to interpret the results with greater validity (e.g. heart rate may be elevated due to stress rather than physical activity).

From a practitioner perspective, heart rate telemetry and accelerometry may be most useful when a precise quantification of physical activity is required or any other structured intervention. Data from the instruments would then be downloaded from a relatively small number of participants and the activity contribution of the intervention analysed and reported. In one study (Ridgers et al., 2005, 2006) activity levels were monitored in primary school playgrounds using both heart rate and accelerometry. This was entirely appropriate as the physical activity had a clear focus (play), it occurred in one setting and involved a group (young children) whose accurate recall of the frequency, intensity, duration and mode of activity is generally problematic. Moreover, the data could be analysed by discrete time periods across a school morning or lunch break.

Pedometers

Many physical activity interventions and health promotion messages promote walking as a healthy and free form of physical activity available to all those physically able to take advantage of it. Pedometers can provide useful information on ambulatory walking however there are a number of problems with their use. Individual data such as stride length, body weight and age can be input into some pedometers. However, data are sometimes rounded to the nearest 1 kg or 10 cm, causing an immediate source of inaccuracy. The incorrect input of stride length is arguably the largest cause of error in estimating physical activity energy expenditure and distances covered during walking. The best use of pedometers is for recording steps and pedometers should always be manually checked for counts by using a calibrated shaker table or by hand (by counting each shake – 1, 2, 3, etc., and checking against the display). For representative data to be obtained participants need to wear a pedometer for 3 days (Tudor-Locke et al., 2005).

Pedometers are a low-cost method of generating accurate and reliable data (depending on the quality of the pedometer). A range of pedometers can be viewed at a number of different Web sites (www.walking.about.com; www.polygondirect.com). The recent range of newly developed piezo-electric pedometers are probably best for research and evaluation purposes (www.new-lifestyles.com).

The daily target for physical activity is 10000 steps per day (Tudor-Locke and Bassett, 2004). However 15000 and 12000 steps have been recommended for boys and girls respectively (Tudor-Locke and Bassett, 2004). The key aspect for activity intervention is not necessarily the debate over number of steps but whether total steps increase as a result of engaging in an activity intervention. Recent pedometer evaluations in schools have suggested that pedometers work as motivational tools (Butcher *et al.*, 2007) and stimulate increases in physical activity (see also Chapter 8).

Systematic observation

Systematic observation involves a trained observer coding predetermined physical activity behaviours (sitting, walking, running) in various settings, (playgrounds, parks, homes, etc.) undertaken by participants over set time intervals. McKenzie has designed a number of systematic observation systems and some methods (SOPLAY, SOFIT) are available on the Internet (www-rohan.sdsu.edu/faculty/sallis/measures.html). One of the most comprehensive instruments to assess walking and cycling is the SPACES system (Systematic Pedestrian and Cycling Environmental Scan; Pikora *et al.*, 2002). Systematic observation requires specific training of observers and can be undertaken live or by reviewing video media. This technique is extremely time consuming and should only be used on small groups in specific settings. Systematic observation tools are accessible for practitioners as they provide powerful data by combining both context and behaviour.

Recent technologies (GPS, mobile telephones)

Recently, geographic position system (GPS) and mobile phone technology have been proposed as tools for physical activity measurement. The Nokia 500 Sport has a pedometer integrated into the phone and can also be used to develop physical activity interventions. Sending prompting SMS messages to participants enrolled on interventions to remind them to walk at lunch break or to take the stairs and not the lift is also a good way of promoting physical activity in a cost-effective manner.

The Garmin System is a GPS monitor that detects outdoor activity and geographic positioning. The GPS system is useful for calculating distances and speeds as well as the location of activity. The integration of the system with appropriate software also allows mapping of activity, for example use of a skate park by skateboarders. The data from the GPS system provided evidence of the geographical location of the skateboarders, their distance travelled and speeds attained not only whilst at the venue but also during the travel to and from the venue. The limitation of GPS is that it only works outside and in areas where interference (cloud cover, trees, high-rise buildings) is at a minimum. GPS can be used in conjunction with other measurement methods such as activity diaries and accelerometers.

Cognitive and psycho-social measures

Control over exercise and physical activity (Kerner and Grossman, 2001), enjoyment of exercise (Kendzierski and De Carlo, 1991), cost benefit (Marcus *et al.*, 1992), intention to exercise (Kerner and Grossman, 2001), self-efficacy and social support are also susceptible to change as a result of participating in an activity intervention and are worth considering for use within physical activity interventions.

Physical environment measures

There are many useful measures of physical environments relevant to physical activity. The Neighbourhood Environment Walkability Scale (NEWS; Saelens *et al.*, 2003), Home Environment Scale (Sallis *et al.*, 1997), Perceived Environment Scale (Ball *et al.*, 2001), Awareness of Physical Activity Facilities Scale (Leslie *et al.*, 1999), and Personal, Media, External Environments and Local Opportunity Scales (Stahl *et al.*, 2001), all are readily available and, after familiarisation, are appropriate tools for practitioners to use in their evaluation.

Other outcome measures

Changes in physical fitness scores, height, weight, body mass index (BMI), skin fold measures, blood pressure, run/walk times, weight lifted, flexibility and ratings of perceived exertion may also be useful evaluation measures within specific interventions such as exercise referral. Health outcomes such as perceived health status, increased feelings of well-being and improved mental health can also provide useful evidence of programme impact (Bowling, 1997).

Qualitative evaluation techniques

Physical activity is a complex behaviour that is difficult to measure accurately. Qualitative research techniques allow behaviour to be studied in depth and in an ongoing manner. In order to enhance the rigour of qualitative research, various techniques can be employed such as triangulation (where quantitative and qualitative data are used together in an evaluation design), purposive sampling (where specific cases are selected) and sampling until saturation is reached (i.e. no new themes are emerging when you interview more people).

Qualitative evaluation techniques: one-to-one interviews and focus groups

Interviews are useful for tracking and exploring complex issues. A semi-structured interview format is often the best approach as it allows enough focus for specific questions to be asked by the evaluator however, it allows enough scope for the interviewee to give free-ranging opinions on unintended benefits and outcomes of the intervention under investigation. Focus groups (Morgan and Krueger, 1998) are a type of group interview, usually comprising about eight people, which allow very specific questions to be explored. These are a useful tool to measure ongoing processes during an intervention, or as a reflective tool to look back retrospectively on an experience of an intervention.

Image-based techniques: videos, video-diaries and disposable cameras

Images are increasingly being used to measure health-related behaviour as they allow the reality of the ongoing behaviour to be captured (Bauer and Gaskell, 2000). They can also be used by the participants themselves and hence provide an insider perspective on an intervention. Pictures and images are a powerful mechanism for getting participants to reflect on behaviour and they can also be used as a trigger for a focus group conversation. Drawings (e.g. draw and write method) are a useful tool to use with children to engage them in the research process and overcome language barriers.

Stage three – data analysis

Data should be organised according to the type of response.

Qualitative analysis

If qualitative responses are generated, then these will need to be coded. Coding is where similar thematic areas arising from within the textual evidence (interview transcript) are grouped together; e.g. all factors relating to barriers to physical activity could be grouped as one thematic area. Coding allows patterns within the data to be defined and described. This data can be organised by a paper-based or electronic method. Key points for respondents will be recorded from which themes related to activity behaviour will emerge.

Quantitative analysis

When handling quantitative data a spreadsheet or database will have to be designed, into which the data can then be input. From this, statistical analyses can be performed, and general descriptive statistics produced (means, ranges, standard deviations) on the outcome measure (physical activity). These data may be related to sub groups (sometimes called independent or grouping variables) such as gender, age and SOA (Super Output Area-Post Code). Any use of data should conform to the Data Protection Act (www.data-protection-act.co.uk), where individual identity and related data should be coded appropriately and kept in different electronic files. These data will then be available for use in an overall evaluation of sport/physical activity programming.

Stage four – dissemination

In order to ensure action results from the evaluation it is vital that all data collected during the evaluation is analysed, interpreted and disseminated in an appropriate and timely manner. Recent use of geographic information systems (GIS) may enable some data to be mapped. A balance of both positive and negative aspects should be highlighted. Examples of good practice such as case studies, qualitative quotes or photographs may improve the utility and quality of the report.

Case study: Getting Our Active Lifestyles Started! (GOALS[1]) – Phase 1

Outline of project: The GOALS project was set up to establish the feasibility of a family-based, community lifestyle intervention for obese children in Liverpool. The project has undergone several phases, the first of which is outlined in the following case study. The phase that followed (Phase 2) is discussed in Chapter 8.

Evidence is beginning to emerge that suggests management of childhood obesity requires a whole family approach, a focus on lifestyle change and input from a number of disciplines, namely physical activity, nutrition and behaviour change (Edwards *et al.*, 2005; Sacher *et al.*, 2005; Rudolf *et al.*, 2006). However, very little is known about the process of childhood obesity management and much of the how to information remains absent from current guidelines (SIGN, 2003; NICE, 2006b).

A family-focused childhood obesity intervention involves a complex and dynamic interplay between a number of components (e.g. intervention content, delivery style and environment, group dynamics, family relationships, etc.). Such complexity does not lend itself well to traditional scientific methods of evaluation [such as randomised controlled trials (RCTs) which require standardization, control and isolation of components], particularly when little is known about the phenomena in question. An alternative phased approach to evaluation was recommended by the Medical Research Council (MRC, 2000), with preliminary feasibility phases employing qualitative methodology to explore process aspects of an intervention. Too often seen as peripheral to quantifiable outcome data, it is these how and why questions that allow identification of the key components of an intervention, and therefore permit policy makers and practitioners to turn evidence into practice (Blamey and Mutrie, 2004). Following the feasibility phases, objective measures can then be drawn upon to trial the intervention's effectiveness.

Evaluation design: In line with the recommendations of the MRC (2000), Phase 1 of the GOALS project employed an action research approach to evaluation, working in collaboration with local families to develop an intervention to meet their needs. An initial structural outline was drawn from elements of the North American-based Committed to Kids (CTK) intervention (Sothern et al., 2000), which involves the whole family, is delivered in a group environment and focuses on lifestyle change (physical activity, healthy eating and behaviour modification) over a sustained period (a year). A range of qualitative methods were then used to inform the weekly development of the intervention and to identify the key components needed to build a successful lifestyle intervention for obese children in a UK community setting.

The year-long feasibility phase involved eight families attending a 2-hour weekly group session at a local community secondary school. Each family unit was made up of at least one child who was obese (aged 6–12 years) and one adult carer, though other family members were encouraged to attend. Each week the intervention covered nutrition (Fun Foods), health behaviour (Target Time) and physical activity (Move It!) through interactive, solution-focused group sessions (Sharry, 2001). The final session each week was a practical 45-minute physical activity class for the whole family, with an emphasis on fun and sustainable activities that can be practiced at home.

Figure 4.2 provides an outline of the evaluation protocol, and highlights the means through which qualitative data was collected and used throughout the year. To explore the process of behavioural change over time, each family took part in three to four semi-structured interviews during the course of the year. These were designed to explore the family's activity levels, dietary behaviour and associated feelings, and thus provided a means of tracking each family's personal experience throughout the intervention. Each participant also took part in two focus groups, designed to explore the families' shared experiences of the intervention and create a forum through which negative and positive process aspects could be discussed (e.g. recruitment, content, structure, length, method of delivery, group dynamics, aims and approaches). The interviews and focus groups were underpinned by an ongoing ethnographic exploration of the families' experiences (for a discussion of ethnography, see Hammersley and Atkinson, 1995), through which the researcher

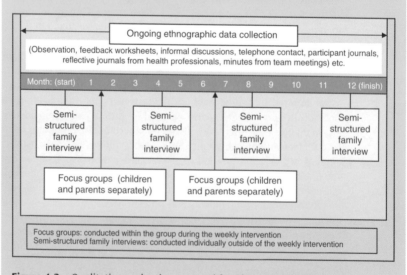

Figure 4.2 Qualitative evaluation protocol for Phase 1 of GOALS project.

collected data from a variety of sources, including observation of and participation in the weekly sessions, informal discussions with families, and reflective journals from delivery staff.

Outcomes of evaluation: Four families completed the full year of the intervention. However, qualitative data from all eight families was used to demonstrate the complexities of lifestyle change for obese children. Several themes emerged that were used to refine the intervention to trial on a larger scale across Liverpool (see Phase 2 case study, Chapter 8).

Long-term engagement: The families who completed the year felt the sustained engagement had contributed to the changes they were able to make. Others commented how a 6-month programme may have reduced the drop-out rate, but how it was important to plan an exit strategy of follow-up support.

> 'I think the fact that they [the changes] were introduced over quite a long period, nearly a year, means they're more embedded on a day to day basis. I think if it was a six week programme, I don't think it would have worked in the same way'. (Parent of 7-year-old boy)

Small, realistic steps: Families were encouraged to make small gradual steps towards their goals, with an emphasis on realistic changes they could fit into their daily lives and sustain forever. Participants reported this to be the key in forming new habits.

> 'You do need to have targets, and you do need to recognize realistic goals. Rome wasn't built in a day. Small changes work and they are commendable. If in the whole year you only change three things this is still better than nothing, and if the changes stay with you for the future then you have cracked it'! (Parent of 9-year-old girl and 11-year-old boy)

Whole family approach: A unique aspect of the GOALS approach was the inclusion of the whole family. Adult family members and non-overweight siblings were encouraged to join in the sessions, and a crèche was provided on site for younger siblings. The focus on lifestyle change for the whole family, rather than weight management for the obese child, led to a feeling of empowerment for some of the children.

> 'I come to GOALS to feel better about myself … if you go to any other programme they do more of an adult routine and like "teach the kids this, teach the kids that". But in GOALS it's like helping the adults as well as the children'. (11-year-old girl)

Open, non-judgmental approach: Although the focus of GOALS was on lifestyle change, parents highlighted the importance of acknowledging the issue of weight management. Parents noted they would be more likely to pick up a flyer if it openly stated the intervention was for overweight children (rather than general healthy lifestyles), and acknowledged that 'molly-coddling' the children might do them more harm than good; advocating a sensitive, open approach to the issue.

> 'I know we all say " fat" is not very nice but "overweight" is alright … trying to hide it and sort of molly coddle them is stupid, and they're not stupid

children, they know why they're there ... Concentrate on the positive ... say "yeh, you've done really well" and praise them'.   (Parent of 9-year-old boy)

Focus on fun – combining group and individual support: One of the key elements of the GOALS intervention was that families enjoyed attending. The group approach allowed families to learn from each other, and empowered them to challenge ideas and come up with their own solutions to support their lifestyle change. At the same time, it was found that families needed individual time to work through personal goals. During the year, skills were imparted through fun, interactive activities such as cooking sessions and active games. This is particularly important when working with children who are obese, who may have already developed a poor self-perception in relation to physical and social activities.

Application to practice: The involvement of participants in intervention design and implementation is advocated by the growing body of international health promotion literature (Popay and Williams, 1994; Rootman *et al.*, 2001). By working with local communities through a bottom-up approach, the above case study demonstrates how qualitative methodology can be used to inform the development of a larger-scale intervention. In a climate where there is increasing pressure to deliver, yet insufficient evidence of best practice delivery models, this alternative approach to evaluation allows practitioners to bridge the gap between research and practice.

Conclusion: implications for practice

To date the application of rigorous intervention design and evaluation in the field of physical activity promotion has been limited. This is due to a lack of widespread understanding of evaluation practice. The aim of this chapter was to deconstruct and demystify the process of evaluation development, giving practitioners some simple guidelines to follow when planning to evaluate an intervention. Descriptive evaluations involve straightforward analysis and reporting of data. In descriptive designs numbers/percentages of participants, and quotes from interviews may be reported, whereas complex designs involve more advanced statistical content analysis of quantitative and qualitative data respectively. In descriptive evaluations expertise within your organization or partnership may be sufficient whereas for complex designs, external support and expertise may be required. Table 4.2 (adapted from Bauman *et al.*, 2006) summarises the evaluation process. A simple, focused and rigorously executed evaluation that results in the production of informative data is the ultimate aim, rather than an overly elaborate evaluation design which may be difficult to analyse and interpret.

Finally, it is important to remember that practitioner-based, evaluation research should go beyond a process of data collection and analysis.

Table 4.2 A review of the evaluation process (taken from Dugdill and Stratton, 2007; adapted from Bauman *et al.*, 2006).

Programme stages	Level of measurement	Stages of measures	Examples of measures
	Design of physical activity programme	Formative evaluation measures	Responses of target groups prior to testing of physical activity messages or programme materials, perceptions of stakeholders of programme's likely success
Programme started	Population reached	Process and implementation measures	The proportion of people attending the programme event: or % of health professionals participating The programme was delivered as intended Environmental changes were carried out as planned; inter-agency planning/partnerships materialise and are maintained
	Proximal effects	Individual level measures	Awareness of physical activity health benefits Cognitive changes such as self efficacy Intention to be more active, beliefs Social supports; enhanced social influences; social environment; social capital
		Inter-individual measures	Physical activity behavioural changes – increased walking
		Individual level measures	Increased moderate and vigorous activities; Decreased sedentary behaviour or screen time; Increases in incidental physical activity, active transport
	Health promotion impact measures	Physical environmental measures	Changes to physical environments implemented/completed
Programme sustainability		Community level changes	Policies developed and implemented Programme elements institutionalised, programme elements self-sustaining without the presence of programme initiators

(Continued)

Table 4.2 (Continued).

Programme stages	Level of measurement	Stages of measures	Examples of measures
Programme derived policy	Long-term outcomes		Reduced disease incidence or mortality from inactivity related conditions; improved well-being/quality of life/ social capital
Dissemination		Other (non health outcomes)	Environment which facilitates physical activity better, such as improved public transport, better parks, urban planning, cultural norms and values changed to demand physical activity infrastructure. Sustained policy changes to facilitate physical activity enhancements Spread of physical activity promoting culture and its policy and resources for effective programmes to all regions where inactivity is a problem

It must produce data and which is both 'useful, usable and used' (Boaz and Hayden, 2002, p. 440) in order to effect change within that programme, or as Patton (1997) would define, utilization-focused evaluation. It is the continued learning from evaluation that can inform practice, delivery and the content of intervention processes, which ultimately will improve both their quality and effectiveness.

Acknowledgements

The authors thank the following people in the production of this chapter: Jackie Brennan (Regional Health and Physical Activity Coordinator, North West Public Health Group); Shileen Tarpey (Sport, Physical Activity and Health Manager, Sport England, North West); the Children's Fund and Neighbourhood Renewal Fund for funding the GOALS project; all participants in the GOALS project, Liverpool and the GOALS delivery team.

Note

1. GOALS Phase 1 was a partnership between Liverpool John Moores University, Liverpool City Council, University of Salford, Alder Hey Children's Hospital, Liverpool Community Dietetics Department and Leeds Trinity and All Saints College.

References

Ball, K., Bauman, A, Leslie, E. and Owen, N. (2001) Perceived environmental aesthetics and convenience and company are associated with walking for exercise among Australian adults. *Preventive Medicine*, 33: 434–440.

Bauer, M.W. and Gaskell, G. (Eds) (2000) *Qualitative Researching with Text, Image and Sound*. Sage, London.

Bauman, A., Phongsavan, P., Schoeppe, S. and Owen, N. (2006) Physical activity measurement – a primer for health promotion. *IUHPE – Promotion and Education*, 13: 92–103.

Blamey, A. and Mutrie, N. (2004) Changing the individual to promote health-enhancing physical activity: The difficulties of producing evidence and translating it into practice. *Journal of Sport Sciences*, 22: 741–754.

Boaz, A. and Hayden, C. (2002) Pro-active evaluators: Enabling research to be useful, usable and used. *Evaluation*, 8(4): 440–453.

Bowling, A. (1997) *Research Methods in Health: Investigating Health and Health Services*. OUP, Buckingham.

Butcher, Z., Fairclough, S., Stratton, G. and Richardson, D. (2007) The effect of feedback and information on children's pedometer step counts at school. *Pediatric Exercise Science*, 19(1): 29–38.

Craig, C.L., Marshall, A.L., Sjostrom, M., Bauman, A., Botth, M.L., Ainsworth, B.E., Pratt, M., Ekelund, U., Yngve, A., Sallis, J.F. and Oja, P. (2003) International Physical Activity Questionnaire: 12 country reliability and validity. *Medicine and Science in Sport and Exercise*, 29: 1381–1395.

Crocker, P.R., Bailey, D.A., Faulkner, R.A., Kowalski, K.C. and McGrath, R. (1997) Measuring general levels of physical activity: Preliminary evidence for the Physical Activity Questionnaire for Older Children. *Medicine and Science in Sport and Exercise*, 29: 1344–1349.

Department of Health (2004) *At Least Five a Week. Evidence of the Impact of Physical Activity and its Relationship to Health. A Report from the Chief Medical Officer.* HMSO, London.

Department of Health (2005) *Choosing Activity: A Physical Activity Action Plan.* Department of Health Publications, London.

Dugdill, L. (2001) *Evaluation Supplement: Framework for Action.* Health Development Agency. London.

Dugdill, L., Graham, R. and McNair, F. (2005) Exercise referral: The public health panacea for physical activity promotion? A critical perspective of exercise referral schemes; their development and evaluation. *Ergonomics*, 48(11–14): 1390–1410.

Dugdill, L. and Stratton, G. (2007) *Evaluating Sport and Physical Activity Interventions: A Guide for Practitioners.* Salford University Press, Salford.

Edwards, C., Nicholls, D., Croker, H., van Zyl, S., Viner, R. and Wardle, J. (2005) Family-based behavioural treatment of obesity: Acceptability and effectiveness in the UK. *European Journal of Clinical Nutrition*, 60(5): 587–592.

Ekelund, U., Sepp, H., Brage, S., Becker, W., Jakes, R., Hennings, M. and Wareham, N.J. (2006) Criterion-related validity of the last 7-day, short form of the International Physical Activity Questionnaire in Swedish adults. *Public Health Nutrition*, 9(2): 258–265.

Flores, K.S. (2008) *Youth Participatory Evaluation.* Jossey-Bass, California.

Gidlow, C., Johnston, L.H., Crone, D. and James, D.V.B. (2008) Methods of evaluation: Issues and implications for physical activity referral schemes. *American Journal of Lifestyle Medicine*, 2(1): 46–50.

Goodstadt, M.S., Hyndman, B., McQueen, D.V., Potvin, L., Rootman, I. and Springett, J. (2001). Evaluation in health promotion: Synthesis and recommendations. In: *Evaluation in Health Promotion: Principles and Perspectives* (Eds I. Rootman., M. Goodstadt., B. Hyndman., D. McQueen., L. Potvin., J. Springett. and E. Ziglio.), pp. 517–533. WHO Regional Publications, Denmark.

Hammersley, M. and Atkinson, P. (1995) *Ethnography: Principles in Practice* (2nd Edn). Routledge, London.

Health Survey for England (2003) http://www.sportengland.org/2003_health_survey_for_england_sport_and_walking.pdf (accessed 07/10/07).

Kendzierski, D. and DeCarlo, K.J. (1991) Physical Activity Enjoyment Scale: Two validation studies. *Journal of Sport and Exercise Psychology*, 13(1): 50–64.

Kerner, M.S. and Grossman, A.H. (2001) Scale construction for measuring attitude, attitude, beliefs, perception of control, and intention to exercise. *Journal of Sports Medicine and Physical Fitness*, 41(1): 124–31.

Leslie, E., Owen, N., Salmon, J., Bauman, A., Sallis, J.F. and Kai Lo, S. (1999) Insufficiently active Australian college students: Perceived personal, social, and environmental influences. *Preventive Medicine*, 28: 20–27.

Marcus, B.H., Rakowski, W. and Rossi, J.S. (1992) Assessing motivational readiness and decision-making for exercise. *Health Psychology*, 11: 257–261.

Medical Research Council (2000) A Framework for Development and Evaluation of RCTs for complex interventions to improve health. Discussion document drafted by members of the MRC Health Services and Public Health Research Board.

Morgan, D.L. and Krueger, R.A. (1998) *The Focus Group Kit*. Sage, London.

National Institute for Health and Clinical Excellence (2006a) *Public Health Guidance: Development Process and Methods*. NICE, London.

National Institute for Health and Clinical Excellence (2006b) *Obesity: Guidance on the Prevention, Identification, Assessment and Management of Overweight and Obesity in Adults and Children (Clinical Guideline 43)*. NICE, London.

Ovretveit, J. (1998) *Evaluating Health Interventions*. Oxford University Press, Buckingham.

Patton, M.Q. (1997) *Utilization-Focused Evaluation* (3rd Edn). Sage, London.

Pereira, M.A., FitzerGerald, S.J., Gregg, E.W., Joswiak, M.L., Ryan, W.J., Suminski, R.R., Utter, A.C. and Zmuda, J.M. (1997) A collection of physical activity questionnaires for health-related research. *Medicine and Science in Sports and Exercise*, 29: S1–205.

Pikora, T.J., Bull F.C.L., Jamrozik, K., Knuiman, M., Giles-Cortie, B. and Donovan, R.J. (2002) Developing a reliable audit instrument to measure the physical activity environment for physical activity. *American Journal of Preventive Medicine*, 23(3): 187–194.

Popay, J. and Williams, G. (Eds) (1994) *Researching the People's Health*. Routledge, London.

Ridgers, N.D. and Stratton, G. (2005) Physical activity during school recess – The Liverpool Sporting Playgrounds Project. *Pediatric Exercise Science*, 17: 281–290.

Ridgers, N.D., Stratton, G. and Fairclough, S.J. (2006) Assessing physical activity during recess using accelerometry. *Preventive Medicine*, 41: 102–107.

Rootman, I., Goodstadt, M., Hyndman, B., McQueen, D.V., Potvin, L., Springett, R.J. and Ziglio, E. (Eds) (2001) *Evaluation in Health Promotion: Principles and Perspectives*. WHO Regional Publications, Denmark.

Rudolf, M.C.J., Christie, D., McElhone, S., Sahota, P., Dixey, R., Walker, J. and Wellings, C. (2006) Watch it: A community based programme for obese children and adolescents. *Archives of Disease in Childhood*, 91: 736–739.

Rutten, A., Vuillemin, A., Ooijendijk, W.T., Schena, F., Sjostrom, M., Stahl, T., Vanden Auweele, Y., Welshman, J. and Ziemainz, H. (2003) Physical activity monitoring in Europe. The European Physical Activity Surveillance System (EUPASS) approach and indicator testing. *Public Health Nutrition*, 6: 377–384.

Rzewnicki. R., Vanden Auweele, Y. and De Bourdeaudhuij, I. (2003) Addressing over-reporting on the International Physical Activity Questionnaire (IPAQ) telephone survey with a population sample. *Public Health Nutrition*, 6: 299–305.

Sacher, P.M., Chadwick, P. and Wells, J.C.K. (2005) Assessing the acceptability and feasibility of the MEND intervention in a small group of obese 7–11 year old children. *Journal of Human Nutrition and Diet*, 18: 3–5.

Saelens, B.E., Sallis, J.F., Black, J.B. and Chen, D. (2003) Neighborhood-based differences in physical activity: an environment scale evaluation. *American Journal of Public Health*, 93(9): 1552–1558.

Sallis, J.F., Johnson, M.F., Calfas, K.J., Caparosa, S. and Nichols, J.F. (1997) Assessing perceived physical environmental variables that may influence physical activity. *Research Quarterly for Exercise and Sport*, 68(4): 345–351.

Scottish Intercollegiate Guidelines Network (2003) *Management of Obesity in Children and Young People: A National Clinical Guideline*. Edinburgh: SIGN. http://www.sign.ac.uk (accessed 15/12/07).

Sharry, J. (2001) *Solution-Focused Groupwork*. Sage, London.

Sothern, M.S., Udall, J.N. Jr., Suskind, R.M., Vargas, A. and Blecker, U. (2000) Weight loss and growth velocity in obese children after very low calorie diet, exercise and behavior modification. *Acta Paediatrica*, 89(9): 1036–1043.

Ståhl, T., Rütten, A., Nutbeam, D., Bauman, A., Kannas, L., Abel, T., Lüschen, G., Rodriquez, D.J.A., Vinck, J. and van der Zee, J. (2001) The importance of the social environment for physically active lifestyle – results from an international study. *Social Science and Medicine*, 52: 1–10.

Stratton, G., Ridgers, N.D., Gobbii, R., and Tocque, K. (2005) *Physical Activity Exercise, Sport and Health: Regional Mapping for the North-West*. http:// www.nwph.net/pad/ (accessed 13/3/07).

Stratton, G. (2006) *Ethics: A Primary Consideration for BASES Members. The Exercise Scientist*. BASES, Leeds.

South, J. and Tilford, S. (2000) Perceptions of research and evaluation in health promotion practice and influences on activity. *Health Education Research*, 15:(6): 729–741.

Tudor-Locke, C. and Bassett, D.R. Jr. (2004) How many steps/day are enough? Preliminary pedometer indices for public health. *Sports Medicine*, 34: 1–8.

Tudor-Locke, C., Burkett, L., Reis, J.P., Ainsworth, B.E., Macera, C.A. and Wilson, D.K. (2005) How many days of pedometer monitoring predict weekly physical activity in adults? *Preventive Medicine*, 40: 293–8.

Welk, G.J. (Ed) (2002) *Physical Activity Assessments for Health-related Research*. Human Kinetics, Champaign, IL.

Wimbush, E. and Watson, J. (2000) An evaluation framework for health promotion: theory, quality and effectiveness. *Evaluation*, 6(3): 301–321.

Part II   Interventions in physical activity practice

Drawing on the key concepts discussed in Part I, Part II explores the evidence base and current practice for interventions in different settings and for a variety of population groups. Chapters 5 through 10 present a contemporary review of evidence, a case study of evidence-based practice from the UK, and recommendations and implications for practice in the future. The penultimate chapter provides an international perspective of physical activity promotion for public health. The book concludes with an insightful perspective on physical activity promotion for health, in the future.

5 Physical activity promotion in primary health care

Chris Gidlow and Rebecca Murphy

Introduction

A range of global and international health policy documents demonstrate the significance of healthy lifestyle promotion to public health in the twenty-first century (Department of Health, 2004a, 2004b, 2005; House of Commons Health Committee, 2004; Wanless, 2004; World Health Organisation, 2004; Hillsdon *et al.*, 2005). In the UK, the importance of the National Health Service in providing leadership in the promotion of physical activity is evident. The government has called for an active health care system (Department of Health, 2004b, 2005); one in which health care professionals offer physical activity advice, both opportunistically and routinely, and work closely with local government, private and voluntary organisations (Department of Health, 2005). Consequently, primary health care has commonly been used as a setting for physical activity promotion. The present chapter considers some of the advantages and disadvantages of this practice, and outlines the rationale behind the exercise referral approach, which is considered in more detail.

Learning outcomes

The aims of this chapter are to:

1. explain the political requirements, advantages and challenges of promoting physical activity from within the primary health care setting
2. analyse the effectiveness of exercise referral programmes (ERPs) as a public health intervention
3. critically discuss the relative qualities and importance of different methodological approaches (experimental, non-experimental quantitative and qualitative) for determining programme effectiveness

4. explain how evidence derived from different methodological approaches can be used pragmatically to inform best-practice at an operational level
5. provide a case study of a non-experimental quantitative evaluation of an exercise referral programme based in a largely rural county, to improve understanding of evidence-based practice

Why use the primary care setting?

Primary care has been considered an appropriate setting for physical activity promotion for two main reasons. Firstly, three-quarters of the UK population visit their family doctor (GP) at least once a year (Health Education Authority, 1994). This provides a unique level of access to a large and diverse population enabling physical activity promotion within the general patient population and, if appropriate, targeted towards those with existing disease or an elevated risk of lifestyle disease (Simons-Morton et al., 1998). Secondly, health professionals are often regarded as credible sources of lifestyle advice (Stathi et al., 2003) and can be important agents for promoting behaviour change in adult and patient populations (Lewis and Lynch, 1993).

Despite the advantages, there are also problems associated with using the primary care setting for physical activity promotion. Most relate to a reliance on health professionals to deliver physical activity interventions; not least because GPs, the most likely candidates for delivery, already face the substantial workload pressures of providing health care to most of the population (Eaton and Menard, 1998; Department of Health, 2004c). There are also longstanding doubts regarding health professionals' abilities to identify suitable patients and promote physical activity in an appropriate and effective manner (Gould et al., 1995; Hillsdon, 1998). Indeed, health professionals' positive attitudes towards physical activity promotion (Gould et al., 1995; McKenna et al., 1998; Smith, 1998; Steptoe et al., 1999; Douglas et al., 2006a; 2006b) appear to be offset by inconsistencies in knowledge and perceived ability (Steptoe et al., 1999). Additional organisational barriers include limited time, inadequate training, and lack of financial incentive for health professionals to promote physical activity (McKenna et al., 1998; Taylor, 2003; Douglas et al., 2006a). These themes identified by UK health professionals have been echoed internationally (King et al., 1992; Devereaux Melillo et al., 2000; Gribben et al., 2000; King, 2000; Taylor, 2003).

A number of physical activity promotion strategies have been implemented within the primary care setting, from brief opportunistic advice and provision of health promotion literature to office-based counselling and exercise referrals (Biddle *et al.*, 1994; Fox *et al.*, 1997). However, evaluations of such interventions have often been inconclusive, reporting, at best, short-term increases in physical activity (Imperial Cancer Research fund OXCHECK study group, 1995; Chambers *et al.*, 2000; Smith *et al.*, 2000; Hillsdon *et al.*, 2002; Lowther *et al.*, 2002). The aforementioned limitations associated with a health professional-delivered model for physical activity promotion make a case for intervention delivery outside of primary care by those with the necessary expertise and resources. This effectively describes the exercise referral approach, which combines the advantages of the primary care setting for identifying participants and initiating interventions, with delivery by qualified exercise professionals at local leisure facilities.

Exercise referral programmes (ERPs)

Since the inception of the first exercise referral programmes (ERP; exercise referral been referred to as 'exercise on prescription', 'GP exercise referral', 'exercise referral' and 'physical activity referral schemes') in 1990 (Taylor, 1999), they have proliferated rapidly across the UK (Fox *et al.*, 1997) from approximately 200 in 1994 (Biddle *et al.*, 1994) to over 800 ERPs distributed throughout 89% of primary care trusts (Dr Foster Limited, 2003). A common model of exercise referral was outlined in the National Quality Assurance Framework (NQAF) (Department of Health, 2001). There are many variants of the ERP model (Fox *et al.*, 1997), but they typically involve collaboration between health professionals and local exercise professionals (Figure 5.1). The first step in the referral process is identification of suitable participants by the health professional. Most commonly, this is a GP or practice nurse within primary care, although referrals can be initiated from tertiary-based programmes (e.g. cardiac rehabilitation, hospital physiotherapy department), and occasionally, patients initiate referrals themselves (Lord and Green, 1995; Taylor *et al.*, 1998; Hardcastle and Taylor, 2001). Participants are then referred to an exercise professional. The exercise professional uses relevant medical information to devise a suitable programme of activity lasting between 8 and 14 weeks (Singh, 1997). Activity programmes tend to be delivered at local leisure facilities such as leisure centres, health clubs or alternative community settings. They involve attendance at a set number of exercise sessions (1–2 per week), which may be provided free of charge or at subsidised rates. A typical ERP targets participants with cardiovascular risk factors (e.g. hypertension, raised cholesterol, smoker), or other medical conditions that would benefit from engaging in regular physical activity (e.g. arthritis, obesity).

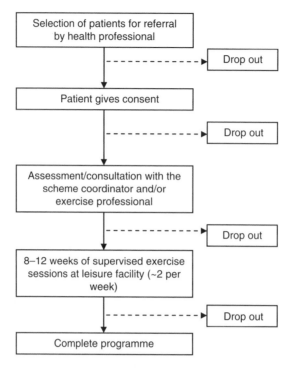

Figure 5.1 Typical referral process (adapted from Gidlow *et al.*, 2008).

Determining the effectiveness of ERPs as a public health intervention

Despite their apparent popularity with participants, professionals (Fielder *et al.*, 1995; Fox *et al.*, 1997), and a history of government endorsement (Health Education Authority, 1996; Department of Health, 2005), the public health contribution of ERPs has been the subject of much review and debate (Iliffe *et al.*, 1994; Riddoch *et al.*, 1998). Many leisure and health agencies measure the success of ERPs on scale alone; that is the number of participants who pass through a scheme each year (Iliffe *et al.*, 1994; Riddoch *et al.*, 1998; Wright Foundation Conference, 2003). The limitation of this approach is that issues of quality (i.e. experiences of participants) and sustainability (long-term adherence) are ignored. Experience shows that practitioners often design ERPs in an 'off the shelf' fashion, basing the content and delivery of their own localised programme on existing schemes. However, many operational ERPs in the UK are never evaluated and, by inference, never improved. Others gather data which are of limited use, either because the measures used are inappropriate, or are never fed back to the stakeholders. The National Institute of Health and Clinical Excellence (NICE), established in 1999 as part of the National Health Service, has the remit of providing participants, health professionals and the public with authoritative, robust and reliable guidance on current best practice. Consequently, evidence based practice has become a requirement for Primary Care Trusts (PCTs). As a service delivery mechanism, ERPs have come under greater scrutiny, which has increased pressure on scheme implementers for rigorous evaluation.

Evaluations of ERPs have included experimental trials (Munro, 1997; Stevens et al., 1998; Taylor et al., 1998; Harland et al., 1999; Harrison et al., 2005b), non-experimental quantitative evaluations (Fielder et al., 1995; Lord and Green, 1995; Smith et al., 1996a; Hammond et al., 1997; Singh, 1997; Martin and Woolf-May, 1999; Tai et al., 1999; Day and Nettleton, 2001; Carrol et al., 2002; Crone et al., 2004; Thurston and Green, 2004; Dugdill et al., 2005; Harrison et al., 2005a; Johnston et al., 2005; Gidlow et al., 2007; James et al., 2008), qualitative investigations (Singh, 1997; Crone-Grant and Smith, 1999; Hardcastle and Taylor, 2001; Stathi et al., 2003; Wormald and Ingle, 2004; Crone et al., 2005) and systematic and non-systematic reviews (Biddle et al., 1994; Fox et al., 1997; Riddoch et al., 1998; Gidlow et al., 2005; Hillsdon et al., 2005; Morgan, 2005). The remainder of this chapter will consider the different types of evidence and their respective roles for informing evidence based practice in ERPs.

Experimental evaluations

A number of randomised controlled trials (RCTs) have attempted to determine whether or not ERPs can effectively increase physical activity levels in the short and long term (Stevens et al., 1998; Taylor et al., 1998; Harland et al., 1999; Harrison et al., 2005b), and/or promote positive physiological changes associated with increased physical activity. Researchers have commonly reported short-term increases in physical activity in the intervention versus control participants (post-intervention), which are attenuated at subsequent follow-ups (Taylor et al., 1998; Harland et al., 1999; Harrison et al., 2005b). Evidence of physiological improvements (e.g. reduced body fatness, reduced blood pressure, improved self-reported health) has been similarly weak, and only associated with high attendance (Munro, 1997; Taylor et al., 1998).

Although RCTs have been similar in terms of recruitment methods, intervention duration and target patient group, there has been diversity in how closely experimental trials have adhered to the typical ERP operational processes, the nature of the intervention, and how researchers have defined success. This heterogeneity combined with some methodological weaknesses (e.g. apparent control group contamination) make it difficult to reach conclusions regarding the effectiveness of ERP.

A review by NICE examined the effectiveness of ERPs in promoting physical activity in adults (NICE, 2006). Studies were included if they were experimental, controlled and measured physical activity or physical fitness outcomes at baseline and six weeks post-intervention. Based on findings from the four RCTs that met the inclusion criteria, the review concluded that ERP can have positive effects on physical activity in the short term (6–12 weeks), but are ineffective in increasing physical activity levels in the longer term (over 12 weeks) or the very long term (over 1 year). This led reviewers to recommend:

> 'Practitioners, policy makers and commissioners should only endorse exercise referral schemes to promote physical activity that are part of a properly designed and controlled research study to determine effectiveness'.   (NICE, 2006, p. 37)

The RCT is a valuable evaluative approach because of the internal validity that enables isolation of intervention effects (Evans, 2003; Rothwell, 2005). However, internal validity is achieved at the expense of external or ecological validity; that is the extent to which evaluations replicate practice and the subsequent relevance of findings to the practice setting (Dugdill et al., 2005; Rothwell, 2005). Consequently, the use of experimental methods as a means of evaluating physical activity interventions (Riddoch et al., 1998; Strean, 1998; Department of Health, 2001) and complex community interventions (Bowler and Gooding, 1995; Goodstadt et al., 2001) has become a contentious issue (Blamey and Mutrie, 2004; Dugdill et al., 2005). Information obtained from experimental trials can provide information about what works in ideal conditions, but transferring the operational characteristics of efficacy trials into real-world situations, where resource and funding become a limitation, is problematic (Bowler and Gooding, 1995).

With one exception (Harrison et al., 2005a), experimental research to date, has manipulated the operational processes that are characteristic of UK ERPs in terms of recruitment strategies, exclusion criteria, and the nature of support provided for participants. Subjects have been recruited by researchers through postal invitation (Stevens et al., 1998; Taylor et al., 1998) or within a practice setting (Harland et al., 1999). There is evidence that GPs are regarded as credible sources of health advice, making them potential determining factors in behaviour change (O'Neill and Reid, 1991; Hardcastle and Taylor, 2001; Stathi et al., 2003). Therefore, it is important to consider the likely differences in people's responses to an invitation (from a researcher) to participate in a study compared with a recommendation made by their GP; clearly this has potential implications for sample representativeness in ERP trials (Gidlow et al., 2008). The use of specific inclusion/exclusion criteria that are not used in practice can be similarly detrimental for sample representativeness. For example, recruiting adults of middle-to-early old age (Stevens *et al.*, 1998; Taylor *et al.*, 1998; Harland *et al.*, 1999) might ensure adequate numbers within the target group. However, as such specific age limits are rarely applied in practice, ecological validity is compromised (Gidlow *et al.*, 2008). Finally, a common feature of experimental evaluations has been a lack of supervised exercise sessions and limited participant support beyond health professional advice, yet support for exercise following referral is the key characteristic of UK ERPs (Department of Health, 2001).

Non-experimental quantitative evaluations

A number of non-experimental, quantitative, longitudinal evaluations have attempted to understand elements of the exercise referral process without manipulating operational aspects of ERPs. By adhering to the operational processes of the scheme under evaluation, this approach concedes some of the internal validity associated with controlled experimental trials in order to maximise their relevance and applicability to practice. Such studies are, nevertheless, relevant to the effectiveness debate surrounding ERPs. An ecologically valid approach is required to understand the types of people who get referred to schemes and (un)successfully attend in practice, which in turn, will influence how successful they are. An earlier review of British ERPs revealed a lack of in-depth evaluation of who is referred, who removes themselves from the scheme at different stages and who attends or successfully completes the exercise programmes (Gidlow *et al.*, 2005). Indeed, known socio-demographic correlates of physical activity (Trost *et al.*, 2002) have been given limited consideration in relation to both uptake and attendance.

Published evidence from this kind of longitudinal evaluation has provided valuable information on rates and patterning of referral, uptake and programme completion in ERPs. Evidence derived from non-experimental quantitative evaluations and qualitative investigations provides knowledge of the population groups most suited to the exercise referral process, offering better insight into the public health role of ERPs. Rates of referral uptake have been variable (43–79%; Dugdill and Graham, 2005; Harrison *et al.*, 2005a), and rates of sustained attendance or programme completion often low (<20–42%: Lord and Green 1995; Dugdill and Graham, 2005). However, poor reporting and monitoring of participant characteristics in relation to referral, uptake and attendance, in addition to variation in ERP interventions, have previously limited how much we can learn about the most appropriate participants and specific characteristics of successful schemes (Gidlow *et al.*, 2005).

More recent population-based longitudinal ERP evaluations have identified marked socio-demographic patterns (Harrison et al., 2005a; Gidlow et al., 2007). As discussed in the chapter case study, referral patterns that largely mirror the socio-demographics of primary care consultations suggest relative equity in access to ERP, but patterns of referral uptake and programme attendance appear more closely related to well-established correlates of participation in physical activity and related research/interventions (Harrison et al., 2005a; Gidlow et al., 2007). Therefore, data from non-experimental ERP evaluations suggest that the ERP model is less appropriate for certain population groups, which must be considered when designing and targeting schemes.

Limitations of RCT/quantitative data – challenging the quality of delivery

Positivist research methodologies have dominated review articles concerning the evaluation of ERPs (Riddoch et al., 1998; Hillsdon et al., 2005; Morgan, 2005). The limitations of relying solely upon experimental methods to determine the effectiveness of ERP are linked to a wider debate concerning what constitutes evidence in health promotion and the most appropriate methodologies to derive such evidence (Baum, 1995; Goodstadt et al., 2001; Springett, 2001; Coote et al., 2004; Dugdill et al., 2005). There is a contradiction between the RCT approach and the underlying philosophy of health promotion. In contrast to the expert driven ideology of the RCT, health promotion aims to empower participants by engaging them in the process (World Health Organisation, 1986; Peersman, 2001). Artificial randomisation of participants to a non-intervention control group can be questioned on ethical grounds (Dugdill et al., 2005) and is often compromised by contamination of control participants (Nutbeam, 1998; Hardman, 1999).

Research design strategies associated with positivistic research doctrines, in particular the RCT, are considered the gold standard within Sport and Exercise Science (Hillsdon et al., 1995; Sparkes, 1995; Hillsdon and Thorogood, 1996; Ashenden et al., 1997; Eaton and Menard, 1998; Hillsdon et al., 2005). Yet, health behaviours, including physical activity, are complex and deeply embedded within and influenced by a range of social, environmental and political factors (Morrow, 2001). Likewise, physical activity initiatives such as ERPs are multidisciplinary in nature and conceptually utilise principles of practice drawn from disciplines including both health promotion/evaluation and sport and exercise sciences. Therefore, to understand physical activity as both a health behaviour and public health intervention, it is necessary to consider evidence from a range of areas and disciplines (e.g. behavioural sciences, sociology and psychology), using a variety of research methods. Unlike Sport and Exercise Science, health promotion, as a discipline, has embraced alternative research methodologies ranging from rigidly structured experimental or quasi-experimental designs, to less structured, more participative forms of enquiry (Nutbeam, 1998).

The major challenge facing health and exercise professionals, and organisations concerned with health development and policy target delivery, is how to facilitate long-term behaviour change in the population (McKay et al., 2003). However useful, quantitative outcomes alone provide a somewhat incomplete picture by describing what is happening in practice. The role of qualitative research in providing a more in-depth understanding of why certain patterns or behaviours are observed should not be underestimated. Despite featuring in the national guidance document in 2001 (Department of Health, 2001), the need to base practice on both quantitative and qualitative evidence has only come to prominence relatively recently. Only in recent years has the value of studies using alternative research methods gained recognition within the published literature. Evidence from qualitative research provides valuable information concerning the effective promotion of physical activity and may be the most effective means by which to describe the processes that underpin physical activity interventions (McKenna and Mutrie, 2003).

A number of review articles have embraced research that has used methods other than experimental trials; i.e. non-experimental (Gidlow et al., 2005) and qualitative evaluations (Thurston and Green, 2004). Thurston and Green (2004) propose that sociological principles should be considered when attempting to understand exercise behaviour in relation to an ERP. The authors suggest that 'any study of adults' propensity towards sustainable physical activity needs to be viewed as an aspect of their lives in the round' (p. 379) and advocate the synthesis of different perspectives in order to understand participant experiences. This viewpoint is unique to a field of research that has predominantly used principles of practice drawn from psychological and physiological disciplines.

Qualitative evaluations

Understanding peoples' experiences and the social contexts that strengthen and support physical activity behaviour is important for successful replication and dissemination of information (Nutbeam, 1998). Qualitative research methods have been used to explore the experiences of ERP participants and the specific factors that influence such experiences (Singh, 1997; Crone-Grant and Smith, 1999; Hardcastle and Taylor, 2001; Stathi et al., 2003; Wormald and Ingle, 2004; Crone et al., 2005). Referring professionals' perspectives of the exercise referral process (practice nurses, general practitioners and practice managers) have also been examined, albeit to a lesser degree (Smith et al., 1996b).

Results from qualitative investigations have revealed that participants of ERP are a complex and heterogeneous group in terms of reasons for adopting exercise behaviour, reasons for adhering to the programme, explanations for exercise behaviour post-intervention and perceived health improvements. A wide range of factors that affect participants' decisions to adopt and adhere to ERPs have been identified. These include factors related to the exercise programme (e.g. supervision and advice), participants' perceptions of their health status (both present and future) and the psycho-social environment in which the exercise takes place. Advice from a health professional is a key reason for participants to start an ERP (Stathi et al., 2003). In addition, a positive approach and attitude from exercise professionals appears important during both the early (Stathi et al., 2003) and latter stages of the programme (Wormald and Ingle, 2004). Social support from exercise instructors, family and fellow exercisers has emerged as an important component of participants' experiences of ERPs (Hardcastle and Taylor, 2001; Wormald and Ingle, 2004). Wormald and Ingle (2004), reported that the personalised, supportive and supervised nature of the intervention promoted adherence.

In addition to the anticipated physiological and behavioural benefits of engaging in an ERP, a broad range of outcomes of personal importance to participants have been identified through qualitative evaluation. These include improvements in physiological, functional, social and mental health. Specifically, improvements in physiological indices, mood and well-being (Stathi et al., 2003; Wormald and Ingle, 2004), social integration, personal development and ability to perform daily functional tasks (Crone-Grant and Smith, 1999; Hardcastle and Taylor, 2001; Stathi et al., 2003) have been reported. In this sense monitoring processes utilised by health and exercise professionals must account for the wide-ranging benefits that are experienced and, perhaps more importantly for long-term exercise behaviour change, valued by participants. Currently, the promotion of exercise at a practical level is directed by exercise guidelines (Wimbush, 1994; Sallis and Owen, 1999). Guidance for designing an exercise programme based upon pathology, physical capacity and medication is readily available to exercise professionals. However, there is less evidence available to support exercise professionals in considering the broader influences on exercise behaviour. The importance and influence of psychosocial factors in relation to participants' exercise levels, both in the short and long term, need to be recognised in the ERP context.

Health professional perspectives and partnership working

Partnership working is an underlying principle of the Public Health White Paper Choosing Health: Making healthier choices easier (Department of

Health, 2004b). Similarly, the National Quality Assurance Framework for ERP suggested that 'a scheme is more likely to demonstrate best practice if all of those involved understand their roles and commit to the process and there is partnership working with an identified lead from either primary care or leisure services' (Department of Health, 2001, p. viii). Health professionals are the primary gatekeepers for patients entering the exercise referral process and, therefore, play a pivotal role in current programme delivery. However, concerns over health professionals' abilities to appropriately identify and refer participants to an ERP have been raised (Fielder *et al.*, 1995; Riddoch *et al.*, 1998; Johnston *et al.* 2005). An examination of the reasons why, and the mechanisms of how health professionals refer participants to an ERP is essential to successful programme implementation (Taylor, 2003). Information obtained, in terms of operation and programme processes (including partnership working) at the primary care level, may have implications for health professional involvement and subsequent improvement/ modification of the referral model. At present, however, this remains a relatively under-researched aspect of ERP effectiveness.

Inter-professional partnership working can be problematic and complex due to the different training experiences and subsequent competencies articulated by professional groups (Richards *et al.*, 2000). Some evidence suggests a lack of communication and connectedness between exercise referral officers, exercise professionals based in leisure settings, and health professionals based in primary care settings (Graham *et al.*, 2005). Health professionals are also a heterogeneous group in terms of their attitude, opinion, and knowledge concerning exercise promotion in primary health care and, not surprisingly, show disparity in referring practices. All parties should be involved in the development and design of the programme. Despite the importance of the health professionals' role in initiating the referral process, they appear to have a relatively small role to play (if any), in decisions concerning the design or the delivery of the programme.

Case study: The ProActive exercise referral programme

Outline of project: Established in 1994, the ProActive ERP is a countywide collaboration between the Somerset Physical Activity Group (SPAG), Somerset Primary Care Trust, and formerly, Sheffield Hallam University (2005–2006) and the University of Gloucestershire (2000–2004). ProActive operates within a largely rural county and involves the referral of patients by primary health care professionals for a programme of supervised exercise sessions with recognised local leisure providers. Leisure providers are mostly leisure centres or health clubs located within Somerset's main towns that provide subsidised programmes of twice-weekly exercise sessions lasting between eight and 12 weeks. ProActive manages in excess of 1500 referrals per year, predominantly from GPs (>70%), and covering a broad range of medical conditions (James *et al.*, in press).

Following an earlier evaluation (Grant, 1999), changes were made to the ProActive set up to facilitate evaluation, in keeping with the current recommendations (Riddoch *et al.*, 1998) and later released national guidance (Department of Health, 2001): firstly, the Central Referral Mechanism (CRM) was introduced; secondly, scheme management was contracted out to an educational institution (Crone *et al.*, 2004). The CRM is a central database designed to keep a record of all people referred to ProActive. Central storage of all participants' details by a central coordinator overcame the common problem of incomplete information on participants who, once referred, fail to begin their physical activity programme (or take up referral) (Dugdill and Graham, 2005; Gidlow *et al.*, 2005). In addition, by recording participants' attendance levels (monitored by supervising exercise professionals), the CRM provides a log of participants from the point of referral, until the end of their involvement with the scheme. ProActive's affiliation with the University of Gloucestershire, and subsequently Sheffield Hallam University, secured the time, resource and expertise necessary for quality evaluation (Crone *et al.*, 2004).

Evaluation design: A population-based longitudinal evaluation, employing epidemiological methods was used to determine: (i) who gets referred to ProActive and (ii) socio-demographic characteristics associated with subsequent participation.

Socio-demographic characteristics included age, gender, and neighbourhood deprivation based on participants' home postcodes. Neighbourhoods were defined as Output Areas (OA), the smallest geographical unit for area level socio-economic data (mean 300 residents per area). The Townsend score of material deprivation was derived from Census 2001 data on car ownership, housing tenure, economic activity, and household occupancy (Townsend *et al.*, 1988). Dichotomous (urban–rural) and four-category variables (urban, small town/ fringe, village, and hamlets/isolated dwellings) were used to reflect 'rurality' of participant neighbourhoods (Bibby and Shepherd, 2004). The largely rural context of ProActive distinguished this evaluation from most published ERP research, the urban centeredness of which is a likely consequence of their dependence upon leisure facilities. Given the established link between access to, and use of, leisure facilities (Sallis *et al.*, 1990, 1997; Linenger *et al.*, 1991; Giles-Corti and Donovan, 2002), and potential access issues faced by Somerset's rural residents (52% live in rural areas, 32% in villages or hamlets/isolated dwellings), the inclusion of a rurality variable was considered important. Moreover, the need for physical activity intervention may in fact be greater in rural areas. The few studies that have made the comparison, report lower activity levels in rural versus urban and suburban residents (Morgan *et al.*, 2000; Wilcox *et al.*, 2000; Parks *et al.*, 2003; Martin *et al.*, 2005), a finding supported by studies looking at physical environmental characteristics in relation to non-recreational activities (Berrigan and Troiano, 2002; Craig *et al.*, 2002; Ewing *et al.*, 2003; Saelens *et al.*, 2003; Leslie *et al.*, 2005).

Outcomes of evaluation: When those referred to ProActive ($n = 3568$) were compared with the county population, socio-demographic differences initially indicated bias at the point of referral. A higher proportion of women

(61.1 vs. 51.4%), middle-aged and older adults (67.4 vs. 37.8% aged 40–69 years), and residents of more deprived areas (29.8 vs. 25.0% within most vs. least deprived quartile) suggested that health professionals were *over*-referring groups commonly reported as less active or having poorer health outcomes. However, similar socio-demographic patterns observed in primary care consultation rates (Goddard and Smith, 2001) suggest that neither discrimination nor targeting were taking place at the point of referral. With the exception of the over-70s, those groups who visit their GP most frequently were more frequently referred for physical activity.

Patterns that emerged from logistic regression analysis ($n = 2864$) of participant progression and attendance following referral were more in keeping with the accepted epidemiology of physical activity and related research. Firstly, residents of more deprived and rural areas were more likely to remove themselves from the scheme at the earliest opportunity. Compared with the least deprived, those within the most deprived quartile had a 42% reduced likelihood of progression, whereas urban dwellers had a 36% increased likelihood of progressing than rural dwellers. In relation to referral uptake (attending ≥1 session) the negative influences of deprivation and rural residency were again evident, in addition to a strong positive age effect. The odds of participants taking up referral increased in sequentially higher age groups (up to 70 years), such that participants aged 60–69 years were more than twice as likely to take up referral than the under-thirties. In participants who took up referral, the odds of programme completion (≥80% attendance) was approximately 18% lower in women than men, and increased with age, with a threefold difference between the youngest and oldest age groups.

Together, these findings indicate that factors negatively associated with general physical activity (Trost *et al.*, 2002) and related research/interventions (Chinn *et al.*, 2006) only manifested post-referral, once participants were away from the influence of the referring health professional.

***Application to practice*:** As a result of these findings and those from a parallel investigation (James *et al.*, 2008), changes to practice involved localising the ProActive setup. To reduce potential time and access barriers associated with facility-based exercise, and which disproportionately affect younger adults (Allied Dunbar *et al.*, 1992), women (Allied Dunbar *et al.*, 1992; Sallis and Owen, 1999), deprived (Sallis *et al.*, 1997; Coggins *et al.*, 1999; Giles-Corti and Donovan, 2002) and rural residents (Sallis *et al.*, 1990, 1997; Linenger *et al.*, 1991; Cox, 1998), the countywide CRM has been replaced. Five local referral mechanisms now operate, one in each District Council area. Each has a designated Active Lifestyles Officer who is better positioned to find and link up with a greater number and range of activities in the local area, to an extent that was simply not possible with a central coordinator for the whole county. The aim is to afford greater flexibility in terms of activity type, location, timing of sessions, cost, and so on, thus reducing potential barriers to participation (e.g. competing work/family commitments, transport issues and dislike of typical gym-based programmes).

Substantial dropout prior to uptake (35%) indicated that many people who agreed to an exercise referral when suggested by the health professional were not ready, lacked genuine interest or perceived insurmountable barriers to participation. Consequently, changes were made to the referral form to encourage health professionals to further consider the appropriateness of the referral; not only in terms of participants' health, but their motivation to undertake a structured programme of physical activity (Johnston et al., 2005). By promoting greater engagement and consultation at the point of referral, it is hoped that barriers to participation could be revealed at the point of referral.

Adapting the scheme in an attempt to reduce barriers to participation is worthwhile and future evaluation can confirm whether the modifications to ProActive have altered the socio-demographic profile of successful participants. Exercise referral programmes like ProActive that operate in rural areas undoubtedly present different/additional environmental barriers for participants, and potential measurement and methodological challenges for those evaluating schemes. Nevertheless, the issues raised and the way that they have been used to inform practice are relevant to, and warrant further exploration in alternative urban and rural contexts to help provide a more complete picture of factors associated with ERP participation that relate to the design and targeting of schemes.

In the context of evidence based practice, this case study illustrates how the scheme designers and implementers can not only facilitate quality evaluation, but use findings to modify schemes in an ongoing process of evaluation and improvement. It also demonstrates the value of the population-based approach (Gidlow et al., 2005; Harrison et al., 2005a), strengthening the case against delimiting ERP and other physical activity research to controlled trials of effectiveness (NICE, 2006), which by their very nature, can answer only some of the important questions (Dugdill et al., 2005; Rothwell, 2005).

Summary and implications for practice

Exercise referral programmes have emerged as the most common primary care physical activity intervention in the UK. Randomised controlled trials and non-experimental quantitative evaluations have advanced our understanding of primary care based physical activity promotion based upon quantifiable outcomes. Such evidence has identified that ERPs are effective in the short but not the long term (Taylor et al., 1998; Harrison et al., 2005b), that rates of attrition are high (Gidlow et al., 2005) and level of uptake and adherence varies in accordance with participant characteristics (Harrison et al., 2005a; Gidlow et al., 2007; James et al., 2008). A large body of evidence has come out of ERP research using a wide range of methodological approaches, which can be used to better inform current opinion regarding their effectiveness and make recommendations for best practice. However, it seems that studies not adopting a RCT approach tend to be excluded from reviews upon which such recommendations are made. Therefore, despite the abundance of ERP, and many positive and informative outcomes from uncontrolled research (qualitative and qualitative), the dearth of robust RCT evidence has raised serious questions regarding the value of schemes.

Links between physical activity and health are widely recognised (Department of Health, 2004). The resulting introduction of exercise guidelines to direct physical activity promotion (Department of Health, 1996) has led to a variety of different physical activity interventions being employed. Yet, there remains concern about the apparent lack of improvement in physical activity behaviour at a population level (Department of Health, 2003; Hillsdon et al., 2004). From a public health perspective it is important that research remains focused on improving current understanding of effective methods of physical activity promotion and intervention delivery (McKay et al., 2003). In order to replicate effective interventions this must include understanding of the processes underlying their success (Kemm, 2001). The focus of experimental research has been to determine *if* the intervention increases physical activity and not *how* this has been achieved. This inability to explain (in) effectiveness (Wimbush and Watson, 2000) is a key limitation of experimental evaluative approaches. By combining the strengths of the various methodological approaches outlined in this chapter, it is possible to utilise existing data to focus upon both outcomes and processes to determine, not only if, but also how ERP are effective.

Information synthesised and outlined in this chapter has implications for both researchers and practitioners. From a research perspective, to optimise the success of ERPs as a public health intervention, the diversity and value in alternative evaluation approaches demands greater recognition. Typically, attendance statistics and basic physiological data are collected for the purposes of programme evaluation (Department of Health, 2001). To capture broader, more holistic benefits that accrue from such programmes, a range of measures are needed to monitor patient progress and outcomes whilst on the programme. These could include the measurement of psychological parameters, social parameters, in addition to behaviour change, rather than focusing on physiological outcomes. Practitioners have a fundamental role in accurately and reliably collecting and recording data (Gidlow et al., 2005), the nature of which (and processes for doing so) must be clearly established by those involved in the design and implementation of ERP. If time and resources permit, practitioners may also engage in more rigorous and in-depth practitioner-based evaluation. Dugdill et al. (2005, p. 1398) provide a framework for such an approach, stating that:

> 'Practitioner-based evaluation research goes beyond mere measurement. It must, above all, produce data and information which are meaningful and appropriate for the purposes of effecting change within that programme …. If change and modification of the programme (to improve quality of delivery and not health outcomes) are not achieved, the evaluation will have failed'.

The suggestion that certain socio-demographic groups are less suited to ERPs despite having better access, helps confirm that schemes should not be perceived as *the* physical activity promotion intervention

(Dugdill *et al.*, 2005). Rather the role of traditional ERPs could be to provide local personalised support in a safe, supervised environment for those who require it. There are some recent examples that demonstrate a move to incorporate less facility-based alternatives within exercise referral, such as 'green exercise' (e.g. Natural England's Walk the Way to Health) and cycling referral programmes (Tierney and Cavill, 2005). Clearly, adding this kind of diversity has the potential to broaden the appeal of ERP, their role within public health and, no doubt, will bring a new set of challenges for evaluation. Regardless of setting, however, to maximise the public health potential of ERPs and other types of physical activity intervention will require further input from the different types of research described to ensure that practice is based on the best available evidence.

References

Allied Dunbar National Fitness Survey (1992) Sports Council and Health Education Authority.

Ashenden, R., Silagy, C. and Weller, D. (1997) A systematic review of the effectiveness of promoting lifestyle change in general practice. *Family Practice*, 14: 160–176.

Baum, F.E. (1995) Researching public health: Behind the qualitative-quantitative methodological debate. *Social Science and Medicine*, 40: 459–468.

Berrigan, D. and Troiano, R. (2002) The association between urban form and physical activity in U.S. adults. *American Journal of Preventive Medicine*, 23(2S): 74–79.

Bibby, P. and Shepherd, J. (2004) *Developing a New Classification of Urban and Rural Areas for Policy Purposes: The methodology*. DEFRA ODPM ONS Welsh Assembly Government and The Countryside Agency, London.

Biddle, S., Fox, K.R. and Edmunds, L. (1994) *Physical Activity in Primary Health Care in England*. Health Education Authority, London.

Blamey, A. and Mutrie, N. (2004) Changing the individual to promote health enhancing physical activity: The difficulties of producing evidence and translating it into practice. *Journal of Sports Sciences*, 22(8): 741–754.

Bowler, I. and Gooding, S. (1995) Health promotion in primary health care: The situation in England. *Patient Education and Counselling*, 25: 293–299.

Carrol, R., Ali, N. and Azam, N. (2002) Promoting physical activity in South Asian Muslim women through 'exercise on prescription'. *Health Technology Assessment*, 6: 1–99.

Chambers, R., Chambers, C. and Campbell, I. (2000) Exercise promotion for patients with significant medical problems. *Health Education Journal*, 59: 90–98.

Chinn, D.J., White, M., Howel, D., Harland, J.O.E. and Drinkwater, C.K. (2006) Factors associated with non-participation in a physical activity promotion trial. *Public Health*, 120(4): 309–319.

Coggins, A., Swanston, D. and Crombie, H. (1999) *Physical Activity and Inequalities: A Briefing Paper*. Health Education Authority, London.

Coote, A., Allen, J. and Woodhead, D. (2004) *Finding Out What Works. Building Knowledge about Complex, Community based Initiatives*. Kings Fund Publications, London.

Cox, J. (1998) Poverty in rural areas: Is more hidden but no less real than in urban areas. *British Medical Journal*, 316(7133): 722.

Craig, C.L., Brownson, R.C., Cragg, S.E. and Dunn, A.L. (2002) Exploring the effect of the environment on physical activity. *American Journal of Preventive Medicine*, 23(2S): 36–43.

Crone, D., Johnston, L. and Grant, T. (2004) Maintaining quality in exercise referral schemes: A case study of professional practice. *Primary Health Care Research and Development*, 5(5): 96–103.

Crone, D., Smith, A. and Gough, B. (2005) 'I feel totally at one, totally alive and totally happy': A psycho-social explanation of the physical activity and mental health relationship. *Health Education Research*, 20: 600–611.

Crone-Grant, D. and Smith, R.A. (1999) Broadening horizons: A qualitative inquiry on the experience of patients on an Exercise Prescription Scheme. *Journal of Sports Sciences*, 17: 12.

Day, F. and Nettleton, B. (2001) The Scottish Borders general practitioners exercise referral scheme (GPERS). *Health Bulletin*, 59(5): 343–346.

Department of Health (1996) *Strategy Statement on Physical Activity*. The Stationery Office, London.

Department of Health (2001) *Exercise Referral Systems: A National Quality Assurance Framework*. The Stationery Office, London.

Department of Health (2003) *Health Survey for England 2003 Volume 2: Risk Factors for Cardiovascular Disease*. The Stationery Office, London.

Department of Health (2004a) *At Least Five a Week: Evidence on the Impact of Physical Activity and its Relationship to Health*. The Stationery Office, London.

Department of Health (2004b) *Choosing Health: Making Healthy Choices Easier*. The Stationery Office, London.

Department of Health (2004c) *Choosing Health? Choosing Activity: A Consultation on how to Increase Physical Activity*. The Stationery Office, London.

Department of Health (2005) *Choosing Activity: A Physical Activity Action Plan*. The Stationery Office, London.

Devereaux Melillo, K., Crocker Houde, S., Williamson, E. and Futrell, M. (2000) Perceptions of nurse practitioners regarding their roles in physical activity and exercise prescription for older adults. *Clinical Excellence for Nurse Practitioners*, 4(2): 108–116.

Douglas, F., Torrance, N., van Teijlingen, E., Meloni, S. and Kerr, A. (2006a) Primary care staff's views and experiences related to routinely advising patients about physical activity. A questionnaire survey. *BMC Public Health*, 6: 138.

Douglas, F., van Teijlingen, E., Torrance, N., Fearn, P., Kerr, A. and Meloni, S. (2006b) Promoting physical activity in primary care settings: Health visitors' and practice nurses' views and experiences. *Journal of Advanced Nursing*, 55(2): 159–168.

Dr Foster Limited (2003) *Obesity Management in the* UK. http://www.drfoster.co.uk/library/reports/obesityManagement.pdf. (accessed 12/12/05).

Dugdill, L. and Graham, R. (2005) Promoting physical activity: Building sustainable interventions. In: *Exercise in the Prevention and Treatment of Disease* (Eds J. Gormley and J. Hussey), pp. 240–255. Blackwell, Oxford.

Dugdill, L., Graham, R.C. and McNair, F. (2005) Exercise referral: The public health panacea for physical activity promotion? A critical perspective of exercise referral schemes; their development and evaluation. *Ergonomics*, 48(11): 1390–1410.

Eaton, C.B. and Menard, L.M. (1998) A systematic review of physical activity promotion in primary care office settings. *British Journal of Sports Medicine*, 32: 11–16.

Evans, D. (2003) Hierarchy of evidence: A framework for ranking evidence evaluating healthcare interventions. *Journal of Clinical Nursing*, 12(1): 77–84.

Ewing, R., Schmid, T.L., Killingsworth, R., Zlot, A. and Raudenbush, S. (2003) Relationship between urban sprawl and physical activity, obesity, and morbidity. *American Journal of Health Promotion*, 18(1): 47–57.

Fielder, H., Shorney, S. and Wright, D. (1995) Lessons from a pilot study on prescribing exercise. *Health Education Journal*, 54(4): 445–452.

Fox, K., Biddle, S., Edmunds, L., Bowler, I. and Killoran, A. (1997) Physical activity promotion through primary health care in England. *British Journal of General Practice*, 47: 367–369.

Gidlow, C., Johnston, L., Crone, D. and James, D. (2005) Attendance of exercise referral schemes in the UK: A systematic review. *Health Education Journal*, 64(2): 168–186.

Gidlow, C., Johnston, L.H., Crone, D. and James, D.V.B. (2008) Methods of evaluation: Issues and implications for physical activity referral schemes. *American Journal of Lifestyle Medicine*, 2(1): 46–50.

Gidlow, C., Johnston, L.H., Crone, D., Morris, C., Smith, A., Foster, C. and James, D.V.B. (2007) Socio-demographic patterning of referral, uptake and attendance in Physical Activity Referral Schemes. *Journal of Public Health*, 29: 107–113.

Giles-Corti, B. and Donovan, R.J. (2002) Socioeconomic status differences in recreational physical activity levels and real and perceived access to a supportive physical environment. *Preventive Medicine*, 35: 601–611.

Goddard, M. and Smith, P. (2001) Equity of access to health care services: Theory and evidence from the UK. *Social Science and Medicine*, 53: 1149–1162.

Goodstadt, M.S., Hyndman, B., McQueen, D.V., Potvin, L., Rootman, I. and Springett, J. (2001) Evaluation in health promotion: Synthesis and recommendations. In: *Evaluation in Health Promotion: Principles and Perspectives* (Eds I. Rootman., M.S. Goodstadt., B. Hyndman., D.V. McQueen, L. Potvin., J. Springett. and E, Ziglio), pp. 517–533. World Health Organisation, Denmark.

Gould, M.M., Thorogood, M., Iliffe, S. and Morris, J.N. (1995) Promoting physical activity in primary care: Measuring the knowledge gap. *Health Education Journal*, 54: 304–311.

Graham, R.C., Dugdill, L. and Cable, T. (2005) Health practitioner perspectives in exercise referral: Implications for the referral process. *Ergonomics*, 48(11): 1411–1422.

Grant, T. (1999) ProActive: Increasing physical activity through a community-based intervention: A study to assess the effectiveness of the Somerset Physical Activity Referral Scheme. Unpublished report. Somerset Health Authority, Somerset.

Gribben, B., Goodyear-Smith, F., Grobbelaar, M., O'Neill, D. and Walker, S. (2000) The early experience of general practitioners using Green Prescription. *New Zealand Medical Journal*, 113(1117): 372–373.

Hammond, J.M., Brodie, D.A. and Bundred, P.E. (1997) Exercise on prescription: Guidelines for health professionals. *Health Promotion International*, 12(1): 33–41.

Hardcastle, S. and Taylor, A.H. (2001) Looking for more than weight loss and fitness gain: Psychosocial dimensions among older women in a primary-care exercise-referral program. *Journal of Aging & Physical Activity*, 9(3): 313–328.

Hardman, A.E. (1999) Physical activity intervention studies with health-related outcomes: Some issues. *Journal of Sports Sciences*, 17: 685–687.

Harland, J., White, M., Drinkwater, C., Chinn, D., Farr, L. and Howel, D. (1999) The Newcastle exercise project: A randomised controlled trial of methods to promote physical activity in primary care. *British Medical Journal*, 319: 828–832.

Harrison, R.A., McNair, F. and Dugdill, L. (2005a) Access to exercise referral schemes – a population based analysis. *Journal of Public Health Medicine*, 27(4): 326–330.

Harrison, R.A., Roberts, C. and Elton, P.J. (2005b) Does primary care referral to an exercise programme increase physical activity one year later? A randomized controlled trial. *Journal of Public Health*, 27(1): 25–32.

Health Education Authority (1994) Health screening: The facts. *Healthlines* April(8).

Health Education Authority (1996) *Promoting Physical Activity in Primary Health Care: Guidance for the Primary Health Care Team*. HEA, London.

Hillsdon, M. (1998) Promoting physical activity: Issues in primary health care. *International Journal of Obesity*, 22(2): S52–S54.

Hillsdon, M., Foster, C., Naidoo, B. and Crombie, H. (2004) *The Effectiveness of Public Health Interventions for Increasing Physical Activity Among Adults: A Review of Reviews.* Health Development Agency, London.

Hillsdon, M., Foster, C. and Thorogood, M. (2005) Interventions for promoting physical activity. *The Cochrane Database of Systematic Reviews* (Issue 1): Art. No.: CD003180. pub2. DOI: 10.1002/14651858.CD003180.pub2

Hillsdon, M. and Thorogood, M. (1996) A systematic review of physical activity promotion strategies. *British Journal of Sports Medicine*, 30: 84–89.

Hillsdon, M., Thorogood, M., Anstiss, T. and Morris, J. (1995) Randomised controlled trials of physical activity promotion in free living populations; A review. *Journal of Epidemiology and Community Health*, 49: 448–453.

Hillsdon, M., Thorogood, M., White, I. and Foster, C. (2002) Advising people to take more exercise is ineffective: A randomised controlled trial of physical activity promotion in primary care. *International Journal of Epidemiology*, 32: 808–815.

House of Commons Health Committee (2004) *Obesity: Third Report of Session 2003–2004*, Vol. 1. The Stationery Office, London.

Iliffe, S., Tai, S.S., Gould, M., Thorogood, M. and Hillsdon, M. (1994) Prescribing exercise in general practice. *British Medical Journal*, 309(6953): 494.

Imperial Cancer Research fund OXCHECK study group. (1995) Effectiveness of health checks conducted by nurses in primary care: Final results of the OXCHECK study. *British Medical Journal*, 310: 1099–1104.

James, D., Johnston, L., Crone, D., Sidford, A., Gidlow, C., Morris, C. and Foster, C. (2008) Factors associated with physical activity referral uptake and participation. *Journal of Sports Sciences*, 26(2): 217–224.

Johnston, L.H., Warwick, J., De Ste Croix, M., Crone, D. and Sidford, A. (2005) The nature of all 'inappropriate referrals' made to a countywide physical activity referral scheme: Implications for practice. *Health Education Journal*, 64(1): 58–69.

Kemm, J. (2001) Evaluation and health promotion: Seeking the common ground in different approaches: A discussion paper. *International Journal of Health Promotion*, 39: 76–79.

King, A.C. (2000) Role of exercise counselling in health promotion. *British Journal of Sports Medicine*, 34(2): 80–81.

King, A.C., Blair, S.N., Bild, D.E., Dishman, R.K., Dubbert, P.M., Marcus, B.H., Oldridge, N.B., Paffenbarger, R.S., Powell, K.E. and Yeager, K.K. (1992) Determinants of physical activity and interventions in adults. *Medicine and Science in Sports and Exercise*, 24(6): 221–236.

Leslie, E., Saelens, B., Frank, L., Owen, N., Bauman, A., Coffee, N. and Hugo, G. (2005) Resident perceptions of walk ability attributes in objectively different neighbourhoods: A pilot study. *Health and Place*, 11(3): 227–236.

Lewis, B.S. and Lynch, W.D. (1993) The effect of physician advice on exercise behaviour. *Preventive Medicine*, 22: 110–121.

Linenger, J.M., Chesson, C.V. and Nice, S.D. (1991) Physical fitness gain following simple environmental change. *American Journal of Preventive Medicine*, 7(5): 298–310.

Lord, J.C. and Green, F. (1995) Exercise on prescription: Does it work? *Health Education Journal*, 54: 453–464.

Lowther, M., Mutrie, N. and Scott, E.M. (2002) Promoting physical activity in a socially and economically deprived community: A 12 month randomized control trial of fitness assessment and exercise consultation. *Journal of Sports Sciences*, 20: 577–588.

Martin, C. and Woolf-May, K. (1999) The retrospective evaluation of a general practitioner exercise prescription programme. *Journal of Human Nutrition & Dietetics*, 12(1): 32–42.

Martin, S.L., Kirkner, G.J., Mayo, K., Matthews, C.E., Durstine, J.L. and Hebert, J.R. (2005) Urban, rural, and regional variations in physical activity. *Journal of Rural Health*, 21(3): 239–244.

McKay, H.A., Macdonald, H., Reed, K.E. and Khan, K.M. (2003) Exercise interventions for health: Time to focus on dimension, delivery, and dollars. *British Journal of Sports Medicine*, 37(2): 98–99.

McKenna, J. and Mutrie, N. (2003) Emphasizing quality in qualitative papers. *Journal of Sports Sciences*, 21: 955–958.

McKenna, J., Naylor, P.-J. and McDowell, N. (1998) Barriers to physical activity promotion by general practitioners and practice nurses. *British Journal of Sports Medicine*, 32: 242–247.

Morgan, K., Armstrong, G.K., Huppert, F.A., Brayne, C. and Solomou, W. (2000) Healthy ageing in urban and rural Britain: A comparison of exercise and diet. *Age and Ageing*, 29: 341–348.

Morgan, O. (2005) Approaches to increase physical activity: Reviewing the evidence for exercise-referral schemes. *Public Health*, 119: 361–370.

Morrow, V. (2001) Using qualitative methods to elicit young people's perspectives on their environments: Some ideas for community health initiatives. *Health Education Research*, 16: 255–268.

Munro, J. (1997) A randomised controlled trial of exercise in over-65-year olds: Experience from the first year. In: *Proceedings of the 4th International Conference on Physical Activity, Ageing and Sports* (Ed G. Huber), pp. 264–267, Health Promotion Publications, Hamburg.

National Institute for Health and Clinical Excellence (2006) Four Commonly Used Methods to Increase Physical Activity: Brief Interventions in Primary Care, Exercise Referral Schemes, Pedometers and Community-based Exercise Programmes for Walking and Cycling: Public Health Intervention Guidance no. 2. NICE, London.

Nutbeam, D. (1998) Evaluating health promotion – progress, problems and solutions. *Health Promotion International*, 13: 27–44.

O'Neill, K. and Reid, G. (1991) Perceived barriers to physical activity by older adults. *Canadian Journal of Public Health*, 82: 392–396.

Parks, S.E., Housemann, R.A. and Brownson, R.C. (2003) Differential correlates of physical activity in urban and rural adults of various socioeconomic backgrounds in the United States. *Journal of Epidemiology and Community Health*, 27: 29–35.

Peersman, G. (2001) Promoting health: Principles of practice and evaluation. In: *Using Research for Effective Health Promotion* (Eds S. Oliver and G. Peersman), pp. 3–15. Open University Press, Buckingham.

Richards, A., Carley, J., Jenkins-Clarke, S. and Richards, D.A. (2000) Skill mix between nurses and doctors working in primary care-delegation or allocation: A review of the literature. *International Journal of Nursing Studies*, 37: 185–197.

Riddoch, C., Puig-Ribera, A. and Cooper, A. (1998) *Effectiveness of Physical Activity Promotion Schemes in Primary Care: A Review*. Health Education Authority, London.

Rothwell, P.M. (2005) External validity of randomised controlled trials: 'To whom do the results of this trial apply?' *The Lancet*, 365(9453): 82–93.

Saelens, B.E., Sallis, J.F., Black, J.B. and Chen, D. (2003) Neighbourhood-based differences in physical activity: An environmental scale evaluation. *American Journal of Public Health*, 93(9): 1552–1558.

Sallis, J.F., Hovell, M.F., Hofstetter, R.C., Elder, J.P., Hackley, M., Caspersen, C.J. and Powell, K.E. (1990) Distance between homes and exercise facilities related to frequency of exercise among San Diego residents. *Public Health Reports*, 105(2): 179–185.

Sallis, J.F., Johnson, M.F., Calfas, K.J., Caparosa, S. and Nichols, J.F. (1997) Assessing perceived physical environmental variables that may influence physical activity. *Research Quarterly for Exercise and Sport*, 68(4): 345–351.

Sallis, J.F. and Owen, N. (1999) *Physical Activity & Behavioural Medicine*. Sage. London.

Simons-Morton, D.G., Calfas, K.J., Oldenburg, B. and Burton, N.W. (1998) Effects of interventions in health care settings on physical activity or cardiorespiratory fitness. *American Journal of Preventive Medicine*, 15(4): 413–430.

Singh, S. (1997) Why are GP exercise schemes so successful (for those who attend)? Results from a pilot study. *Journal of Management in Medicine*, 11(4): 233–237.

Smith, B.J., Bauman, A.E., Bull, F.C.L., Booth, M.L. and Harris, M.F. (2000) Promoting physical activity in general practice: A controlled trial of written advice and information materials. *British Journal of Sports Medicine*, 34: 262–267.

Smith, P., Illfe, S., Gould, M. and Tai, S.S. (1996a) Prescription for exercise in primary care: Is it worth it? *British Journal of Health Care Management*, 2: 324–327.

Smith, P.A., Gould, M.M., Tai, S.S. and Iliffe, S. (1996b) Exercise as therapy? Results from group interviews with general practice teams involved in an inner-London 'prescription for exercise' scheme. *Health Education Journal*, 55: 439–446.

Smith, R.A. (1998) Health professionals' attitudes towards promoting physical activity. Communications of the Annual Conference of the British Association of Sports and Exercise Sciences (BASES), University College of Ripon and York. *Journal of Sports Sciences*, 16: 104.

Sparkes, A. (1995) Writing people: Reflections on the dual crises of representation and legitimisation in qualitative research. *Quest*, 47: 158–195.

Springett, J. (2001) Appropriate approaches to the evaluation of health promotion. *Critical Public Health*, 11: 139–151.

Stathi, A., McKenna, J. and Fox, K.R. (2003) The experiences of older people participating in exercise referral schemes. *Journal of the Royal Society for the Promotion of Health*, 123(1): 18–23.

Steptoe, A., Doherty, S., Kendrick, T., Rink, E. and Hilton, S. (1999) Attitudes to cardiovascular health promotion among GPs and practice nurses. *Family Practice*, 16(2): 158–163.

Stevens, W., Hillsdon, M., Thorogood, M. and McArdle, D. (1998) Cost-effectiveness of a primary care based physical activity intervention in 45–74 year old men and women: A randomized controlled trial. *British Journal of Sports Medicine*, 32: 236–241.

Strean, W.B. (1998) Possibilities for qualitative research in sport psychology. The *Sport Psychologist*, 12: 333–345.

Tai, S.S., Gould, M., Smith, P. and Iliffe, S. (1999) Promoting physical activity in general practice; should prescribed exercise be free. *Journal of the Royal Society of Medicine*, 92: 65–67.

Taylor, A. (2003) The role of primary care in promoting physical activity. In: *Perspective on Health and Exercise* (Eds J. McKenna and C.Riddoch), pp. 153–173. Palgrave Macmillan, Basingstoke.

Taylor, A.H. (1999) Adherence in primary care exercise promotion schemes. In: *Adherence Issues in Support of Exercise* (Ed S.Bull), pp. 47–74. J. Wiley, Chichester.

Taylor, A.H., Doust, J. and Webborn, N. (1998) Randomised controlled trial to examine the effects of a GP exercise referral programme in Hailsham, East Sussex, on modifiable coronary heart disease risk factors. *Journal of Epidemiology and Community Health*, 52: 595–601.

Thurston, M. and Green, K. (2004) Adherence to exercise in later life: How can exercise on prescription programmes be made more effective. *Health Promotion International*, 19: 379–387.

Tierney, I. and Cavill, N. (2005) *Health on WHEELS: A Guide to Developing Cycling Referral Projects*. Available at http://www.cyclingengland.co.uk/viewer.php?fd=4 (accessed 28/01/08).

Townsend, P., Phillimore, P. and Beattie, A. (1988) *Health and Deprivation*. Croom Helm Ltd, Kent.

Trost, S.G., Owen, N., Bauman, A.E., Sallis, J.F. and Brown, W. (2002) Correlates of adults' participation in physical activity: Review and update. *Medicine and Science in Sports and Exercise*, 34(12): 1886–2001.

Wanless, D. (2004) *Securing Good Health for the Whole Population*. The Stationery Office, London.

Wilcox, S., Castro, C., King, A.C., Housemann, R.A. and Brownson, R.C. (2000) Determinants of leisure time physical activity in rural compared with urban older and ethnically diverse women in the United States. *Journal of Epidemiology and Community Health*, 54: 667–672.

Wimbush, E. (1994) A moderate approach to promoting physical activity: The evidence and implications. *Health Education Journal*, 53: 322–336.

Wimbush, E. and Watson, J. (2000) An evaluation framework for health promotion: Theory, quality and effectiveness. *Evaluation*, 6: 301–321.

World Health Organisation (1986) *Ottawa Charter for Health Promotion*. World Health Organisation, Geneva. Available at http://www.opha.on.ca/resources/charter.pdf

World Health Organisation (2004) *Global Strategy on Diet, Physical Activity and Health*. Available at http://www.who.int/dietphysicalactivity/strategy/eb11344/strategy_english_web (accessed 28/01/08).

Wormald, H. and Ingle, L. (2004) GP exercise referral schemes: Improving the patient's experience. *Health Education Journal*, 63(4): 362–373.

Wright Foundation Conference (2003) *4th National GP Referral Conference*. NEC, Birmingham.

6 Physical activity interventions in the community

Diane Crone and Colin Baker

Introduction

This chapter provides a review of UK-based physical activity interventions within the community and concludes with a contemporary case study, an example of a way of working which may dominate physical activity promotion for many years to come. The chapter explains the nature of interventions in the community and their variety, both in design and target population. It then explores a contemporary approach to the promotion of physical activity within the community currently being adopted by the government and implemented at county level within England. The development of County Sports Partnerships across England attempts to draw together, all the relevant organisations and agencies who are involved in the development and delivery of sport and physical activity in an attempt to raise physical activity levels by 1% per annum, within the community (Sport England, 2004).

Learning outcomes

The aims of this chapter are to:

1. present an historical perspective of physical activity interventions within the community since 1997
2. explain the political developments that have led to the establishment of Community Sports Partnerships throughout England
3. describe and critique the role, function and potential effectiveness of these Partnerships for physical activity levels within England

---

Physical activity interventions in the community: an historical perspective in the UK

Since the epidemiological evidence regarding the role of physical activity for health has been accepted, and international bodies such as the World Health Organisation and national governments in the Western world included its promotion within policy documents, physical activity initiatives have proliferated and are now widespread in both their number and variety of design.

Many interventions, for example in Scotland, have been led by a national physical activity strategy (Scottish Executive, 2003); however, in England it has more commonly been through partnerships between local government and primary and secondary care health authorities (for an example of partnership approach to exercise referral schemes, see Crone et al., 2004). As a consequence of a localised response to the development of interventions, these have varied in design, delivery, funding and evaluation protocol. As such, the quality of these interventions in terms of design, delivery and effectiveness has also been wide ranging (Gidlow et al., 2008). Subsequently, the evaluation and development of an evidence base underpinning these interventions has also been varied and not necessarily conclusive regarding their potential role in striving to increase physical activity levels within the community (Gidlow et al., 2008).

Despite these problems, example of interventions in the community are widespread and include, for example, the following:

- walking programmes for people with mental health problems
- community based cardiac rehabilitation programmes
- football programmes for people with special needs
- exercise referral schemes to address health inequalities
- exercise and weight management programmes for people who are over weight or obese
- falls prevention exercise classes for the elderly

A brief explanation of these programmes is provided in Table 6.1. The diversity of funding sources and partners involved (from the examples provided) highlights the variety in intervention practice across the country. Furthermore, they identify a contrast between the central government's acknowledgement of their worth in public health documents and a lack of mainstream funding for physical activity projects. Numerous policy documents, since 1997 (when the Labour Government were elected), have been produced extolling the benefits of physical activity for health (Department of Health, 2004a), recommending its use in the maintenance and promotion of health and treatment of poor health (Department of Health, 2004b) and to address health inequalities (Department of Health, 1999). Furthermore, many of these documents have given community interventions as examples of good practice. All of these facts point to a fundamental issue that lies at the heart of developing effective physical-activity-based interventions where there is a clear intention

Table 6.1 A summary review of example community interventions.

Name of Intervention	Key organisations involved	Target group	Funding source	Description of intervention
Walking back to health	South Somerset and Taunton Deane Primary Care Trusts, Somerset Sports and Activity Partnership, Somerset Partnership National Health Service (NHS) Mental Health Trust, University of Gloucestershire	People with long-term mental health problems	Somerset Sports and Activity Partnership	The project targeted service users and involved a monthly walk in the countryside. Participants were picked up by minibus at arranged rendezvous points, usually their supported living residence or day centre. The group travelled to the location of the walk, which was pre planned and arranged by the project coordinator. Locations for the walks included both picturesque and educational settings, e.g. Areas of Outstanding Natural Beauty and land owned or managed by organisations such as Somerset Wildlife Trust and the Royal Society for the Protection of Birds (RSPB). Walks often included educational talks from guides about a range of interests including wildlife, the herbal usage of plants, and fauna and flora. They also included a range of locations ranging from trails in woods, lakes and on coastlines [see Crone (2007) for a review of the findings]
Stepping stones	Mendip District Council, Mendip Social Services, Western Community Leisure, Adult Learning	People with special needs living in the community	Somerset County Council	The aim of the project was to offer taster sessions to adults with learning disabilities with a view to them accessing mainstream leisure provision. Taster sessions included 'Flexercise' (a chair based activity programme) sports and activity sessions in both day care and Leisure Centre settings with activities including circuit training, badminton, bowls, tennis, basketball, and Health Walks. In addition to the taster sessions a 'Buddy Scheme' was developed where registered volunteers acted as a buddy and joined in a whole host of leisure activities with service users to facilitate access to a whole range of activities including carriage riding and dog walking. Between 200 and 300 adults with learning difficulties were introduced to physical activity per year – simultaneously encouraging staff and carers to join in too!

Community-based Phase III and IV Cardiac Rehabilitation	Mendip Primary Care Trust (PCT), Mendip District Council	People who have experienced a cardiac event such as a myocardial infarction	Mendip PCT	The aim of the initiative was to initially develop Phase III cardiac rehabilitation in a rural area of Somerset. Previously Phase III Cardiac Rehabilitation was only available though the county hospitals which were more than 20 miles away from this District. The local PCT funded the Fitness Instructor training programmes for local instructors to become qualified British Association for Cardiac Rehabilitation Phase IV instructors. Once the Fitness Instructors were qualified they developed, in partnership with health care professionals, to establish both Phase III and IV classes in the local community in leisure centres and community centres. Sustainability has been assured through leisure centres managing and running these sessions, and through participant contributions for attendance
Obesity Management in Somerset	Somerset Sports and Activity Partnership, District Councils (Mendip, Taunton Deane, Somerset Coast, South Somerset), Primary Care Trusts, General Practitioner (GP) Practices, Leisure Services, Fitness Professionals	People who are either overweight or obese	Active England (Sport England Opportunity Fund)	The aim of the referral scheme was to enable people who had a BMI of 40+ (with no co-morbidities) or a BMI of between 28 and 40 (with co-morbidities) to access lifestyle counselling, a support group and physical activity sessions from trained and experienced fitness professional. Lifestyle counselling took place within the GP practice and participants were referred to both a support group within the practice, and exercise sessions within the local community, when they were deemed 'ready' to start. Further counselling and support to facilitate behaviour change were provided by the fitness professionals, through the support group and in partnership with the health professionals

(Continued)

Table 6.1 (Continued).

Name of intervention	Key organisations involved	Target group	Funding source	Description of intervention
Healthwise Physical Activity Referral Scheme	Greenwich Leisure Limited, Greenwich Teaching Primary Care Trust, Greenwich Council, University of Gloucestershire	People with known health inequalities within the borough of Greenwich	Single Regeneration Budget funding	The main aim was to ensure that affordable, accessible opportunities are provided for people to become more physically active to improve the health and well-being of the local population and reduce health inequalities. Patients were referred from health professionals. The scheme utilised five leisure centres in the Greenwich area for exercise options such as gym-based supervised sessions, circuit training and exercise to music sessions. A facilitator was assigned to the patient to assess and oversee their progression. The scheme was provided at a subsidised rate to the referred patients. The scheme's duration was between 12 and 26 weeks, depending on the patient's progress (see Mills *et al.*, in press, for a description of the project)
PROGESS (Programme of Referral to Exercise, Safety and Support)	Mendip, Taunton Deane, Somerset Coast, South Somerset Primary Care Trusts, Leisure Services, Fitness Professionals	Older people who were at risk from falling	Department of Trade and Industry	The project had two aims: ■ to provide a nationally recognised training course for fitness professionals and physiotherapist to lead safe and effective falls prevention exercise classes ■ to deliver a six month intervention of falls prevention exercise classes for people at risk from falling Participants were referred from primary care, usually a falls clinic, to a programme of structured exercise at a local leisure centre. The classes were specifically designed to prevent falls, led by one of the trained fitness professionals and the project also included a home exercise pack [see Stathi and Crone (2005), and Crone and Stathi (2005), for a summary of the evaluation of the project]

to promote better public health but uncertainty over the methods to achieve this.

Part of the reason the management and implementation of community physical activity interventions has been shared by a wide range of organisations is because within England the responsibility for the promotion and leadership of sport has traditionally been the remit of Sport England (previously The Sports Council). For many years their remit has not included the concept of physical activity. However, in 2001 there was a significant shift in the perspective taken by the government when they published Game Plan: A Strategy for Delivering Government's Sport and Physical Activity Targets (Department for Culture, Media and Sport [DCMS]/Strategy Unit, 2002). This was the first document published by a British government that combined the promotion of sport, from grass routes participation to elite performance, with the promotion of community based physical activity promotion for health improvement. Boldly, this document set targets for the improvements in baseline physical activity levels. This document was significant in that it combined, for the first time, the promotion of sport and physical activity for England. It also charged Sport England, along with partners in health, local government and the community, to contribute towards increasing national physical activity participation levels, currently 30%, to a target of 70% by 2020, of the population undertaking physical activity for at least 30 minutes of moderate activity per day, on a minimum of 5 days of the week. This ambitious target has since been amended to 50% by 2011 (Department of Health, 2005). Despite these targets being set, however, there was still no mention of significant funding for physical activity promotion until after the publication of the Chief Medical Officer's (CMO) report on the relationship between physical activity and health (Department of Health, 2004a). The CMO's report, similar to the CMO Report, again highlighted the low proportion of people not taking part in recommended levels of physical activity and as a consequence the Department of Health, the Countryside Agency and Sport England funded the LEAP (Local Exercise Action Pilots) project. The LEAP project aimed to develop and evaluate interventions designed for people with poor health, who were not meeting the national recommendations for physical activity (Leeds Metropolitan University, 2007). Ten sites within the country were identified situated in Primary Care Trust areas and each site piloted more than one physical activity intervention, for example exercise referral, peer mentoring, motivational interviewing and so on. Findings from the evaluation regarding increases in physical activity levels were mixed (for further information on the projects and evaluation, see Leeds Metropolitan University, 2007, and Dugdill and Muirhead, 2007). Although the funding of the LEAP project was commendable, it was unfortunately not available to all areas of the country. This shortfall highlighted that although there are ample references concerning the need to promote physical activity in policy and even in the setting of targets, little has been provided nationally, in terms of financial support and profile, especially when compared to that of the smoking cessation or healthy eating campaigns that have occurred in recent years.

The ambitious targets set out in Game Plan established the long-term vision for participation in sport and physical activity. In addition to setting targets, the document adopted a prescriptive approach in terms of how the conditions for increased participation could be created. This was with a view to increasing participation in sport and physical activity within all sectors of society, an approach that had not previously been adopted within government policy in the UK. Although the relative merits of sport have long been recognised in terms of their positive effect on people and communities little consideration had been devoted to developing strategies and systems to deliver these benefits long term. Game Plan was unique in that it adopted an evidence-based approach concerning the positive impact of participation and sought to integrate this directly into a comprehensive framework in order to deliver positive outcomes to all parties. This necessarily placed emphasis on reform that considered end users of sport and physical activity initiatives as fundamental to policy and planning. Game Plan recognised the need to address the lack of joined up working between public and private sectors, which had developed due to the previously ad hoc nature of policy development and the emergence of physical activity interventions within the community. Neither had appeared to be effective in, either informally or strategically, drawing private and public bodies together to share strategies on issues that crossed the boundaries of health and social welfare. As a result, across an array of contrasting strategies, local authorities developed facilities and interventions that provided opportunities for participation without necessarily developing the means to sustain this long term, or with appropriate evaluation methods at the heart of their development. Consequently, partnership working has been highlighted as a critical component in the sustainable provision of facilities and wider initiatives for participation. Alongside this is the challenge to establish criteria against which performance can be measured and evaluated in order to develop evidence for best working practices. In response to Game Plan, statutory and non governmental bodies overhauled the system for delivering sport and physical activity in the community. This has led to a new emphasis on joined up policy making, investment and delivery processes whereby partners share collective responsibility for end user experiences and share accountability for public spending.

Sport England is the main springboard for population-wide participation in community sport because it is poised between high level government and local communities in England. Although embedded in a sporting context, concepts of physical activity are implied within the overall Sport England strategy which recognises that participating in sport does not necessarily appeal to all sectors of society. In 2004 it published The Framework for Sport in England (Sport England, 2004) as a direct response to Game Plan and sought to establish the means by which organisations could develop successful sports and physical activity strategies within local areas. In doing so it aligned the outcomes of partnership working with increases in participation as criteria for success. In line with the recommendations made in Game Plan this framework document avoided focusing on developing whole-scale structures for delivering sport and instead sought to streamline working practices and coordinate decision making within existing sport structures where possible. This reflected a desire to better utilise local resources for traditional sports development initiatives as well as providing a conduit by which small scale physical activity projects could be developed and evaluated. The drive to develop collaborative working practices is not only indicative of a desire to improve cost-effectiveness and financial accountability but also of a relatively weak evidence base regarding nebulous concepts of physical activity. The integration of increasing physical activity participation as a distinctive component within the framework is significant because it will allow practitioners to develop greater knowledge and understanding of what works within non-sport based initiatives. It is anticipated that by using collaborative approaches that transcend professional boundaries the framework is the best means by which to increase and sustain participation in all forms of physical activity, including traditional sport initiatives. The framework (Sport England, 2004) is supported by the establishment of nine new Regional Sports Boards and Whole Sport Plans developed by the National Governing Bodies (NGBs) of 32 priority sports (identified by Sport England in 2003), and, as such, for the first time, has focused strategic planning for community sport *and* physical activity in England, at the heart of which lie County Sports Partnerships.

County Sports Partnerships: organisation and purpose

County Sports Partnerships (CSPs) were launched by Sport England in 2005 with the intention of developing more effective means of drawing together local stakeholders, such as further education colleges, local authorities and Primary Care Trusts, involved with raising participation in physical activity and sport in England. CSPs are key local agencies tasked with coordinating resources effectively to meet nationally determined objectives and locally identified priorities. Because physical activity and sport initiatives cut across many policy areas such as social care and the environment, these functions constitute an important part of local health agendas. As such, successful projects can contribute significantly to the Audit Commission's Comprehensive Performance

Assessment (CPAs), part of a public services management framework used to monitor standards within policy areas managed by local authorities (Local Area Agreements). Forty-nine such partnerships exist within England providing strategic direction, financial management and performance measurement. Essential to their role is the ability to determine at a local level the best means by which to achieve national objectives for sport and physical activity participation [Public Service Agreement (PSA) 1 and PSA 3], outlined by the Department for Culture, Media and Sport in 2005 (DCMS, 2005). This is achieved through communication with NGBs at the local level and Community Sports Networks, which consist of organisations directly involved with the delivery of sport and physical activity in communities, particularly Local Authority bodies. These networks are a fundamental link in the chain that ensures elements of financial accountability and cost effectiveness at the point of delivery are satisfied concurrent with Government safeguards on public spending. The function of CSPs is to deliver lasting change in local areas by providing open channels for communication between regional partners, such as the education sector, and those at the community level, such as sports clubs. This is a direct consequence of the recommendations for improved partnership working at the strategic level made in Game Plan. Essentially, CSPs act as high-level decision making bodies capable of overseeing the development of various local initiatives whilst remaining firmly embedded in the nationwide network of Sport England.

Essential to the operation of CSP's is the role performed by dedicated Sport England teams. These specialist teams consisting of professional managers, coaches and administrators form a central hub which link with local partners. At the time of writing, CSPs function as coordinators for sub-regional strategy, funding, and advocacy for sport and physical activity within their respective areas and develop essential administrative and business systems to facilitate this. Funding is received from a combination of Exchequer and Lottery sources with additional support from local authorities, Primary Care Trusts, NGBs and businesses. Many of these teams are still in their infancy and rely on a small number of staff to perform the day to day business functions with financial and operational support coming from partner organisations. This reflects an incremental top-down bottom-up approach that attaches significance to shared objectives between partners engaging together in the development of strategy from its inception and joint responsibility for its delivery.

The Single Delivery System

The organisational ethos of contemporary partnership working is firmly embedded within the Single Delivery System, seeking to devolve power to communities whilst maintaining a central administrative hub as the main point of contact. Within this context lies the potential for progressive and considered local initiatives that appreciates the complexity of contemporary sport delivery. This reflects exactly the sentiments of Lord Carter who identified a lack of joined up working as a fundamental barrier in effective sports provision and an unnecessary duplication of resources (Lord Carter of Coles, 2005).

The adoption of partnership working as a fundamental aspect of the sport and physical activity agenda in England is a genuine attempt to develop initiatives that are driven by local needs. As a consequence the myriad of organisations, clubs and other bodies involved in decision making rely on a complex set of relationships to produce meaningful outcomes. This represents a serious challenge to the ways in which organisations function and the ways in which their representatives think. At best these relationships may produce cost-effective initiatives that reach target populations with a high rate of success. Alternatively, as Newman suggests, partnerships may create illusory units masking fundamental differences in power and resources characterised by elements of tension and conflict (Newman, 2001). Thus a fundamental issue facing partnership working is the question of identity. Partnerships challenge organisations to understand their position within a broader health perspective that espouses the merits of participation without losing sight of their traditional perceptions of identity and purpose. CSPs play a critical role in developing links with partners that encourage openness between partners and a commitment to the values that lie at the core of Sport England's framework for delivery. The Single Delivery System is a significant role in this aspect in that it clarifies relationships between different agencies and organisations by highlighting their relative positions and facilitates cohesive relationships so that notions of partnership working may become manifest in real and purposeful action. This system seeks to ensure:

▪ a single strategy for sport
▪ an evidence-based approach
▪ rigorous performance management
▪ effective targeting of investment
▪ joined-up working practice

The basic tenets of this system of working (e.g. the implied equity of relationships between partners) stem from a fundamental assumption that only through equitable partnerships can equitable outcomes be developed (for an exploration of equity in health, see Rootman et al., 2001). Such is the potential diversity of members within the system that the contribution of sports partnership initiatives may be felt across broad health and social agendas. Partnership working, as a tool for engagement, develops opportunities for contrasting sectors (e.g. education and health), to maximise the use of resources by effectively aligning agendas where appropriate. This is a consequence of the pervasive political requirement for the public sector to collaborate with society at large in order to achieve genuine, citizen-centred services (Coulson, 2005). The Single Delivery System eschews the dangers of an inwards-looking 'silo' mentality (Walter *et al.*, 2003) in favour of a doctrine that is receptive to the idea of working with a variety of sectors. This parallels recommendations and ways of working within other government agencies (Department of Health, 2000a, 2004b; DfES, 2005; NICE, 2006), and facilitates the meeting of key health, education and local authority representatives working towards the common objective of improving public health across all sectors of society.

Ultimately, this system seeks to develop accountability through shared action with partners who are able to understand their role within the framework for sport in England. As such the system is integral to the functioning of partnerships between high level political institutions, lower-level strategic bodies and the participants in sport and physical activity. It lends itself to be a useful tool for identifying opportunities and problems because there is no delineation with regard to specific organisations, sports or population groups. The benefits of this are twofold. Firstly, this flexibility adds value to the provision sport and physical activity in England because users at all levels are able to employ it within planning, development and delivery stages regardless of the nature of activity. This may be defining a working process, designing strategies or developing links between local organisations. Secondly, it underpins and supports defined pathways in other sporting areas (such as the Youth Sports Trust and UK Sport) by encouraging and supporting the conditions for sporting success without redesigning systems already in place in these specific organisational areas (see Figure 6.1).

Perhaps the singularly most challenging issue facing the successful implementation of the Single Delivery System is the lack of evidence concerning the effectiveness of targeted interventions and how best to evaluate them. Although the efficacy of sport and physical activity for health is now accepted (Department of Health, 2004a), the methods by which these benefits are delivered successfully into communities are at best ad hoc and at worst ineffectual. This may be the result of the variances in quality and type of advice being offered to health professionals involved with developing local strategies (Dugdill *et al.*, 2005; Dugdill and Stratton, 2007). In the case of contemporary partnerships, there exists a danger that the political rhetoric of joined-up working is not being matched by a corresponding understanding of how to deliver successful outcomes at the local level (Halliday *et al.*, 2004). As a consequence, resource-intensive interventions may neither improve health status nor provide cost-effective designs. Within the context

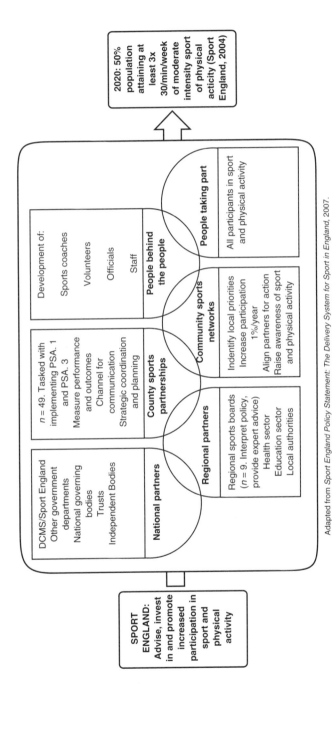

Figure 6.1   The overlapping links in the Single Delivery System.

Adapted from *Sport England Policy Statement: The Delivery System for Sport in England*, 2007.

of sport in England, the Active People Survey (Sport England, 2006) sought to redress the lack of evidence concerning population scale participation by developing a large scale database of sport and physical activity habits across England. It is anticipated this data will assist partner organisations in understanding local trends in sports participation and better enable them to develop opportunities that deliver long-term effects. Given the relative infancy and continuing emergence of local partnerships, it is unlikely that this information will impact outcomes in any significant way until the methods by which to employ it are developed across the regions. However, in terms of understanding population level trends and local patterns of participation, the Active People Survey is a significant step forward and develops an ongoing tool for performance measurement by establishing key evaluation criteria. Possible barriers to its future usefulness are outlined further below.

Within public service mechanisms such as the Single Delivery System, it is recognised that there are inherent risks that have the potential to stifle efficiency and effectiveness of partnerships (Audit Commission/ National Audit Office, 2006). A lack of clarity between partners concerning desired outcomes potentially gives rise to situations where resources are insufficiently aligned for the desired effects to take place. As such, there is a new imperative for research that seeks to determine the nature and effects of factors within partnerships. Current safeguards within the delivery system formalise partnership agreements in order to develop measures of accountability between those involved. This provides a potent tool for maintaining the collective focus of partners during the development and implementation of interventions and initiatives. These include criteria that must be met by potential partners and actions plans outlining the use of resources to effect change. The relative differences in stages of partnership development currently mean that these safeguards may vary in strength and nature across England. Within this operational context at every stage is the fundamental issue of how best to define effective partnership working practices.

Although government policy has for some time recommended that organisations develop ways of working together towards common objectives within the health agenda (Department of Health, 1999, 2004b), there is a danger that the relative benefits of partnerships are assumed without necessarily being incorporated into practice in any meaningful way. This is because evidence tends to be based on studies focusing on the principles of partnership processes rather than assessing the outcomes they generate (Boydell and Rugkåsa, 2007). This emphasis should serve to remind organisations that alongside the diversity that partnerships embrace sit difficult methodological questions in determining their true validity within sport and physical activity provision. The current research agenda by implication must distinguish investigations pertaining to the outcomes of partnership working and the outcomes of interventions and initiatives (El Ansari and Phillips, 2001). In response to the current gaps in knowledge concerning the efficacy of partnerships, McDonald (2005) calls for more contextual analysis to determine not prescriptive models of practice but theories capable of distinguishing between types of partnerships. This approach has value in that it may develop a more realistic understanding of the benefits, potential contradictions and processes involved within partnerships. Considering that valuable data already exists concerning population level participation there is an urgency to develop and refine mechanisms and approaches with which to make use of it. It is likely that until the role, relevance and contextual dynamics of partnerships are better understood, partnerships seeking to address issues of participation and non participation may have limited effectiveness. The case study below explores this in more detail.

Case study: Active Gloucestershire – an effective partnership to increase community participation?

The following case study profiles local aspects of the delivery system and seeks to demonstrate the practicalities involved in establishing partnerships for community health improvement.

Demographic profile of Gloucestershire (Gloucestershire County Council, 2005)

- The population figure for Gloucestershire in mid-2005 was estimated as 575 200 people, which represented an average increase of 0.49% or 2 614 people per year since 1991 although this growth is slowing.
- There was an overall trend of falling fertility rates at county and district level and despite anomalies in 2005 this continued to be below the required replacement fertility level, reflecting the national trend.
- The majority of population growth across the county over this period was attributable to net in-migration, which accounted for over 86% of the increase.
- The latest life expectancy estimates increased slightly to 77.7 years for men and to 81.7 years for women. This mirrors national trends in which life expectancy has increased for men and women (to 76.5 years and 80.9 years respectively).
- There is a trend towards an ageing population. The growth of the elderly population continues to outpace that of the young population. Between 1991 and 2005 the proportion of pensioners in the county increased from 19.8% to 20.6%. The proportion of children aged under 16 decreased from 19.6% to 19.0%.

Active People Survey results (Sport England, 2006)

Active Gloucestershire serves the central administrative role for the County Sports Partnership in Gloucestershire. It is tasked with increasing and sustaining participation in sport and physical activity across the County. Partners include local authorities, the primary care trust and public and private organisations. Active Gloucestershire is part of the South West Regional Sports Board and shares its vision for physical activity and sport participation laid out by the DCMS with all English counties. To achieve the necessary 1% year-on-year increase in sport and physical activity participation required to meet the government objectives (DCMS/Strategy Unit, 2002), an additional 188,809 individuals need to be engaged in this region by 2012 to meet interim targets. Within Gloucestershire this figure equates to an additional 21 246 people undertaking regular activity. The county was measured against Key Performance Indicators (KPIs) set out by Sport England. These sought to develop a picture of the rates of physical activity and sport participation in England, and the type of people that were engaged with various activities.

KPI 1 (Sport England, 2006) measured participation against the current minimum recommendations for health enhancing activity (Department of Health, 2004a, p. 3):

> 'For general health benefit, adults should achieve a total of at least 30 minutes a day of at least moderate intensity physical activity on 5 or more days of the week.'

Results of the Active People Survey identify that in the South West in 2006 21.9% of the adult population participated in 30 minutes of moderate intensity activity three times per week. This figure is higher than the national average of 21%.

Table 6.2 breaks down the local picture of activity into local districts within the County. Approximately half of the adult population in Gloucestershire do not participate in any sport or physical activity.

Although the results for Gloucestershire tended to be at least the national average or above, there were results that indicated some areas suffered from lower participation rates. The results for Gloucester City for KPI 1 are considerably lower than the rest of the County. Gloucester City is in the bottom 25% of all local

Table 6.2 Active People Survey results for Gloucestershire districts.

	Zero days	1 to 3 days [nearly 1 × 30 minutes per week]	4 to 7 days [1 × 30 minutes per week]	8 to 11 days [2 × 30 minutes per week]	12 or more days [3 × 30 minutes per week]
LA Area	%	%	%	%	%
Cheltenham	42.84	10.36	14.25	10.03	22.52
Cotswold	48.37	7.44	11.34	8.35	24.49
Forest of Dean	51.36	8.06	11.89	6.59	22.10
Gloucester	51.71	9.69	11.57	8.11	18.93
Stroud	48.12	9.19	11.09	7.67	23.92
Tewkesbury	48.09	8.72	12.34	8.35	22.51

Source: Active People Survey (Sport England, 2006).

authorities in England although the data identified a trend of low-level physical activity (one to two sport or physical activity sessions per week). Nearly 52% of the adult population in this area reported as not engaging in any sport or physical activity in contrast with Cheltenham, a town only 8 miles away that has the lowest level of self-reported non-participation in the South West Region (42.84%). This poses serious challenges to local partnerships to work effectively in understanding local variations in participation and opportunities. It is precisely this kind of localised discrepancy, in an ethnically diverse and economically deprived area, that partnerships are considered most effective at addressing.

Active Gloucestershire's relevance in this context is its role in the development and expansion of Community Sport Networks (CSNs). The development of Community Sport and Physical Activity Networks (CSPANs) within the county is a model for partnerships that Sport England has endorsed in order to increase the effectiveness of local interventions. After the successful application of local action plans to Sport England, initial CSPAN funding is being drawn from Community Investment Funds (CIF) and contributions from the South West Regional Sports Board, whilst longer term funding is likely to be drawn from public and private sectors (Sport England, 2007). Essentially, these networks are CSNs but have been titled in such a way as to appeal to the whole spectrum of sport and physical activity partners and, as such, are not distinct from CSNs identified in the Single Delivery System. Under the current government funding cycle, CSPANs are able to obtain financial support to develop better strategic plans through staff training and communication systems that, it is hoped, deliver on promises of increased community participation. This demonstrates Sport England's fundamental objective to target resources at specific interventions rather than funding ill-defined and general interventions. However, as stated previously, the affirmation of partnerships as the critical factor in local strategy is a potentially insidious issue in that evidence concerning their effectiveness is still not conclusive. Thus, it is only anticipated that financially supporting the sharing of knowledge and skills within partnerships will develop and entrench strong strategic alliances capable of effectively delivering sport and physical activity in the community. Whether this transpires in long-term success is unclear. Despite this, in late 2007 Active Gloucestershire is involved with meeting representatives of each district with a view to establishing CSPANs throughout the county, eventually with the aim of establishing CSPAN forums that will operate as a central information channel for all districts. It is envisaged that this will provide a window through which local authorities are able to view the impact of partnership projects on the health and social agenda of the local strategic partnership.

The challenge facing these new CSPANs is to manage the developent of partnerships so that they work effectively to deliver sport and physical activity projects. No reliable template currently exists within Active Gloucestershire or any other county organisation that accounts for the unique composition and purpose of these partnerships or ways in which to fill the gaps in knowledge within them. As such, Active Gloucestershire is working closely with the University of Gloucestershire to develop research into the nature and outcomes of this type of approach to deliver health improvement within local communities. It is anticipated that this will serve to generate evidence concerning both the effectiveness of the interventions and the effectiveness of the partnerships themselves. Given the proliferation of partnerships and the increasing reliance on their success for community health improvement, evidence must be gathered that not only proves their effectiveness through sound evaluation, but also that promotes the further development of certain working practices. This may have two significant outcomes vital to the long term success of interventions and partnerships themselves. Firstly, from a funding perspective this may allow for better informed decision making when making funding applications to the South West Regional Sports Board and when distributing funds to local projects. For county sport partnerships such as Active Gloucestershire, this may improve efficiency in an area where relatively little funding is guaranteed for new small scale physical activity projects in comparison to more established agendas elsewhere in community sport, such as school sports participation. Secondly, from a partnership perspective evidence that informs better working practices must be underpinned by high quality research standards (El Ansari and Weiss, 2006). This is needed in order to develop a more holistic impression of what constitutes a successful partnership and should combat the potentially harmful effects of the contradictions and conflict inherent in contemporary local delivery systems.

Conclusion

As Active Gloucestershire seeks to roll out CSPANs across the county it is likely that some organisations will carry more influence in decision making for reasons of organisational experience and political clout. By its very nature the Sport England delivery system may potentially encourage power imbalances because it urges organisations to lead and evolve partnerships in order to maintain focus on interventions and good practice. The challenge to the emerging CSPANs is to both develop and contribute towards systems that safeguard equality at the decision making level and minimise the effects of traditional hierarchical partnerships that still dominate the sport agenda (McDonald, 2005). In essence this is the precise point at which friction is created where the top-down bottom-up approach to community health improvement meets. The challenge to Active Gloucestershire is to facilitate and act on the goodwill of organisations to think in new ways about how to best tackle the community health agenda. With the first conclusive Active People Survey results now in the public domain, adopting a realistic and evidence-based understanding that partnership working is necessarily complex may help to reinforce a commitment to finding solutions through intelligent compromise between partners.

Summary and conclusion

Despite the lack of specific evidence that partnership working in physical activity development is an effective way of working there is support from policy and in practice for this way of working in health promotion as an effective method to achieve changes in population behaviour change. Furthermore, since the Labour government were elected in 1997 they have always proposed a partnership approach to tackling health inequalities. For example, their first white paper, 'Saving Lives: Our Healthier Nation' (Department of Health, 1999), extolled the value of individuals, communities and government working together to improve the health of the nation in England. Their supplementary texts, too, followed this with specific support and advice for the development and implementation of partnership working (e.g. Department of Health, 2000c). The development of these current 'Partnerships' within each county in England are an opportunity, if they are to be evaluated, to establish the effectiveness of partnership working for the promotion of physical activity and ultimately whether they have an impact on the physical activity levels of the nation. Eclectic research and evaluation approaches and methods that investigate not only which interventions are effective but also what makes them effective, in terms of a way of working and the partnership processes involved within their implementation, are therefore essential. They are important not only to establish if Sports Partnerships are an effective way of increasing the physical activity levels of the nation but also in the development of a situation-specific evidence base (Geanellos, 2004). This will further support the current ways of working but also provide successive governments with the necessary evidence base to develop working practices upon, in the future.

References

Audit Commission/National Audit Office (2006) *Delivering Efficiently: Strengthening the Links in Public Service Delivery Chains*. The Stationery Office, London.

Boydell, L.R. and Rugkåsa, J. (2007) Benefits of working in partnership: A model. *Critical Public Health*, 17(3): 217–228.

Coulson, A. (2005) A plague on all your partnerships: Theory and practice in regeneration. *International Journal of Public Sector Management*, 18(2): 151–163.

Crone, D., Johnston, L. and Grant, T. (2004) Maintaining quality in exercise referral schemes: A case study of professional practice. *Primary Health Care Research and Development*, (5): 96–103.

Crone, D. (2007) Walking back to health: A qualitative investigation into service users experiences of a walking project. *Issues in Mental Health Nursing*, 28(2): 167–184.

Crone, D. and Stathi, A. (2005) A qualitative evaluation of older peoples experiences of the progress falls prevention exercise programme. *ISSP 11th World Congress of Sport Psychology*, 15–19 August, Sydney, Australia.

DfEE (Department for Education and Skills) (2005) *14–19 Education and Skills*. The Stationery Office, London.

Department of Health (1999) *Saving Lives – Our Healthier Nation: A Contract for Health*. The Stationery Office, London.

Department of Health (2000a) *National Service Framework for Coronary Heart Disease*. The Stationery Office, London.

Department of Health (2000b) *The NHS Plan: A Plan for Investment a Plan for Reform*. The Stationery Office, London.

Department of Health (2000c) *Working in Partnership: Developing a Whole Systems Approach*. The Stationery Office, London.

Department of Health (2004a) *At Least 5 a Week: Evidence on the Impact of Physical Activity and Its Relationship to Health*. The Stationery Office, London.

Department of Health (2004b) *Choosing Health: Making Healthier Choices Easier*. The Stationery Office, London.

Department of Health (2005) *Choosing Activity: A Physical Activity Action Plan*. Department of Health, London.

DCMS/Strategy Unit (2002) *Game Plan: A Strategy for Delivering Government's Sport and Physical Activity Targets*. Cabinet Office, London.

Department for Culture, Media and Sport (2005) *Five Year Plan: Living Life to the Full*. Department for Culture, Media and Sport, London.

Dugdill, L., Graham, R.C. and McNair, F. (2005) Exercise referral: The public health panacea for physical activity promotion? A critical perspective of exercise referral schemes; their development and evaluation. *Ergonomics*, 48(11–14): 1390–1410.

Dugdill, L. and Muirhead, A. (2007) *Wigan's Local Exercise Action Pilot (LEAP) Programme Stepping Out 2004–2006*. http://www.ihscr.salford.ac.uk/CPHR/LEAP_report.pdf (accessed 05/10/07).

Dugdill, L. and Stratton, G. (2007) *Evaluating Sport and Physical Activity Interventions a Guide for Practitioners*. http://www.sportengland.org/evaluating_sport___physical_activity_interventions.pdf (accessed 01/11/2007).

El Ansari, W. and Phillips, C.J. (2001) Partnerships, community participation and intersectoral collaboration in South Africa. *Journal of Interprofessional Care*, 15(2): 119–132.

El Ansari, W. and Weiss, E.S. (2006) Quality of research on community partnerships: Developing the evidence base. *Health Education Research*, 21(2): 175–180.

Geanellos, R. (2004) Nursing based evidence: Moving beyond evidenced based practice in mental health nursing. *Journal of Evaluation in Clinical Practice*, 10(2): 177–186.

Gidlow, C., Johnston, L.H., Crone, D. and James, D.V.B. (2008) Methods of evaluation: Issues and implications for physical activity referral schemes. *American Journal of Lifestyle Management*, 2: 46–50.

Gloucestershire County Council (2005) Gloucestershire population monitor. Chief Executive's Support Unit, Gloucestershire County Council.

Halliday, J., Asthana, S.N.M. and Richardson, S. (2004) Evaluating partnership the role of formal assessment tools. *Evaluation*, 10(3): 285–303.

Leeds Metropolitan University (2007) *The National Evaluation of Leap: Final Report of the National Valuation of Local Exercise Action Pilots*. The Stationery Office, London.

Lord Carter of Coles (2005) *Review of National Sport, Effort and Resources*. http://www.culture.gov.uk/NR/rdonlyres/083C36AF-DFF9-4C7A-9B25-06DF941E5AFB/0/Carter_report.pdf (accessed 12/09/07).

McDonald, I. (2005) Theorising partnerships: Governance, communicative action and sport policy. *Journal of Social Policy*, 34(4): 579–600.

Mills, H., Crone, D. and El Ansari, W. (in press) Key concept 22: Physical activity and public health. In: *Fifty Key Concepts in Public Health* (Eds S. Watkins and A. Mabhala). Sage, London.

NICE (2006) *Public Health Intervention Guidance No. 2 Four Commonly Used Methods to Increase Physical Activity: Brief Interventions in Primary Care, Exercise Referral Schemes, Pedometers and Community-Based Exercise Programmes for Walking and Cycling*. National Institute for Health and Clinical Excellence, London.

Newman, J. (2001) *Modernising Governance: New Labour, Policy and Society*. Sage, London.

Rootman, I., Goodstadt, M., Hyndman, B., McQueen, D.V., Potvin, L., Springett, J. and Ziglio, E. (Eds) (2001) *Evaluation in Health Promotion*. WHO Regional Publications, Copenhagen.

Scottish Executive (2003) *Let's Make Scotland More Active: A Strategy for Physical Activity*. Scottish Executive, Edinburgh.

Sport England (2006) *Active People Survey*. http://www.sportengland.org/index/get_resources/research/active_people/aps_results.htm (accessed 20/09/2007).

Sport England (2004) *The Framework for Sport in England Making England an Active and Successful Sporting Nation: A Vision for 2020*. http://www.sportengland.org/national-framework-for-sport.pdf (accessed 05/09/2007).

Stathi, A. and Crone, D. (2005) The impact of a community-based falls prevention programme onto the functional ability and quality of life of frail older adults. *ISSP 11th World Congress of Sport Psychology*, 15–19 August, Sydney, Australia.

Walter, I., Davies, H. and Nutley, S. (2003) Increasing research impact through partnerships: Evidence from outside health care. *Journal of Health Services Research and Policy*, S2: 58–61.

7 Developing physically active workplaces

Lindsey Dugdill and Margaret Coffey

Introduction

During the last 30 years, daily levels of physical activity have decreased although active leisure has increased in England (Department of Health, 2004a). In part this is due to the more sedentary nature of work, alongside increasing use of the car compared with methods of active transport (walking and cycling). Physical activity also decreases markedly with increasing age (Health Survey for England, 2003). The UK workforce tends to spend more hours at work than most other EU countries and have less paid leave per annum (Bishop, 2004; The Work Foundation, 2005), which has a detrimental effect on physical activity as lack of time is a key barrier to adults being active (Sallis and Owen, 1999). Although, the workplace setting affords great potential as a setting for promoting physical activity, managers in the UK have been slow to respond to these opportunities.

> 'For people in employment, work is a key part of life. The environment we work in influences our health choices and can be a force for improving health – both for individuals and the communities they are part of'. (Department of Health, 2004b, p. 153)

Research indicates that having a job is better for your health than not having a job although the relationship between work and health is complex (Naidoo and Wills, 2002; Wilkinson and Marmot, 2003; Department of Health, 2004b). Firstly, having a job is necessary for maintaining income, with income levels determining a wide range of life chances, including socio-economic status (Marmot and Wilkinson, 2003). Secondly, the achievement of occupational status is a means through which personal growth and development are realised (Marmot and Wilkinson, 2003). Thirdly, the type and quality of ones occupation is a strong influence on attitudes and behavioural patterns that are not directly work related, for example leisure time activity, family life, political activity and education (Kohn and Schooler, 1973, cited in Marmot and Wilkinson, 2003). Finally, given the amount of time spent at work (approximately 60% of adult life), exposure to adverse or noxious job conditions (physical or psycho-social) carries a risk of ill health.

The cost of physical inactivity in England, including direct costs of treatment for the major lifestyle-related diseases, and the indirect costs caused through sickness absence from work, has been estimated at £8.2 billion a year (Department of Health, 2004a). Despite varied opportunities for promoting physical activity at work (e.g. through walking/cycling programmes, building re-design, health incentive schemes, active commuting) the lack of a clear evidence base of effectiveness (Dugdill *et al.*, 2007, 2008) has slowed progress in terms of programme implementation and managers are yet to be convinced of the cost–benefit of such programmes.

Learning outcomes

The aims of this chapter are to:

1. explain the diverse nature of the workplace
2. describe how work influences health and ill health
3. explain the 'settings-based' approach to workplace health promotion
4. clarify and explain review level evidence of effectiveness for physical activity interventions in the workplace

---

The nature of contemporary workplaces in the UK

The UK workforce is very diverse in its nature, due to the different types of sector (public, private and voluntary): size of organisation (small, medium and large) and employment contract (e.g. part-time, full-time, self-employed) operating within it. In 2007, 29.01 million people were employed in the UK and the employment rate for people of working age was 74.3% (National Statistics, 2007). The total number of hours worked per week was 925.9 million, which was split between full-time workers, 21.57 million, and part-time workers, 7.44 million (National Statistics, 2007). Of the full-time workers 13.95 million (65%) were men, and 7.62 million (35%) were women, whilst of the part-time workers, 1.73 million (23%) were men and 5.71 million (77%) were women (National Statistics, 2007).

Looking at the different sectors, whilst there is no uniform definition, broadly speaking, the private sector represents approximately 80% (23.23 million) of the UK workforce, comprising workplaces established and operating for profit, for example production, services and construction (Black *et al.*, 2004; National Statistics, 2007). The public sector mainly comprises: central government, local government and public corporations; and in March 2007 the number of people employed in the public sector was 5.79 million (National Statistics, 2007), representing almost 20% of the workforce. The smallest sector is the voluntary. The broadest definition of this sector includes not only charities registered with the Charity Commission but also small voluntary groups, housing associations, universities and colleges, schools and places of worship, trade unions and trade associations, sport and recreation clubs and NHS Trusts [National Council for Voluntary Organisations (NCVO), 2006]. Whilst figures for this sector of the workforce are not reported separately in Labour Force Statistics, according to NVCO (2006), there are about 169 000 general charities within the UK employing 608 000 paid workers (231 000 part-time) a further 13.2 million unpaid volunteers and an estimated 750 000 trustees who take responsibility (unpaid) for the governance of individual charities.

The UK workforce is further split into different sized organisations, namely, small, medium and large. The Department of Trade and Industry (DTI, 2006) reported that in 2005 there were an estimated 4.3 million business enterprises in the UK, of which 99.3% were small (0–49 employees), 27 000 (0.6%) were medium (50–249 employees) and 6 000 (0.1%) were large (250 or more employees). This mirrors trends in Europe, where small- and medium-sized enterprises (referred to as SMEs) account for 99% of all businesses (European Commission, 2006). In the UK it is the eighth successive year that SMEs have increased in numbers (DTI, 2006).

Together with the diverse workforce, profound changes have been happening to both the nature of work and the labour market (Marmot and Wilkinson, 2003). Wilkinson and Marmot (2003) describe changes in the nature of work as including jobs being defined more by psychological and emotional demands, rather than physical demands, fewer jobs being in mass production, more in the service sector and more jobs concerned with information. Changes in the labour market stem from the fact that the population is ageing, more women are working, there are changes in working hours, an increase in short-term working and sub-contracting and a growth in job instability. Looking at these in turn, 'by 2050, ever-lengthening lifespans and slumping birthrates mean that Europe's population of working age will drop by 38 million. At the same time, numbers aged 65 and over will rise by 40 million. That will swell the EU's pensioner population to more than 100 million. The number of workers for every individual of 65-plus will fall from more than three to fewer than two' (The Times, 2007).

The short-term working culture began in the UK in the 1980s typified by outsourcing of services (Cooper, 2000). The growth in the number of small firms, spread of subcontracting and privatisation of public services are reported to be major factors that have resulted in 'a fall in the number of workers with access to health and safety professionals from

23 million in 1992 to 7.5 million in 2002' (Trade Union Technical Bureau for Health and Safety, 2003, p. 21). The longer working hours culture developed in the UK (Cooper, 2000). In this respect, full time workers have been reported to work an average of 44 hours per week in the UK compared to an EU average of 40 hours per week (Bishop, 2004). Additionally, although this has declined over the past decade, the UK still has a higher proportion of employees working 45 hours and over per week than France, Denmark and Sweden (Bishop, 2004).

The UK also has a high proportion (42%) of part-time workers [Equal Opportunities Commission (EOC), 2006] who are mostly women (77%) and are mostly prevalent in the service sector; comprising the '5 C's; i.e. cooking, cleaning, cashiering, clerical and caring. This represents an increase for women's employment from about 6 out of 10 to 7 out of 10 (70%) for women of working age (16–59) since 1975 (ONS, 2005a; cited in EOC, 2006). Also notable is the increase in working mothers with dependent children. In 1975 approximately half of mothers with dependent children worked, and the employment rate of mothers of under-fives was 28%, whilst latest figures show two-thirds of mothers and 55% of mothers of under-fives in employment (OPCS, 1990 and ONS, 2005b: cited in EOC, 2006). Whilst the number of women in work, especially part time, has increased there is still a persistent pay gap between women and men. In 2005 for women working full time the average hourly pay was £11.57, compared with £14.08 for men (a gap of 17.1%). 'Part-time women earned £8.68 on average, and comparing this figure with men's average full-time earnings of £14.08 gives a part-time gender pay gap of 38.4%' [OPCS (1990) and ONS (2005b): cited in EOC, 2006, p. 19]. Hutton (1995 cited in Marmot and Wilkinson, 2003) describes Britain as being made up of 40% of the male population being in secure jobs, 30% are not working, whilst 30% have insecure jobs.

Hence, work opportunities and settings in the UK are diverse and provide a challenge for the promotion of physical activity. Furthermore, trends in physical activity by socio-economic group and occupation are also very complex. Participation in sport, exercise and walking is significantly related to social class; for example 42% of men and 33% of women in social class I participated in walking compared with 31% men and 16% women in social class V (National Statistics Office and Medical Research Council of Human Nutrition, 2004).

An analysis of the Health Survey for England (2003) showed that men from the highest socio-economic group (managerial and professional) had lowest self-reported total physical activity, with only 26% taking the recommended amount (at least 30 minutes moderate physical activity on 5 or more days/week) when compared with about 34% for the lowest socio-economic group (semi-routine and routine workers). This difference may be explained by greater levels of occupationally related physical activity in the latter group (i.e. higher manual components). However, sports participation for men was shown to have an opposite relationship with the highest socio-economic group (managerial and professional) having the greatest participation is sport (46% men reported taking part in sport in the last four weeks) compared with only 25% of men in the lowest socio-economic group. Data for women was limited.

Health and ill health at work

The European Foundation for the Improvement of Living and Working Conditions stated that 'exposure to physical hazards at the workplace, intensification of work and flexible employment practices are still a primary cause of health problems for workers in the European Union' (2001, p. 1). In this respect, Coats and Max (2005 cited in Sedgley and Dooris, 2007) highlight that the way work is organised, both within organisations and across society, affects health and well-being in a number of ways. The two main factors appear to be firstly inequalities in terms of relative income and status, which are important in determining societal health, as 'even in the most affluent countries, people who are less well off have substantially shorter life expectancies and more illnesses than the rich' (Wilkinson and Marmot, 2003, p. 7). And secondly, poor quality work, which is associated with low levels of well-being, and a higher incidence of physical and mental illness (see e.g., Marmot, 2004, cited in Sedgley and Dooris, 2007). The recent and rapid increase in the number of migrant workers in the UK, making up approximately 10% of the total working population, has also brought challenges for the promotion of health, amongst a group which is increasingly diverse and transitory in nature (Robinson, 2002).

Given the changes that have been happening to both the nature of work and the labour market, it is perhaps unsurprising that the overall cost of sickness absence increased to approximately £12 billion in 2004/05 [Health and Safety Executive (HSE), 2006], from £11.6 billion in 2003 [Confederation of British Industry (CBI), 2005]. However, absenteeism is not evenly distributed. Younger employees (16–34) and female employees are more likely than other groups to take at least one day off sick (Barham and Begum, 2005). Furthermore public sector absence averages 9.1 days per employee per annum, compared with 6.4 days per private sector employee (CBI, 2005). Data on the voluntary sector is sparse, with Cunningham (2001, cited in Alatrista and Arrowsmith, 2004) stating that academic research almost entirely ignores this sector regarding paid employment. However, where data does exist, absence in this sector is reported to be high (Working Families, 2004). Levels of sickness absence, particularly in the public sector, are of major concern, with the CBI (2005) asserting that that if the absence rate in the public sector could be reduced to the private sector average, absence would fall by more than 20 million days and save the UK taxpayer £1.2 billion.

The main causes of absenteeism in the UK are reported to be: musculoskeletal disorders (MSDs), followed by stress, anxiety or depression, breathing or lung problems and hearing problems (see Health and Safety Commission, 2006). Considering the two main causes of absenteeism (MSDs and stress), there appears to be some association between the two. Parkes *et al.* (2005), in a recent study using the Nordic Musculoskeletal Questionnaire ($n = 321$), reported that in longitudinal analyses, mental health, workload, physical, environment stressors and body mass index predicted MSDs. Also, anxiety and social support were found to be significant factors predicting change in MSDs, and in addition, anxiety (in common with previous findings) predicted the development of MSDs. In the UK, stress is estimated to be costing the economy approximately £3.7 billion each year (HSE, 2006). Psychosocial factors found to be associated with stress comprise: organisation culture and function, role in organisation, career development, decision latitude/control,; interpersonal relationships at work, work environment and work environment, task design; workload/workpace and work schedule (Cox *et al.*, 2000) .

The government's response to ill health at work is evidenced by rapid developments in workplace health strategy in the UK, which has seen the publication of a range of important national reports since 2000, such as:

▩ Strategy for Workplace Health and Safety in Great Britain to 2010 and beyond (2004) (Health and Safety Commission, 2004).
▩ Flexible Working: the right to request and the duty to consider (Department of Trade and Industry, 2003).
▩ Health, Work and Wellbeing – Caring for our Future (Department of Health, the Department of Work and Pensions, and the Health and Safety Executive, 2005).

These are long-term strategies for health and safety and occupational health respectively, which define the workplace as a key setting for improving health. Revitalising Health and Safety (Health and Safety Executive, 2000), although primarily focusing on accident reduction and improving safety at work, does call for the 'promotion of better working environments' (p. 18) and the importance of 'worker involvement' (p. 29). Physical activity and lifestyle change is not directly mentioned in Revitalising Health and Safety but could play a vital role in the rehabilitation agenda; for example MSDs are one of the main causes of sickness absence across the UK, but many of these can be alleviated through appropriate physiotherapy/exercise interventions.

A 'settings-based' approach to health at work

> 'The worksite is one of the key channels for the delivery of inter-
> ventions to reduce chronic diseases among adult populations. It
> provides easy and regular access to a relatively stable population and
> it encourages sustained peer support'.   (Moy *et al.*, 2006, p. 301)

The concept of the workplace as a setting for health was first noted
in the Ottawa Charter for Health Promotion (WHO, 1986), which
asserted that the way society organises work should create a healthy society. More recently, the government's Public Health White Paper, Choosing
Health: Making Healthy Choices Easier (Department of Health, 2004b),
makes a clear commitment to supporting a range of healthy settings,
stating that 'Workplaces are often under-utilised as a setting for promoting health and well-being' (p. 166). Moreover, the recent policy Choosing
Activity: a Physical Activity Action Plan (Department of Health, 2005)
stated that 'Employers, the Government and trade unions all have a role
to play in establishing environments that support healthy choices across
a range of behaviours including better diet, smoke-free environments,
smoking cessation and encouraging activity' (p. 33).
   In this respect, the workplace offers a unique setting in which to
promote health, because adults spend 60% of their waking hours at
work; it gives access to a captive target group of healthy adults; modes of
communication are already set up; and peer support groups are already
established within the working community (Naidoo and Wills, 2002).
Whitelaw *et al.* (2001) assert that the settings approach emerged from
'a perception of an over-reliance on individualistic methods' (p. 339).
The move away from an 'individualistic' approach can be seen in the
three key elements that make up the settings approach, namely, creating
supportive and healthy working and living environments, integrating
health promotion into the daily activities of the setting and recognising that people do not operate in just one setting and that one setting
impacts on other settings and the wider community (Baric, 1994;
cited in Dooris, 2004).

> 'Over the last 10 years settings based health promotion has become
> a central feature of efforts to promote health that recognise the sig-
> nificance of context'.   (Whitelaw *et al.*, 2001, p. 339).

However, Dooris (2004) warns that 'there remains limited consensus
about either theory or practice within the field and there has been a relative absence of critical debate concerning the approach and its potential
contribution to public health investment' (p. 49). In this respect,
rigorous research and evaluation studies are the key to generating
evidence of effectiveness in relation to healthy settings (Dooris, 2005).

Workplace health promotion programmes 'Can be characterised as an integrated approach of a total package of activities, on both organizational and individual levels' (Schreurs et al., 1996, p. 466). Interventions fall broadly into three categories, primary, secondary and tertiary. Primary includes health promotion that acts on the determinants of health to prevent disease occurring; secondary is essentially the early detection of disease, followed by appropriate intervention, such as health promotion or treatment; and tertiary aims to reduce the impact of the disease and promote quality of life through active rehabilitation (Department of Health, 2007). These intervention strategies can be difficult to separate because the categories overlap considerably; for example physical activity can be undertaken as a primary intervention, in order to prevent the onset of health problems, or as a secondary intervention, following the detection of the onset of health problems. However, these three categories fall into two main approaches, that is organisation-oriented and individual-oriented.

Organisational approaches include environmental, legislative or policy changes (e.g. improving the work organisation and work environment by providing facilities for exercise e.g. showers, bike racks, etc., or introducing policies which give workers time to exercise during the working day), whilst individual-oriented approaches include inter-personal (led physical activity sessions/classes) or individual (consultations, fitness assessments, motivational counselling) (Mutrie and Woods, 2003). Historically, the predominant focus has been on individual behaviour change, rather than organisational or environmental change. However, in order to maximise future opportunities there needs to be a more balanced approach to physical activity promotion which incorporates both organisational and individual-oriented approaches in a more comprehensive package, in line with socio-ecological theory.

The interface between work and home settings affords another important opportunity for physical activity through active commuting/travel (walking and cycling). It is generally accepted that the most effective way of increasing physical activity levels is by incorporating it into an individual's lifestyle and active commuting can make a significant contribution to daily levels of physical activity amongst the working population (Sustrans, 2005).

However, the trend towards more sedentary modes of travel is clear. The British Heart Foundation (2005) reported that over the last 30 years, in England the average number of miles per capita travelled by foot fell by a quarter, and by cycle by around a third, whereas the average number of miles travelled per capita by car rose by 70%. The 2002 National Travel Survey (2004) reported that car travel accounted for 80% of the total distance travelled (in 2002) for Great Britain residents. Overall, the distance travelled by car increased by 8% over the last decade, whereas the number of walking trips fell by 20% in the same time period. People in higher socio-economic groups are more likely to have access to a car.

Unfortunately, the evidence suggests that active travel to work in the UK is also decreasing. About 70% of people travelled to work by car or motorcycle, 14% by bus or rail, 3% always worked at home. From this data it can be presumed that 13% (or less) used an active method of travelling to work (bike or foot). The 2002 National Travel Survey (2004) also showed that the percentage of walking trips to work fell from 16% (in 1985/6) to 10% (by 2002); and the percentage of people cycling to work also reduced. The Labour Force Survey 2001 (2003) reported that only 3% of commuters in Great Britain, used a bike to get to work, and women were twice as likely as men to walk to work (15% c.f. 7%). People in the lowest income quintile were more likely to walk (25%) or take the bus (17%) to work.

Evidence of effectiveness of workplace physical activity interventions

The early evidence base for workplace health promotion was derived in the 1960s with the majority of evidence based on research from the US or case studies in practice (Dugdill and Springett, 2001). Early workplace health developments in the UK focused on the implementation of legislation such as the Health and Safety at Work Act (1974) rather than directly promoting workers' health. This approach contrasted with other EU countries such as Sweden, where health promotion efforts focused on the psychosocial work environment, work re-design and organisational development (Karasek and Theorell, 1990). Such approaches were later embraced by UK-based companies such as Nissan UK, who re-organised motor car manufacture (in the 1990s) around team-based models of production rather than traditional production line approaches. This re-organisation led to greater involvement of all workers in the management of key processes, increased autonomy, and improved sickness absence rates and levels of job satisfaction.

There was a growing realisation of the economic benefits of having a healthy workforce (Springett and Dugdill, 1999) and consequently the 1990s saw a diversification of health programmes within UK workplaces with action primarily found in large organisations, with US and other multi-national companies leading the way with such developments. The public sector was also proactive in attempting to promote the health of its workforce as it was seen to be part of the central ethos of its way of working; hence, the evidence base is often dominated by research studies carried out in large, public sector organisations. Where evidence existed, it showed workplace health programmes which were comprehensive, reflected the real needs of the employees and had full management endorsement were the most likely to be effective. Despite the growing dominance of the SME workplace community (in terms of both size and economic importance), there has been little progress in the development of comprehensive health programmes (and concomitant evidence) for either this sector (Dugdill, 2003) or the voluntary sector (Coffey and Dugdill, 2006).

Workplace health interventions were often designed to address managerial rather than employee agendas and were often a reaction to a problem (high sickness absence rates) rather than a systematic attempt to improve conditions for the well-being of all employees, using an established evidence base. The practical skills to promote health at work were often under-developed and not well resourced by the organisation concerned.

A small number of systematic reviews have been undertaken that examine the health impacts of workplace physical activity interventions. Dishman et al. (1998) carried out a rigorous meta-analysis of 26 workplace physical activity intervention studies that aimed to improve physical activity and/or physical fitness and concluded that the typical worksite physical activity intervention had yet to demonstrate a statistically significant increase in physical activity or fitness.

Proper et al. (2003) examined the effectiveness of worksite physical activity programmes on physical activity, physical fitness and health. They concluded that there was sufficient evidence to support the implementation of worksite physical activity programmes for increasing the level of physical activity of employees (however this judgement was made on the basis of only two high quality studies – both randomised controlled trials) and reducing the risk of musculoskeletal disorders but there was limited evidence of effectiveness for fatigue, physical fitness and general health. Both reviews (Dishman et al., 1998; Proper et al., 2003) reported that the methodological quality of the published literature was weak due to poor study design and outcomes being measured solely by self-reported physical activity.

A more recent systematic review of workplace physical activity intervention effectiveness (Dugdill et al., 2007, 2008) revealed that evidence of the effectiveness of stair walking interventions in the workplace was limited and intervention effects were short lived (Marshall et al., 2002; Auweele et al., 2005). Three public sector studies provided evidence that workplace walking interventions using pedometers can increase daily step counts, if accompanied by facilitated goal setting (Chan et al., 2004; Thomas and Williams, 2006), self-complete diaries and self-monitoring (Chan et al., 2004; Murphy et al., 2006; Thomas and Williams, 2006) and advertised walking routes (Gilson et al., 2007). One good-quality study (Mutrie et al., 2002) reported a positive intervention effect on walking to work behaviour (active travel) in economically advantaged, female employees. There was strong evidence from four studies (Talvi et al., 1999; Proper et al., 2003; Aittasalo et al., 2004; Osteras and Hammer, 2006) that workplace counselling influenced physical activity behaviour. Further, well-designed research studies are required to boost the developing evidence base on workplace physical activity interventions. Emphasis needs to be placed on researching workplaces that have so far been under-represented in the SME and voluntary sectors in particular.

With respect to the evidence regarding active travel, the Health Development Agency's evidence briefing (Killoran et al., 2006) reported review-level evidence that programmes (focus was community rather than workplace) which targeted people – who were motivated to change their transport behaviour through individualised marketing – were able to effect a shift from car use to walking and cycling. However, review-level evidence was inconclusive about the effectiveness of publicity campaigns directed at groups in the population including campaigns using travel coordinators as agents of change; engineering measures such as re-design of cycle lanes, traffic calming measures; financial incentives, for example travel subsidies/tolls, and alternative travel services, for example car-share and rail travel, in achieving a shift from car use to walking and cycling.

Pelletier (1996) carried out an extensive review of workplace health interventions (76 studies) which demonstrated a growing body of evidence with respect to cost-effectiveness outcomes. Most evidence in this field has been generated in the US, where the focus has been in large organisations, with respect to medical screening and reduction in associated health care costs. With respect to physical activity programmes, the cost-effectiveness evidence is much more limited as a recent review by Beale et al. (2007) revealed. Seven studies met the inclusion criteria, and only one of which had been published within the last 9 years and none were from the UK. These authors concluded that currently there was no strong economic evidence to support the implementation of workplace physical activity programmes.

In order to address the general lack of evidence in this field, some large-scale workplace evaluation studies are currently being undertaken in the UK. One such study is the Well @ Work programme, which is a workplace health initiative led by the British Heart Foundation (2007) and funded by the Department of Health and Active England, a joint Sport England and Big Lottery Fund funding programme. The £1.6 million programme supports nine national pilot sites for a major national evaluation project. Well @ Work has focused on the promotion of healthy lifestyles in particular, increasing physical activity, smoking cessation, healthy eating and active travel. A variety of interventions are being implemented in each of the pilot settings including walking trails around the worksite and neighbourhood, targeted poster campaigns such as 'Take the Stairs', encouraging cycling, staff use of the on-site gym as well as local fitness facilities, applying a range of complementary therapies, nutritional information displays, healthier food options and pedometer-based activity programmes for staff. The programme is emphasising the importance of providing supportive environments and also developing workplace policy to underpin interventions.

Case study: An evaluation of the Liverpool Corporate Cup (Evans, 2002)

Outline of project: Lifestyle events are frequently used in the UK to raise health awareness within communities; however, there is little evidence to support their implementation; especially evidence of the effectiveness of running events. Evans (2002) designed a multi-method, evaluation study to measure the impact of the Liverpool Corporate Cup (LCC), a 5 km team running event held annually in the city centre of Liverpool, UK. The event recruits employees from across public, private and voluntary sectors and is the biggest event within the North West Corporate Series. The LCC is organised by Liverpool City Council and Healthstart (on behalf of the local Primary Care Trusts) and annually attracts more than 2500 participants. The intervention draws on the concept of social support being an important psychosocial factor when undertaking physical activity, hence the team-based approach (four participants per team). Team cohesion developed during training and competing in the LCC event also has a potential beneficial effect on workplace behaviours (e.g. productivity).

Evaluation design: Most evaluation studies focus measurement at the level of individual behaviour change and fail to assess changes at a higher level of the system. Consequently, the wider benefits of physical activity interventions are often not understood. This research project used a unique ecological evaluation design (Figure 7.1), incorporating quantitative and qualitative studies, to measure the effectiveness of the event from personal, interpersonal, organisational, community, environmental and policy perspectives (Evans, 2002). Participant and stakeholder views were actively sought through a series of focus groups, interviews and questionnaires that were purposively constructed. Answers to a range of questions were sought such as

- *'How does competing in the LCC impact on your long-term physical activity patterns?'*
- *'Has this team-based intervention influenced your behaviour at work?'*
- *'What organisational support do you get from your employer to compete?'*

Evaluation outcome: The evaluation study established that:

- 52% of runners had previously participated in the LCC
- 38% took part for enjoyment

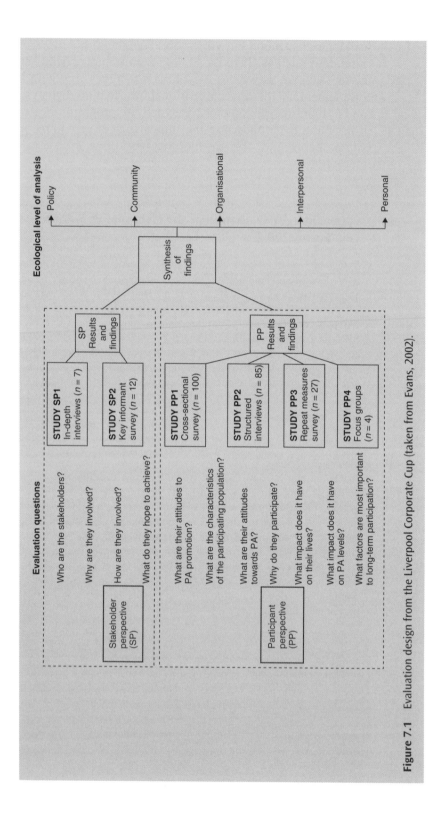

Figure 7.1 Evaluation design from the Liverpool Corporate Cup (taken from Evans, 2002).

- 18% joined in to team build with colleagues
- 12% participated for health and fitness reasons
- 46% said they took part in additional physical activity in order to train for the event

Also, very importantly it was clear that behavioural change had been established in many participants as 96% believed that the Corporate Series helped previously inactive people to become more active and 76% could identify someone who had become more active as a result of taking part. Women runners in particular seemed to benefit from the team-based approach as they gained support from family, friends and work colleagues. Focus group statements clearly illustrated the increase in self-confidence and self-efficacy in female runners:

'I always thought I would never run, ever. When I started I used to feel embarrassed but I don't care now. We do more than just the Corporate Cup events now'.

'The interest we now have in running has taken us further ... after the Corporate Cup we did the women's 10K (Liverpool Women's 10K) and then ... a half marathon and in 1997 a full marathon'.

Participants could recognise the benefit of team-based physical activity interventions and many initially took part solely because they had been asked to do so by a colleague. For many interviewees this then had then lead to participation in further events within the North West Corporate Series and physical activity had become a sustained habit.

Application to practice: In conclusion, this evaluation showed that the Liverpool Corporate Cup was successful in attracting, and sustaining, running behaviour in previously, inactive adults, particularly women. Improving *health* was not a strong motivator for people taking part (only 12% cited this as a reason for participation) – fun, enjoyment and the social aspects were much more important reasons for participation.

Conclusion: implications for practice

This chapter has emphasised both the complexity of the workplace and the diversity of working populations. The implementation of workplace health programmes requires an appreciation of the type of organisation and workforce you are working with and the health needs of this group before proceeding. It is also important to remember that a 'one model fits all' approach is unlikely to lead to success. Interventions should be planned with a thorough understanding of the organisation in mind. Interventions that work well in a large organisation may not be realistic for the SME sector, for example due to resource limitations.

Workplaces are also vital settings for the promotion of physical activity although; the lack of evidence of effectiveness has limited developments in the UK. However, this evidence base is developing rapidly (Dugdill *et al.*, 2007, 2008) and certain workplace physical activity programmes, especially walking to or at work and those supported by counselling and health professional support, can be recommended as effective interventions for employers to offer.

The most progressive workplaces to date have tended to be large, public sector organisations that prioritise the health of their staff in comparison to other sectors. The SME sector could benefit from future investment but this will require a partnership approach, for example with Primary Care Trusts or Community Sports Partnerships, in order for resources to be made available.

Partnerships for delivering physical activity programmes should involve trade unions and workers wherever possible, and seek to understand the complexity/diversity of workforce groups in order to maximise the potential impact of any programme. Management must openly endorse interventions. Practitioners should endeavour to implement well-designed evaluations, which gather objective measures of physical activity behaviour change wherever possible. The case for cost-effectiveness of such programmes in still to be made in the UK and researchers need to focus their efforts in this domain, although evidence from the US is fairly unequivocal in terms of the impact of workplace health programmes on increased productivity and reduced health care costs.

References

Aittasalo, M., Miilunpalo, S. and Suni, J. (2004) The effectiveness of physical activity counseling in a work-site setting. A randomized, controlled trial. *Patient Education and Counseling*, 55: 193–202.

Alatrista, J. and Arrowsmith, J. (2004) Managing employment commitment in the not-for-profit sector. *Personnel Review*, 33(5): 536–548.

Auweele, Y.V., Boen, F., Schapendonk, W. and Dornez, K. (2005) Promoting stair use among female employees: The effects of a health sign followed by an e-mail. *Journal of Sport and Exercise Psychology*, 27: 188–196.

Barham, C. and Begum, N. (2005) Sickness absence from work in the UK. *Labour Market Trends*, April 2005.

Baric, L. (1994) Health promotion and health education in practice: Module 2. *The Organisational Model*. Altrincham, Barns.

Beale, S., Bending, M. and Hutton, J. (2007) Workplace physical activity: how to encourage employees to be physically active: A rapid review of economic literature. University of York, Health Economics Consortium. http://www.nice.org.uk/nicemedia/pdf/Workplace_Physical_Activity_Economics_Review.pdf (accessed 28/01/08).

Bishop, K. (2004) *Working Time Patterns in the UK, France, Denmark and Sweden. Labour Market Division, Office for National Statistics.* http://www.statistics.gov.uk/articles/labour_market_trends/Working_time_patterns.pdf (accessed February, 2007).

Black, O., Richardson, I. and Herbert, R. (2004) *Jobs in the Public Sector – Mid 2003 National Statistics Feature, Labour Market Trends, July.* http://www.statistics.gov.uk/articles/labour_market_trends/public_sector_jobs.pdf (accessed 31/01/08)

British Heart Foundation (2005) *CVD Statistics.* http://www.bhf.org.uk/professionals/uploaded/factsheet2005finalaw.pdf (accessed 14/12/06).

British Heart Foundation (2007) *Well@Work Programme* http://www.bhfactive.org.uk/workplace/evaluation.html (accessed 06/01/08).

Chan, C.B., Ryan, D.A. and Tudor-Locke, C. (2004) Health benefits of a pedometer-based physical activity intervention in sedentary workers. *Preventive Medicine,* 39: 1215–1222.

Coats, D. and Max, C. (2005) *Healthy Work: Productive Workplaces Why the UK Needs More Good Jobs.* Work Foundation and London Commission.

Coffey, M. and Dugdill, L. (2006) Policies alone are not enough: Workplace health development in the public, private and voluntary sector. *Critical Public Health,* 16(3): 233–243.

Confederation of British Industry (2005) *Press Release: May 2005 – Workplace Absence Costs UK £12.2 bn – NEW SURVEY.* http://www.cbi.org.uk/ndbs/press.nsf/0363c1f07c6ca12a8025671c00381cc7/97b8d7895758471f80256fe2005b6fbb?OpenDocument (accessed 31/01/08).

Cooper, C.L. (2000) The psychological implications of the Americanisation of work in the UK. *Stress News,* 12 (2).

Cox, T., Griffiths, A. and Rial-Gonzalez, E. (2000) *Research on Work Related Stress. The European Agency for Safety and Health at Work.* Luxembourg. http://www.isma.org.uk/files/ismaxx0001/images/books_publications/stress-occupational/stress_en.pdf (accessed 08/01/08).

Cunningham, I. (2001) Why research the voluntary sector? *Employee Relations,* 23(3): 223–225.

Department of Health (2004a) *At Least 5 a Week: Evidence on the Impact of Physical Activity and Its Relationship to Health.* A Report from the Chief Medical Officer. DH, London.

Department of Health (2004b) *Choosing Health: Making Healthy Choices Easier.* http://www.dh.gov.uk/en/Publicationsandstatistics/Publications/Publications-PolicyAndGuidance/DH_4094550 (accessed 3/01/08).

Department of Health, the Department of Work and Pensions, and the Health and Safety Executive (2005) *Health, Work and Wellbeing – Caring for our Future.* A strategy published jointly by the Department of Health, the Department of Work and Pensions, and the Health and Safety Executive. http://www.dwp.gov.uk/publications/dwp/2005/health_and_wellbeing.pdf (accessed 3/01/08).

Department of Health (2005) *Choosing Activity: A Physical Activity Action Plan HM Government.* The Stationery Office, London.

Department of Health (2007) *Choosing Health through Pharmacy.* HM Government, The Stationery Office, London. http://site320.theclubuk.com/en/Publicationsandstatistics/Publications/PublicationsPolicyAndGuidance/Browsable/DH_4107796 (accessed 3/01/08).

Department of Trade and Industry (2003) *Flexible Working: The Right to Request and the Duty to Consider. A Guide for Employers and Employees.* DTI, London. http://www.dti.gov.uk/employment/workandfamilies/flexible-working/index.html (accessed 3/12/06).

DTI (Department of Trade and Industry) (2006) *Statistical Press Release – URN 06/92, August.* http://www.dtistats.net/smes/sme/smestats2005-ukspr.pdf (accessed 3/01/08).

Dishman, R.K., Oldenburg, B., O'Neal, H. and Shephard, R.J. (1998) Worksite physical activity interventions. *American Journal of Preventive Medicine,* 15: 344–361.

Dooris, M. (2004) Joining up settings for health: A valuable investment for strategic partnerships? *Critical Public Health,* 14(1): 49–61.

Dooris, M. (2005) Healthy settings: Challenges to generating evidence of effectiveness. *Health Promotion International,* 21(1): 55–65.

Dooris, M. (2007) *Healthy Settings: History and Origins.* Healthy Settings Development Unit. http://www.uclan.ac.uk/facs/health/hsdu/history/introduction.htm (accessed 31/01/08).

Dugdill, L. and Springett, J. (2001) Evaluating health promotion programmes in the workplace. In: *Evaluation in Health Promotion. Principles and Perspectives* (Eds I. Rootman, M. Goodstadt, B. Hyndman, D. McQueen, L. Potvin, J. Springett and E. Ziglio), pp. 285–308. WHO Regional Publications, Denmark.

Dugdill, L. (2003) Understanding workplace health promotion: Programme development and evaluation for the small business sector. In: *The Social Significance of Health Promotion* (Ed. T.H. MacDonald), Routledge, London.

Dugdill, L., Brettle, A., Hulme, C., McCluskey, S. and Long, A.F. (2007) Intervention guidance on workplace health promotion with reference to physical activity and what works in motivating and changing employees' health behaviour. Systematic Review for the National Institute of Health and Clinical Excellence, University of Salford.

Dugdill, L., Brettle, A., Hulme, C., McCluskey, S. and Long, A.F. (2008) Workplace physical activity interventions: A systematic review. *International Journal of Workplace Health Management,* 1(1): 20–40.

EOC (Equal Opportunities Commission) (2006) *Facts about Women and Men in Great Britain.* http://www.eoc.org.uk/pdf/facts_about_GB_2006.pdf (accessed 31/01/08).

European Commission (2006) *Facts and Figures – SMEs in Europe.* http://ec.europa.eu/enterprise/entrepreneurship/facts_figures.htm (accessed 11/08/07).

European Foundation for the Improvement of Living and Working Conditions (Eurofound) (2001) *Ten Years of Working Conditions in the European Union.* http://www.eurofound.eu.int/publications/files/EF00128EN.pdf (accessed 31/01/08).

Evans, L.J. (2002) *Evaluating the Effectiveness of Corporate Running Events in the North West Region.* M.Phil thesis, Liverpool John Moores University.

Gilson, N., Mckenna, J., Cooke, C. and Brown, W. (2007) Walking towards health in a university community: A feasibility study. *Preventive Medicine,* 44: 167–169.

Health and Safety Commission (2004) *Strategy for Workplace Health and Safety in Great Britain to 2010 and Beyond*. http://www.hse.gov.uk/aboutus/hsc/strategy.htm (accessed 31/01/08).

Health and Safety Commission (2006) *Health and Safety Statistics 2005/06 – National Statistics*. http://www.hse.gov.uk/statistics/overall/hssh0506.pdf (accessed 31/01/08).

Health and Safety Executive (1974) *Health and Safety at Work Act*. http://www.hse.gov.uk/legislation/hswa.pdf (accessed 31/01/08).

Health and Safety Executive (2000) *Revitalising Health and Safety – Strategy Statement*. http://www.hse.gov.uk/revitalising/strategy.pdf (accessed 31/01/08).

Health and Safety Executive (2006) *Absence Costs UK Economy £12 Billion Every Year*. Press release E009:06 http://www.hse.gov.uk/PRESS/2006/e06009.htm (accessed 31/01/08).

Health Survey for England (2003) http://www.sportengland.org/2003_health_survey_for_england_sport_and_walking.pdf (accessed 07/10/07).

Hutton, W. (1995) High risk. *Guardian*, 2–3.

Karasek, R. and Theorell, T. (1990) *Healthy Work: Stress, Productivity and the Reconstruction of Working Life*. Basic Books, New York.

Killoran, A., Doule, N., Waller, S., Wohlgemuth, C. and Crombie, H. (2006) *Transport Interventions Promoting Safe Cycling and Walking*. National Institute for Health and Clinical Excellence, London.

Kohn, M. and Schooler, C. (1973) Occupational experiences and psychological functioning: An assessment of reciprocal effects. *American Sociological Review*, 38: 97–118.

The Labour Force Survey 2001 (2003) *Travel to Work in GB: Personal Travel Factsheet 3*. http://www.dft.gov.uk/stellent/groups/dft_transstats/documents/page/dft_transstats_508290.pdf (accessed 14/12/06).

Marmot, M. and Wilkinson, R. (2003) *The Social Determinants of Health*. Oxford University Press, Oxford.

Marmot, M. (2004) *Status Syndrome*. Bloomsbury, London.

Marshall, A.L., Bauman, A.E., Patch, C., Wilson, J. and Chen, J. (2002) Can motivational signs prompt increases in incidental physical activity in an Australian health-care facility? *Health Education Research*, 17: 743–749.

Moy, F., Sallam, A.A.B. and Wong, M. (2006) The results of a worksite health promotion programme in Kuala Lumpur, Malaysia. *Health Promotion International*, 21(4): 301–310.

Murphy, M.H., Murtagh, E.M., Boreham, C.A.G., Hare, L.G. and Nevill, A.M. (2006) The effect of a workplace based walking programme on cardiovascular risk in previously sedentary civil servants. *BMC Public Health*, 6: 136.

Mutrie, N., Carney, C., Blamey, A., Crawford, F., Aitchison, T. and Whitelaw, A. (2002) "Walk in to Work Out": A randomised controlled trial of a self help intervention to promote active commuting. *Journal of Epidemiology and Community Health*, 56: 407–412.

Mutrie, N. and Woods, C. (2003) How can we get people to become more active? A problem waiting to be solved. In: *Perspectives In Exercise and Health* (Eds C. Riddoch and J. McKenna), pp. 131–152. MacMillan, Basingstoke.

Naidoo, J. and Wills, J. (2002) *Health Promotion: Foundations for Practice* (2nd edn). Baillière Tindall in association with the RCN, Edinburgh.

National Council for Voluntary Organisation (2006) *Working in the Voluntary Sector. Working for a Charity.* http://www.wfac.org.uk/?Information:Working_in_the_Voluntary_Sector (accessed 13/07/07).

National Statistics Office and Medical Research Council of Human Nutrition (2004) *National Diet and Nutrition Survey: Adults Aged 19–64 Years.* Stationery Office, London.

National Statistics (2007) *Labour Market Statistics – Headlines,* June 2007. http://www.statistics.gov.uk (accessed 4/11/07).

National Travel Survey (2002 – revised July 2004) *Main Trends.* http://www.dft.gov.uk/stellent/groups/dft_transstats/documents/page/dft_transstats_030036.pdf (accessed 14/12/06).

ONS (2005a) *Labour Market Statistics* – Time Series Data.

ONS (2005b) *Labour Force Survey Spring* 2005 data set.

OPCS (1990) *General Household Survey* 1988.

Osteras, H. and Hammer, S. (2006) The effectiveness of a pragmatic workplace physical activity program on maximal oxygen consumption and the physical activity level in healthy people. *Journal of Bodywork and Movement Therapies,* 10: 51–57.

Parkes, K.R., Carnell, S. and Farmer, E. (2005) Musculo-skeletal disorders, mental health and the work environment. Prepared by the University of Oxford for the Health and Safety Executive. Research Report 316. http://www.hse.gov.uk/research/rrpdf/rr316.pdf (accessed 31/01/08).

Pelletier, K.R. (1996) A review and analysis of the health and cost-effectiveness outcome studies of comprehensive health promotion and disease prevention programmes at the worksite. *American Journal of Health Promotion,* 10(5): 380–388.

Proper, K., Hildebrandt, V., Van Der, B.A. and Green, B.B. (2003) A patient-centred, workplace-based counselling programme may increase workers' physical activity. *Evidence-Based Healthcare,* 7: 138–139.

Robinson, V. (2002) Migrant workers in the UK. A study of the flow of migrant workers by sex age and continent of origin and their participation in the UK economy and society. *Labour Market Trends,* 110(9). http://www.statistics.gov.uk/cci/article.asp?id=306 (accessed 06/11/07).

Sallis, J.F. and Owen, N. (1999) *Physical Activity and Behavioural Medicine.* Sage, London.

Schreurs, P.J.G., Winnubst, J.A.M. and Cooper, C.L. (1996) Workplace health programmes. In: *Handbook of Work and Health Psychology* (Eds M.J. Schabracq, J.A.M. Winnubst and C.L. Cooper). John Wiley and Sons, New York.

Sedgley, L. and Dooris, M. (2007) *North West Regional Workplace Health Strategy.* http://www.gos.gov.uk/497468/docs/508516/NWRegionalWorkplaceStrategy.pdf (accessed 31/01/08).

Springett, J. and Dugdill, L. (1999) *Health Promotion Policies and Programmes in the Workplace: A New Challenge for Evaluation.* European Health Promotion Series No. 7. World Health Organisation /EURO.

Sustrans (2005) *Active Travel and Healthy Workplaces*. Information sheet FH06 http://www.sustrans.org.uk/webfiles/AT/Publications/Active%20travel%20and%20healthy%20workplaces%20final.pdf (accessed 14/12/06).

Talvi, A.I., Jarvisalo, J.O. and Knuts, L.R. (1999) A health promotion programme for oil refinery employees: Changes of health promotion needs observed at three years. *Occupational Medicine*, 49: 93–101.

The Times (2007) Ageing population brings grave problems. Duncan G., 25th June.

The Work Foundation (2005) News release. http://www.prnewswire.co.uk/cgi/news/release?id=143751 (accessed 15/12/06).

Thomas, L. and Williams, M. (2006) Promoting physical activity in the workplace: Using pedometers to increase daily activity levels. *Health Promotion Journal of Australia*, 17: 97–102.

Trade Union Technical Bureau for Health and Safety (2003) *Preventative Services – Special Report, No. 21, June*. http://hesa.etui-rehs.org/uk/newsletter/files/Newsletter-21-en.pdf (accessed 31/01/08).

Whitelaw, S., Baxendale, A., Bryce, C., Machardy, L., Young, I. and Witney E. (2001) 'Settings' based health promotion: A review. *Health Promotion International*, 16(4): 339–353.

Wilkinson, R. and Marmot M. (Eds) (2003) *The Solid Facts: The Social Determinants of Health* (2nd Edn), WHO, Geneva. http://www.euro.who.int/document/e81384.pdf (accessed 31/01/08).

WHO (World Health Organisation) (1986) *Ottawa Charter for Health Promotion*. WHO, Geneva. http://www.who.int/hpr/NPH/docs/ottawa_charter_hp.pdf (accessed 31/01/08).

Working Families (2004) *Balancing Work and Home in the Voluntary Sector*. December. http://www.workingfamilies.org.uk/asp/employer_zone/volsec/BWH_report_Nov04.doc (accessed 31/01/08).

8 Young people and physical activity

Gareth Stratton and Paula Watson

Introduction

The aim of this chapter will be to outline key factors specific to the promotion of youth physical activity, fitness and health. Current evidence for the relationship between physical activity, fitness and health will be discussed, and models of health promotion in young people will be outlined. Further discussion will consider how these models help professionals develop interventions in the field, and how researchers formulate approaches to help detect aspects of interventions that are effective at increasing physical activity behaviours in young people. The chapter concludes with two contrasting case studies of physical activity promotion, and a summary of recommendations for research and practice.

For the purposes of this chapter, the term children will be used for ages 0–11 years and adolescents for ages 12–18 years. Where children and adolescents are referred to collectively, the term young people will be used. Youth refers to the full period of childhood and adolescence (0–18 years).

Learning outcomes

The aims of this chapter are to:

1. discuss the importance of promoting physical activity to children and adolescents
2. debate current physical activity recommendations for young people and the role played by sedentary pastimes
3. apply theoretical models of behaviour change to the promotion of physical activity to young people
4. identify the different levels through which physical activity can be promoted to young people, and compare contrasting evidence-based interventions
5. explain the importance of appropriate evaluation in physical activity promotion, and the difficulties facing researchers in the field

---

Benefits of physical activity for young people

Is physical activity good for the health of young people?

Although the promotion of young people's physical activity is widely regarded as essential for public health (Department of Health, 2004; Strong *et al.*, 2005; Hills *et al.*, 2007), the evidence relating physical activity participation and physical fitness to direct health outcomes is limited. Due to the difficulty of demonstrating negative health outcomes during youth, coupled with the paucity of research employing objective measures of physical activity, the belief that a physically active child is a healthy one is born through a combination of suggestive research, evolutionary instinct, and the extensive literature supporting the beneficial effects of physical activity for adults (e.g. Blair and Cooper, 1997). Beneficial outcomes of physical activity during youth might relate to a young person's current health status, a young person's future health status, or a young person's future physical activity levels (with an indirect impact on their future health status; Blair *et al.*, 1989).

In a recent review, Boreham and Riddoch (2001) reported weak to moderate beneficial associations between youth physical activity and physical parameters of current health status, such as blood pressure, body mass, bone health and aerobic fitness. Furthermore, participation in physical activity during childhood and adolescence has psychosocial benefits, including reduced stress and anxiety, improvements in self-confidence, energy levels and the ability to concentrate (Hills *et al.*, 2007).

By far the most pressing health concern for youth physical activity involves the prevention and treatment of overweight and obesity, and the related reduction of risk for future disease. The Health Behaviour in School-Aged Children (HBSC) study gathered cross-sectional data from over 137 000 young people aged 10–16 years in 34 countries. The survey found a significant negative relationship between physical activity and body mass index [BMI = weight (kg) / height (m^2)] in 88% of the countries studied (Janssen *et al.*, 2005), indicating that physical activity is related to weight status in older children and adolescents. Statistics from the National Centre for Social Research indicate that 13.7% of children aged 2–10 in England were classified as obese in 2003, compared with 9.9% in 1998 (Jotangia *et al.*, 2005). According to recent extrapolations from the UK Foresight Programme (Foresight, 2007), the proportion of obese young people under 20 is predicted to rise to 25% by 2050, with suggestions that 70% of girls could be overweight or obese. Since obesity increases with age, and is a known risk factor for many lifestyle-related diseases (Department of Health, 2004), this rise in childhood obesity has serious long-term implications for public health. Furthermore, being overweight as an adolescent is thought to be a more significant predictor of chronic disease in adulthood than being overweight as an adult (Boreham and Riddoch, 2001). Physical activity is believed to play a key role in the prevention and treatment of childhood obesity (Nowicka and Flodmark, 2007). Guidelines based on the available evidence (SIGN, 2003; NICE, 2006) suggest successful management of the already overweight child must involve interventions that are multi-component (physical activity, nutrition and behaviour change), focus on sustainable lifestyle change and involve the whole family.

Does a physically active child become a physically active adult?

The seeds for an active lifestyle are thought to be sown during childhood and a significant effort has been made to promote activity in young people with a view that activity during the growing years will maintain itself throughout the lifespan. The review of physical activity and health undertaken by the Chief Medical Officer (Department of Health, 2004) reported that tracking of physical activity from childhood to adulthood is weak to moderate (Malina, 1996; Twisk et al., 2000) but that associations increased when the quality of the physical activity experience in childhood is taken into account (Engstrom et al., 1991). A more recent systematic review of adolescent physical activity and health reported a consistent albeit moderate association between physical activity during adolescence and adulthood (Hallal et al., 2006). Similarly, a 21-year tracking study (Telama et al., 2005) reported weak to moderate relationships between adult and child physical activity.

One possible reason for the reported weakness of tracking of physical activity from childhood to adulthood is that physical activity itself is a dynamic concept, influenced by numerous factors over time. Such factors might include life transitions (e.g. starting school, moving house, etc.), peer group and family influences (e.g. whether it is considered fashionable to be active within their current peer group, parents' working hours, etc.), access (e.g. local leisure facilities, ownership of bicycles, access to sports teams, etc.) or cognitive factors (e.g. mood, self-efficacy beliefs, etc.). It is therefore not surprising that recording physical activity scores using one measure and then comparing them over time produces relationships that are weak to moderate.

Recommended levels of physical activity for young people

How much physical activity do young people need?

Much debate surrounds the recommended levels of activity for young people. For the past 20 years recommendations have evolved from expert opinion (Sallis and Patrick, 1994; Department of Health, 2004), with limited scientific evidence to support them. These have ranged from 3 × 20 minutes of continuous, to 30 (minimal) or 60 (optimal) minutes of accumulated moderate to vigorous physical activity (MVPA). The nature of the accumulation of physical activity is open to debate. Consensus suggests 10-minute bouts of continuous MVPA are sufficient to produce health benefits. However, such an arbitrary definition may not be appropriate for young people, for whom 95% of their physical activity is vigorous in nature and lasts for 15 seconds or less (Bailey et al., 1995; Baquet et al., 2007). Andersen et al. (2006) found that by using an accelerometer-determined intensity threshold of 2000 counts per minute, 9- and 15-years-old European children needed to be active for 88 and 116 minutes respectively if they wanted to avoid clustered metabolic risk. This is one and a half to double the most recent recommended amount of physical activity determined by expert opinion (60 minutes daily; Department of Health, 2004; Strong et al., 2005). Therefore 90–120 minutes, as reported by Andersen et al. (2006), may have more influence on future recommendations for the health of children and adolescents. Whilst duration of 90–120 minutes has strong scientific support, there is little data on the appropriate intensity of activity for health maintenance in young people. What is certain, however, is that recommendations for youth need to move away from adult-style guidelines and take young people' natural predisposition for vigorous, intermittent activity into account.

A number of useful studies have used pedometers to report recommended number of steps by gender, age and BMI as well as patterns of steps across the day. Ten thousand steps have been used as an alternate to a duration measure of physical activity in adults. Recently 13 000 and 16 000 steps have been recommended for girls and boys respectively to combat overweight and obesity (Duncan et al., 2007). Tudor-Locke et al. (2006) investigated pedometer step scores across a segmented day in children. In this study boys took significantly more steps per day than girls, and more steps before school, during playtime, lunchtime and after school, but the same number of steps during structured physical education (PE) classes. Lunchtime physical activity represented the most important source of daily physical activity (15–16%) obtained during school hours for both boys and girls, whereas playtime accounted for 8–9% and PE class accounted for 8–11% of total steps per day. Regardless, almost half of daily steps taken were attributable to after school activities.

Sedentary behaviour

Whereas much discussion has revolved around physical activity, recent recommendations have suggested it may be more useful to focus recommendations on limiting sedentary (inactive) behaviours rather than enhancing physical activity; with the rationale that if sedentary behaviour decreases, physical activity will automatically increase (Hills et al., 2007). In their recent review, Hills et al. (2007) found associations between television viewing and lower habitual physical activity, lower cardiorespiratory fitness and increased obesity. This association became more complex, however, when the value of the sedentary behaviours and the extent to which they competed with physical activity was considered (Epstein et al., 2004). The HBSC study gathered cross-sectional data from over 137 000 young people aged 10–16 years in 34 countries. The survey, which included questions on activity, sedentary behaviours and BMI, found that 65% of all countries sampled showed a significant relationship between television viewing and obesity. However, of the 10 countries with the highest prevalence of obesity 46% of young people watched 3 or more hours of television per day, compared to 51% in the leanest 10 countries. As it is believed that physical activity is a contributing factor to obesity (Hills et al., 2007), the observation that those with a lower BMI were actually watching more television suggests that sedentary behaviours might at times co-exist with active behaviours. This view is supported by Marshall et al. (2002), who identified three clusters for both boys and girls. Boys were clustered into techno-actives, non-socialising actives and uninvolved inactives, and girls were in socialising actives, non-socialising actives and uninvolved inactives. Interestingly 40% of boys in the techno-active class also demonstrated above average levels of physical activity. These data demonstrate how active and inactive behaviours do not always displace each other. They can be independent to the point that the same young person may spend an above average proportion of their day being physically active whilst simultaneously spending an above average amount of time engaging in screen-based sedentary activities.

Thus, health professionals should be promoting activity that is moderate to vigorous in nature that is developmentally appropriate for the age and stage of maturation of the young person. Likewise a balance should be drawn between engaging in activity and inactivity depending on the psycho-social disposition of the young person.

How active are children and adolescents in the UK?

The Health Survey for England (Sproston and Primatesta, 2002) provided data on out-of-school and general physical activity levels of children aged 2–15 in the UK. The types of physical activity recorded were sports and exercise, active play and walking whereas children aged 8 and over were asked further questions about active housework and gardening. Activity that was part of the school curriculum was excluded. Young people were categorised according to the following levels:

- high activity levels = 60 minutes of moderate intensity physical activity on 7 days in the last week (the recommended level)
- medium activity levels = 30 to 59 minutes of moderate intensity physical activity on 7 days in the last week
- low activity levels = those that are active at a lower level or not active at all

The survey reported that 70% of boys and 61% of girls achieved the recommended levels of physical activity. Activity declined with age among girls after age 10. By age 15, half of girls compared to 69% of boys engaged in 60 minutes of physical activity on 7 days of the week. Whereas there were no differences in physical activity by social class there were differences between black and minority ethnic (BME) groups for participation in sports and exercise, but not for walking or play.

Although the Health Survey for England data suggests children's physical activity levels are approaching recommended levels (Sproston and Primatesta, 2002), it is important to note these data were gathered using a questionnaire-based approach. Self-report tools, such as questionnaires, are considered highly subjective and their results must be interpreted with caution. More rigorous measures of physical activity include objective tools such as accelerometry, observation, heart rate or pedometry (Dugdill and Stratton, 2007, also see Chapter 4). These can, however, be costly and impractical to administer on a large scale.

Evidence from other sources suggests the physical activity of young people is declining and many children are not accumulating sufficient physical activity to benefit their health. Active travel, especially to school, has a significant part to play in contributing to overall levels of physical activity (Mackett et al., 2005). The National Transport Survey (Department for Transport, 2005) reported that the proportion of primary school children aged 5–10 that walk to school declined from 53% in 1995/97 to 49% in 2005, with an increase from 38% to 43% in the numbers being driven to school during the same period. However, for secondary school pupils the proportion walking to school increased from 42% in 1995/97 to 44% in 2005, despite a corresponding increase in the proportion of secondary school children being driven to school in the same period. Levels of cycling to school have remained extremely low at 1% or 2% of trips.

Arguably the most robust UK data on children's physical activity has recently been reported (Riddoch et al., 2007). The Avon Longitudinal Study of Parents and Children (ALSPAC) reported measures of physical activity in nearly 6000 young people using accelerometry. At age 11 it was found that the majority of young people were insufficiently active according to current recommended levels for health.

Fitness and fatness

There are 11 components of fitness, five of these are health related (body composition, aerobic fitness, strength, muscular endurance and flexibility) and six are skill related (local muscular endurance, power, speed, reaction time, coordination and agility). The two most commonly used measures of fitness in health and activity are body composition and aerobic fitness. While practitioners may find the debate surrounding physical activity confusing, the issues surrounding the utility of fitness measures are also unclear. However field measures of fitness on a population level are useful indicators of changes in performance. For example, the upward trend in overweight and obesity (Bellizi and Dietz., 1999; Cole *et al.*, 2000; Bundred *et al.*, 2001) and downward trend in fitness (Tomkinson and Olds, 2007; Stratton *et al.*, 2007) suggests that children are not active enough to first maintain a healthy weight and, second, to sustain an adequate level of endurance fitness which is protective in adulthood (Blair and Cooper, 1997). Stratton *et al.* (2007) demonstrated that between 1998 and 2004 both BMI and endurance performance (measured by a 20-metre multi-stage shuttle run test) deteriorated. Furthermore, when the population (n~16000) was split into thirds for BMI it was demonstrated that normal, overweight and obese children were losing fitness, and that even the fittest children were becoming more overweight. These findings support the need for whole population interventions to stem the current increase in overweight during the growing years.

In summary, the recommended amount of physical activity and fitness for young people's health remains open to debate. This debate revolves around the frequency, duration, intensity and type of activity, how it is measured, whether different physical activity targets should be used for sub-groups such as boys and girls or categories of overweight, and whether the benefits of physical activity during the growing years carry themselves through to adulthood.

Promoting physical activity to young people

Correlates of physical activity

Researchers and practitioners involved in the promotion of physical activity to young people must first understand the factors that are associated with physical activity for that population; in particular, the factors that can be manipulated to support young people in becoming more active. In order to establish this, several reviews have looked at the correlates of physical activity for young people. In a review of 33 papers on the environmental factors that determine young people's (3–18 years) physical activity, Davison and Lawson (2006) reported that physical activity was predicted by public provision of facilities and access (local facilities, schools), transport infrastructure (cycle pathways, pavements, traffic density) and local conditions (crime, deprivation). Gustafson and Rhodes (2006) completed a 34 study review on the parental correlates of physical activity in children and young adolescents. Significant correlations were found between parental support and child physical activity level, although there were mixed findings between parental and child physical activity levels. In a further review, Ferreira *et al.* (2007) found that for children (age range 4–12), gender (male), self-efficacy, parental physical activity (for boys) and parental support were positively associated with physical activity. For adolescents (age range 13–18), positive associations were found for gender (male), parental education, attitude, self-efficacy, goal orientation/motivation, physical education/school sports, family influences, and friend support. A positive association was also found between gender (male) and sedentary behavior; thus supporting the notion that physical activity and sedentary behaviours can coincide. Ethnicity (Caucasian), socioeconomic status, and parent education were found to be inversely associated with adolescents' sedentary behaviours. For sedentary behaviour, Gorely *et al.* (2004) reported that TV viewing decreased during adolescence, but that high users at young ages were likely to remain high users when older. Interestingly though for children with access to a television set, viewing time did not appear to have increased over the past 50 years. Qualitative work on correlates of physical activity in adolescents provided much the same evidence as the quantitative reviews although a lack of self-efficacy, dislike of physical education, traditional games and competition in team sports all served as detractors from physical activity in girls (Brooks and Magnusson, 2006).

The complexity of physical activity behaviour

For young people physical activity behaviour is not a single, simple behaviour. Marttila *et al.* (1998) identified five different categories of physical activity – occupational activities, lifestyle and commuting activities, fitness activities to maintain health, sports activities undertaken as part of, or in preparation for, competition (Marttila *et al.*, 1998), physical education and play (Stratton, 2000). This suggests that physical activity behaviour is rather more complex than implied by current stage-based activity promotion interventions which generally assume that individuals are in a single, overall, stage of readiness for physical activity. This is further complicated in young people who are continuously growing and developing socially, psychologically and physically. Factors affecting physical activity behaviour in children and young people are different to adults in that they need to be contextualised in relation to growth (increases in quantity/size) and development (increases in quality). One of the key research issues is the ability of younger children to process and understand (cognition) the physical activity promotion messages given to them, have the social skills (affect) to engage with other people and the physical attributes (psychomotor) to undertake the task. As young people move from childhood through to adulthood, they interact in mainly adult designed and controlled environments where they are socialised into increasingly inactive adult-like behaviours. Moreover, children may physically mature at a faster rate than their psychological development. For example, an early maturing girl may be near adult height at age 12 and thus be physically mature. However, the same girl may have an average psychological development score for a 12 year old. The opposite may also be true where a physically immature boy may be psychologically and socially very mature. Promoting physical activity to both the boy and girl described above at the same time is therefore problematic and no physical activity model has yet been designed to understand these complex issues.

To further understand physical activity promotion for young people, it is useful to consider the role of intrapersonal factors in behaviour change. It can be argued that some form of cognitive activity (e.g. perceptions, attitudes, beliefs – conscious or subconscious) underlies all behaviour. Self-efficacy (i.e. confidence in one's abilities) has been associated with physical activity in young people (Ferreira *et al.*, 2007) and intentions to be active, low perceived barriers and high perceived activity competence are consistent correlates of physical activity in this age group (Sallis *et al.*, 2000). Hence, children who believe they are incapable of playing football (poor self-efficacy), do not enjoy football (low enjoyment) and feel they cannot do anything to improve their skill level (an external locus of control) are unlikely to engage with the local football club (low intention). If, however, something can be done to change children's self-perceptions and attitudes towards football, they might have the confidence to join the local team. Therefore it is possible that sustained changes in physical activity behaviour require (or will at least be enhanced by) a change in underlying cognitions. Following this rationale, any physical activity promotion model must consider the long-term impact on the child's physical activity perceptions, attitudes and beliefs. This could occur on a number of levels – through the environment, the child's own behaviour or their social world. There are relatively few studies of social and cognitive variables in relation to child and adolescent physical activity, and further research is required to determine the extent to which children's cognitions determine their short and long-term physical activity behaviour.

Theoretical models of physical activity promotion for young people

The PRECEDE-PROCEED model was developed as a planning framework from which health education and health promotion programs could be designed (Green and Kreuter, 1999). PRECEDE is an acronym for **P**redisposing, **R**einforcing, and **E**nabling Fa**C**tors in **E**ducational **D**iagnosis and **E**valuation. Predisposing factors include knowledge, attitudes, beliefs, personal preferences, existing skills, and self-efficacy toward physical activity. Reinforcing factors include factors that reward or encourage physical activity and enabling factors are psychological/ emotional or physical factors that motivate, or allow, a child to engage in physical activity. PROCEED, which stands for **P**olicy, **R**egulatory, and **O**rganizational **C**onstructs in **E**ducational and **E**nvironmental **D**evelopment, acknowledges the importance of environmental factors in determining physical activity.

Needless to say there are no perfect models that can be applied unreservedly to paediatric populations. The primary model designed with young people in mind is the Youth Physical Activity Promotion Model (YPAPM; Welk, 1999; Figure 8.1). This model is based on the premise that multidimensional and multidisciplinary methods are required to understand physical activity behaviour. Using the PRECEDE-PROCEED approach the model relates physical activity promotion to unique developmental, psychological, and behavioral characteristics of children within a social-ecological framework.

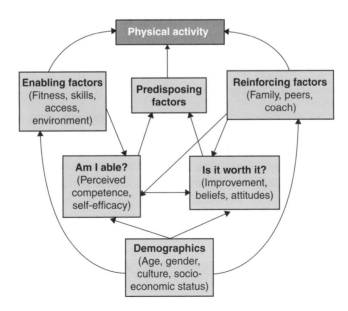

Figure 8.1 The Youth Physical Activity Promotion Model (Welk, 1999).

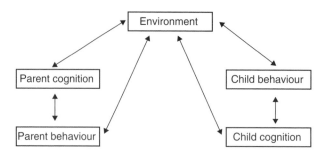

Figure 8.2 A socialisation model of child behaviour (Taylor *et al.*, 1994).

The YPAPM accounts for personal, social, and environmental influences on children's physical activity and acts as a bridge between theory and practice.

In a review of the family determinants of childhood physical activity, Taylor *et al.* (1994) developed a Socialisation Model of Child Behaviour based on Bandura's (1986) Social Cognitive Theory (Figure 8.2). The model suggests that continuous reciprocal interactions occur between the home environment, parental cognitions and behaviours, and child cognitions and behaviours. Any intervention designed to alter a child's physical activity behaviour, therefore, must take into account the complex interactions surrounding the family and home environment. It has been suggested that the way a child perceives their home and local neighbourhood is associated with their participation in different types of physical activity (Hume *et al.*, 2005). Qualitative mapping techniques demonstrated that social space within the family home plays an important role in the lives of children of primary school age, and the home environment may be an important setting in which to enhance the enabling and reinforcing factors for physical activity.

Levels of intervention

One way to deconstruct the complexity of physical activity promotion to young people is to consider interventions from a settings perspective. Figure 8.3 provides examples of interventions at individual, community and population levels. To achieve sustainable behaviour change, the ultimate aim would be to alter children's predisposing factors (or correlates) for physical activity. Therefore, an important distinction must be made between biological predisposing factors and modifiable predisposing factors. Biological factors are those that we are born with, such as age, sex or inherited abilities. Although these may mean we are more or less likely to participate in physical activity, they cannot be altered through intervention and are useful only in targeting populations for intervention (Gustafson and Rhodes, 2006). It is the modifiable predisposing factors that are of most

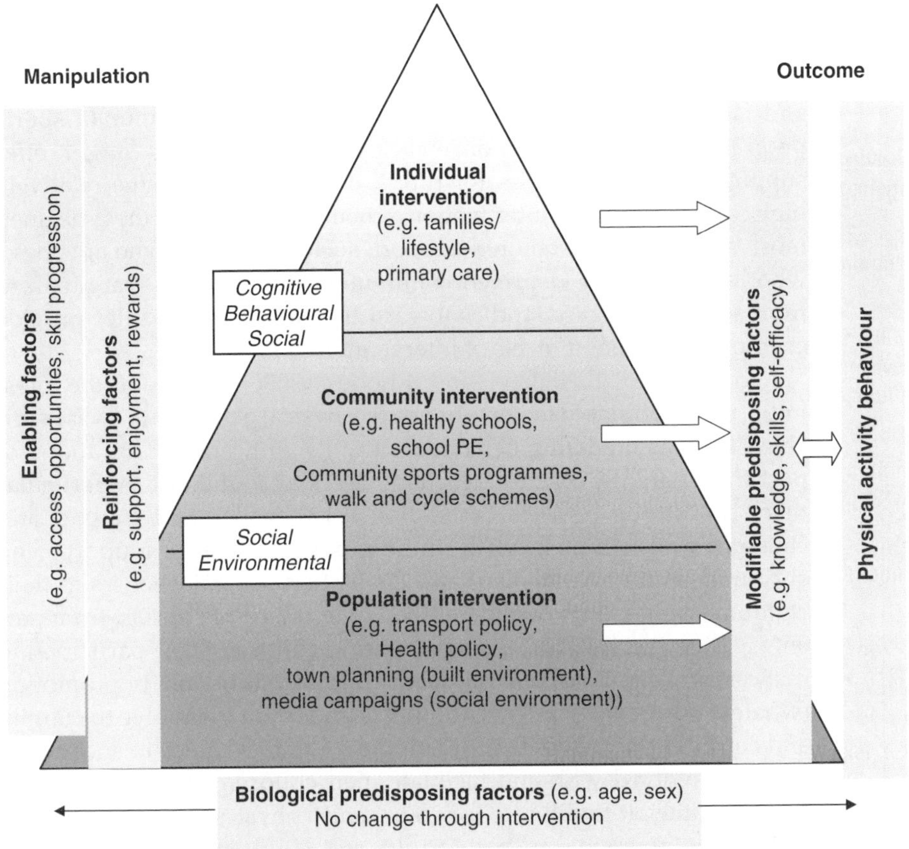
Manipulation
Outcome
Enabling factors
(e.g. access, opportunities, skill progression)
Reinforcing factors
(e.g. support, enjoyment, rewards)
Individual intervention
(e.g. families/ lifestyle, primary care)
Cognitive Behavioural Social
Community intervention
(e.g. healthy schools, school PE, Community sports programmes, walk and cycle schemes)
Social Environmental
Population intervention
(e.g. transport policy, Health policy, town planning (built environment), media campaigns (social environment))
Modifiable predisposing factors
(e.g. knowledge, skills, self-efficacy)
Physical activity behaviour
Biological predisposing factors (e.g. age, sex)
No change through intervention

Figure 8.3 Levels of intervention.

interest (e.g. knowledge, enjoyment, self-efficacy), as these may change as a result of intervention and in turn produce a sustained increase in physical activity.

At whichever level an intervention occurs, the important aspect is that it is enabling and reinforcing physical activity to produce a change in physical activity behaviour. These enabling and reinforcing factors can be broken down further into cognitive variables (e.g. attitudes, beliefs), behavioural variables (e.g. fitness, skills), social variables (e.g. family, peers, coach) and environmental variables (e.g. access, environment). Figure 8.3 illustrates that the type of variables manipulated will depend on the level of intervention. Examples of intervention at a built environmental level might include the provision of cycle lanes, building design of schools, safe walking areas or safe playing fields. At a social environment level, interventions might range from large-scale social marketing campaigns, through media branding of sport, to the less explicit cultural and peer-group norms.

Community intervention for children for the most part will focus around the school day, from active transport to and from school, school physical education, playtime, after school activities, to the school culture and facilities for physical activity. Outside school, community sports programmes, local clubs or walk and cycle schemes might offer support and opportunities for physical activity. Due to the relatively high cost of individual intervention, schemes might target those deemed most 'at risk' to offer tailored support, such as children who are obese, who live in socially deprived communities, or who are marginalized from society. The case studies toward the end of this chapter provide examples of different levels of intervention in practice.

According to Gustafson and Rhodes (2006), some of the most important modifiable factors for youth physical activity are social variables, such as modeling behaviours from significant adults, and support from parents, coaches, teachers, peers and siblings. In particular there is a strong positive correlation between parental support and child physical activity level; the most important forms of support being encouragement, involvement and facilitation. As gatekeepers to their children's behaviours outside of the home, a lack of support from parents can be the sole factor in preventing children from participating in a certain activity. In any model of child physical activity promotion (whatever the level of intervention) it is important to involve the family and consider the factors that determine a parent's choice to encourage, become involved with and facilitate their children's physical activity. Unfortunately, it is still rare for community physical activity interventions to be accessible to both adults and children; most targeted as either a children's sports club or an adult exercise class. With a childhood obesity epidemic looming, however, the family is considered to be a key focus in the establishment of sustainable healthy lifestyles (NICE, 2006).

For sustainable increases in physical activity behaviour, it is likely that multi-level interventions are necessary. In particular, individual and community interventions must be accompanied by wider environmental change. Arguably some of the most significant barriers to physical activity in youth have come about through changes to the physical and social environment in which we live. Technological advances have reduced the level of activity required for everyday tasks and introduced a stream of increasingly attractive sedentary pastimes. More widespread automated transport and media transmission of negative events has provoked anxieties in parents that prevent spontaneous play and active transport in children. As Hills et al. (2007) noted, 'unless interventions are introduced that eradicate the environmental barriers to facilitate and promote an active lifestyle, the problem [reduced physical activity levels in children] is going to get worse' (p. 538).

Evaluating interventions

The previous section described the theoretical basis for intervention in various settings, but what evidence currently exists to support the different approaches to physical activity promotion for young people? In a recent high-quality review, van Sluijs *et al.* (2007) located 57 studies (33 aimed at children and 24 at adolescents) aimed at promoting physical activity to children and adolescents. The review was restricted to published trials that met strict methodological criteria. To be included studies must not have selected participants on the basis of having a specific disease or health problem, must have included a non-physical activity intervention for the control group, and must have statistically analysed an outcome measure related to self-reported or objectively measured physical activity. Effective interventions increased physical education related physical activity by 2.6 minutes, school playtime physical activity by 13 minutes and overall weekly physical activity by 283 minutes. Among children, limited evidence for an effect was found for interventions from low socioeconomic populations, and environmental interventions. Strong evidence was found that school-based with family or community involvement and multi-component interventions increased adolescent physical activity. Unfortunately the authors reported that a lack of high quality evaluations limited conclusions concerning the effectiveness of physical activity interventions, especially among children.

The review by van Sluijs *et al.* (2007) highlights several ongoing problems surrounding evaluation of physical activity interventions. Firstly, the notion of high quality continues to be debated, with traditionalists advocating a number of key criteria that interventions need to meet to be considered for inclusion in credible reviews (e.g. randomisation, control, blinded researchers, etc.). In reality it is extremely difficult to meet all these criteria, where physical activity interventions are largely field based and where it is impossible to isolate components or locate a clearly defined control group (Medical Research Council, 2000; see also Chapter 4). Therefore, many well (albeit not traditionally) evaluated interventions go unreported in the systematic reviews that subsequently inform policy. Secondly, interventions may be successful but may lack the appropriate measures to prove their effectiveness, with delivery costs taking precedence over evaluation. Intervention evaluation is complicated further by a lack of established methods for measuring physical activity levels, particularly in young people (Dugdill and Stratton, 2007). The few objective methods that do exist, such as accelerometry or heart rate measures, are costly to administer and often impractical on a large scale.

In summary, to promote evidence-based practice and allow for replication of successful interventions, designs must include appropriate evaluation protocols that demonstrate changes in behaviour or health-related parameters (such as waist circumference). Practitioners must define clear aims and objectives for their intervention and are urged to adopt multi-method approaches to evaluation, including both quantitative and qualitative methodology (Dugdill *et al.*, 2005). In defining intervention outcomes, sustained changes in physical activity predisposing factors should be given consideration, rather than a focus solely on physical activity behaviour. It must be acknowledged that traditional science cannot simply be lifted from the objective world to the study of human behaviour, and that alternative forms of evaluation (e.g. qualitative designs, non-randomised designs) can offer insightful evidence in the field of physical activity promotion. A process evaluation of any intervention is now almost a necessity.

Case studies

Together the PRECEDE-PROCEED model, the YPAPM and the Socialisation Model of Child Behaviour provide a framework to develop an understanding of physical activity promotion in young people (as summarized in Figure 8.3), and an outline of the different levels at which opportunity for intervention exist. The following case studies demonstrate how different approaches to intervention design and evaluation can be employed to promote sustainable behaviour change in young people. The first targets a wide population through manipulation of the physical environment, the second targets specific individuals through a group family-based intervention. Although the two approaches differ markedly, they are both founded in the PRECEDE-PROCEED model through which they enable and reinforce physical activity for young people.

Case study 1: Changing the environment to promote physical activity – the sporting playgrounds project

Outline of project: As children experience up to 600 playtime periods a year (based on 3 times a day, 5 days a week, 39 weeks a year), the playground offers a unique opportunity to promote children's habitual physical activity levels through unstructured play. Previous short- to medium-term studies have demonstrated that re-designing the physical environment of the playground through markings (Stratton, 2000; Stratton and Mullan, 2005) or providing games equipment (Verstraete *et al.*, 2006) can lead to an increase in children's physical activity levels during school playtime.

Funding (£420 000) was secured from a national £10 million Sporting Playgrounds Initiative, developed by the Department for Education and Skills (DfES) and Nike, to re-design 21 primary school playgrounds in the Liverpool area (North-West of England). Fifteen playgrounds were used for this study, as the completion of the remaining sites was delayed. Located in areas of social and economic deprivation, the dual aims of the initiative were to increase the physical activity of young people, and to tackle social exclusion and playground issues in schools.

The playgrounds were re-designed following the Zoneparc model developed by the Youth Sport Trust (YST) and Nike. The model promoted opportunities for movement and social interaction (Ridgers, 2007) by dividing the playground into three zones, each painted in a distinct colour including markings and structures to encourage different forms of activity. The red sports zone provided a dedicated space for activities such as football, basketball or cricket. In drawing these activities to a confined physical area, this also prevented their domination over the remainder of the playground; thus allowing the less sporty children to have space to engage in other forms of activity. The blue action zone included markings to encourage children to play games and improve their fitness and skills. These were either markings for a specific activity (e.g. hopscotch) or markings that encouraged creativity and active play (e.g. grids, lines, zig-zags, etc.). The yellow chill-out zone encouraged social engagement through less active games such as word games, clapping games or board games.

Evaluation design: The impact of the playground upgrades on children's physical activity was evaluated through a quasi-experimental design (Ridgers *et al.*, 2007a,b). Over 400 children from 26 primary schools across Liverpool took part in the study (15 intervention schools and 11 socio-economic control schools who received no intervention). Activity levels were measured using a rigorous multi-method approach at baseline, 6 weeks after playground re-design and 6 months after playground re-design. Accelerometers, heart rate (HR) monitors and systematic observation were used as objective measures to assess movement (accelerometry), physiological response (HR monitors) and behaviour (systematic observation). Subjective data were collected during meetings with school council focus groups involving children, teachers and parents. Threshold values were determined for the accelerometry and HR measures to represent moderate-to-vigorous (MVPA) and vigorous (VPA) physical activity engagement based on previous research and recommendations (Stratton, 1996; Nilsson *et al.*, 2002).

Outcomes of evaluation: There was a statistically positive intervention effect across time for both MVPA and VPA (Ridgers *et al.*, 2007a,b). Following the playground re-design, the children in the intervention schools were significantly more active than the children in the control schools. This effect was observed at both 6 weeks and 6 months post-intervention (Ridgers *et al.*, 2007b), thus indicating that the intervention was effective at sustaining physical activity increases over time. Although it was found that boys engaged in more overall physical activity during playtime than girls, they experienced comparable increases following the playground re-design (Ridgers *et al.*, 2007a). Interestingly, it was found that the intervention effect was greater for longer playtime duration (HR and accelerometry), for younger children (accelerometry only) and for children who were less active at baseline (HR only; Ridgers *et al.*, 2007b). Qualitative data indicated children, teachers and parents were proud of the playground and children were more alert in class.

Application to practice: Such was the simplicity of the Sporting Playgrounds Project that the approach has now been adopted in schools in France, Holland,

Belgium, Scandinavia and North America. The results from the project demonstrated that manipulation of the playground environment had a positive effect on the levels of physical activity in children, with the greatest effects being observed as the length of available time to play increased. The playground is a unique space that belongs to children, and the importance of playtime is thought to go beyond the physical benefits related to fitness. Pellegrini and Bohn (2005) highlighted the importance of playtime in enhancing cognitive performance and promoting social and emotional development. The fact that children who were less active at baseline saw a greater relative increase in their physical activity levels demonstrated that playground intervention might be an appropriate tool to engage otherwise non-sporty children in physical activity that they enjoy (Ridgers et al., 2007a,b). Further research might explore whether this change in activity behaviour is accompanied by a change in activity-related cognitions (e.g. perceptions of competence, self-efficacy), and whether the benefits of the environmental intervention is enhanced by combining the approach with social reinforcing factors from adults (e.g. use of the space during physical education lessons, or offering rewards for certain activities), or whether in fact this would reduce the appeal of the playground by removing ownership from the children.

Case study 2: A social-cognitive approach to promote physical activity (through the family) – The Getting Our Active Lifestyles Started! (GOALS) Project

Outline of project: The GOALS (GOALS phase 2 was funded by the Neighbourhood Renewal Fund and involved a partnership between Liverpool John Moores University, Liverpool City Council, Liverpool PCT, University of Salford and Alder Hey Children's Hospital) project was set up to develop an evidence-based, community intervention for overweight children (aged 5–16) and their families. Using an action research approach to intervention development (described in detail in Chapter 4), a 19-session intervention was designed to run over three progressive modules. The aim of this intervention was to support families in making gradual, sustainable changes to their eating and activity habits. The majority of sessions were group-based and combined a practical physical activity session (Move It!) with interactive sessions focused on nutrition (Fun Foods) and behaviour change (Target Time). Individual behavioural support was provided through weekly goal-setting, a rewards scheme and a family mentor session at the end of each module. The focus of this case study will be on the physical activity aspect of the intervention.

Promoting activity: The GOALS intervention drew from the theoretical frameworks proposed by Welk (1999) and Taylor et al. (1994) to motivate the participating children and their families to become more physically active. GOALS used a variety of direct and indirect techniques to enable and reinforce physical activity within each family's lifestyle. This was done through the actions of the physical activity coaches [physical activity coaches were employed to lead practical fun-based physical activity sessions for the family groups. Examples of activities included fun games (e.g. cups and saucers, stuck in the mud), relays, sports taster sessions (e.g. basketball, football) and circuit training] during the sessions, through targeted activities to encourage changes in parental cognitions and behaviours, and through fun, engaging activities aimed at positively restructuring the children's physical activity perceptions, attitudes and beliefs.

Coach behaviours: The physical activity sessions during GOALS were focused on fun and enjoyment, with an emphasis on personal improvement (task orientation) rather than competition between individuals (ego orientation). Praise and encouragement were continuous and activities were tailored to be inclusive to the whole group. A can-do culture was encouraged, with a view to enhancing self-efficacy and perceptions of physical activity.

Parent behaviours: Each physical activity session involved the whole family, allowing children to experience both the modelling behaviour of their parents and the enjoyment of being physically active together. Parents were encouraged to take these behaviours home, to set their own goals, and to provide support, encouragement and reinforcement for their children's physical activity achievements; however small.

Parent cognitions: Through a solution-focused approach (Peterson, 2005), parents were encouraged to focus on the controllable, can-do aspects of their lifestyles, such as reorganising their day to fit in time to play with the children, or restructuring the home environment to promote active living. Sessions focused on identifying and overcoming barriers (internal thoughts and feelings that prevent participation in activity) and challenging assumptions and subconscious beliefs (such as the misplaced belief that physical activity is relatively unimportant compared to diet in weight management). In a less direct (though arguably more powerful) manner than the discussion sessions, the opportunity to experience physical activity in a fun, no-pressure environment allowed parents to enjoy and increase their own self-efficacy for activity, thus enhancing the chance of sustaining support for their child.

Child cognitions: Regular, realistic goal-setting (and consequent achievement) allowed the children to experience success. Past success is one of the factors identified by Bandura (1986) as a key contributor to future self-efficacy. If a child has successfully managed to swim 25 metres once, they will believe strongly they can do it again. If they have failed, however, they might develop a belief that they 'can't swim', which in turn may prevent them trying again in the future. At GOALS the opportunity to try out new sports in a safe environment with similar others allowed the children a taste of success and a feeling of achievement; helping to reshape their perception of physical activity and increase the likelihood of their future participation.

Evaluation design: Phase 1 of the project (see Chapter 4) employed qualitative methodology to explore the key components required for a successful lifestyle intervention for overweight children and families. Phase 2 of the intervention was evaluated using a combination of quantitative and qualitative measures. Outcome measures (that provided information about whether the intervention worked) included BMI, waist circumference, lifestyle questionnaires and physical activity diaries. These were taken pre-, post- and 1-year post-commencement of the intervention. Additional information and process data (that provided information about why the intervention worked, or did not work) was collected through qualitative focus groups, feedback sheets and interviews.

Outcomes of evaluation: Qualitative findings from the developmental phase provided evidence for the importance of enjoyment, group support and the participation of the whole family in promoting physical activity.

'My children absolutely loved it [Move It!]. At last they were in someone's team and not 'the fat kid never picked'. All the children were the same. This was the essence of success. Fat children do not dislike exercise, they fear ridicule as do we all. All of the children loved Move It! Especially because Mum joined in. Yes folks your children want to play with YOU and the rougher the better. They like to see you struggle a bit too. It makes them feel that they are not unusual.'   (Parent of 9-year-old girl and 11-year-old boy)

Pre- and post-intervention data from phase 2 suggested families made changes to cognitive predisposing factors for physical activity following participation in the GOALS intervention. At the time of writing follow-up data was not available.

Thirty-three overweight or obese children and their families completed the intervention during the period April 2006–March 2007. In their post-intervention questionnaires three times as many children rated themselves as fit or very fit than in their pre-intervention questionnaires, and far fewer said they 'don't know' or rated themselves as 'unfit'. This data was supported by a significant decrease in waist circumference and a significant increase in perceived social acceptance to their peers [as measured by the social acceptance subscale of Harter's self-perception profile (1985)]. Although the scores on the athletic competence subscale of the questionnaire showed no significant change, the children consistently rated the Move It! (physical activity) session as their favourite. Qualitative data suggested the activity levels of both parents and children had increased and parents considered their children to be more knowledgeable of the importance of physical activity and more confident with regards to participation.

Application to practice: Data from the GOALS intervention demonstrated that a range of techniques (both direct and indirect) can be used to enable and reinforce physical activity within a family, community-based group setting. Through a focus on enjoyment, personal achievement, and a can-do approach, it is possible to enhance self-efficacy for physical activity, which in turn enhances the likelihood of future participation. Although GOALS involved intervention on an individual level, it is important to note it was supported by enabling factors in the local community and environment. The sessions took place at local schools who provided their facilities free of charge and the local council provided free passes for all young people under 17 in Liverpool to attend their leisure facilities.

Conclusion and implications for practice

Physical activity in childhood may be important for adulthood but is also important for positive physical, social and psychological health during the growing phases. Physical activity is linked to health outcomes such as metabolic risk but data from physical activity studies are limited by lack of agreement of a gold standard measure of physical activity. Despite ongoing debate regarding recommended levels, intensity and type of physical activity for young people, body fatness is increasing, fitness is declining and many young people in the UK are insufficiently active to benefit their health. A range of cognitive, behavioural, social and environmental variables are important in enabling and reinforcing physical activity for young people. Two contrasting case studies demonstrated that there is no ideal approach to physical activity promotion, and different levels of intervention can be equally successful in increasing physical activity in young people. The sporting playgrounds study provided an example of a successful environmental intervention, and the GOALS project provided an insight into the successful components of a family-based lifestyle intervention. Both projects were set in real world situations and allowed ecological research and evaluation to take place. To maximise effectiveness it is recommended that interventions do not occur in isolation, but are multi-level in nature, with individual interventions (e.g. motivational interviewing) being supported by community enabling factors (e.g. subsidised leisure facilities) and national policy (e.g. health promotion messages). It is essential that appropriately-evaluated interventions draw on the available evidence to promote physical activity to young people within the family, the community and the wider population.

Acknowledgements

We thank the National Lottery and Gary White, manager of Liverpool Sport Action Zone, for funding the Sporting Playgrounds project, the Neighbourhood Renewal Fund for funding the GOALS project and the participating families and staff that made the intervention possible.

References

Andersen, L.B., Harro, M., Sardinha, L.B., Froberg, K., Ekelund, U., Brage, S. and Anderssen, S.A. (2006) Physical activity and clustered cardiovascular risk in children: A cross-sectional study (The European Youth Heart Study). *Lancet*, 22(368): 299–304.

Bailey, R.C., Olson, J., Pepper, S.L., Porszasz, J., Barstow, T.J. and Cooper D.M. (1995) The level and tempo of children's physical activities: An observational study. *Medicine and Science in Sports and Exercise*, 27: 1033–1041.

Bandura, A. (1986) *Social Foundations of Thought and Action*. Prentice-Hall, Englewood Cliffs, NJ.

Baquet, G., Stratton, G., van Praagh, E. and Berthoin, S. (2007) Improving physical activity assessment in prepubertal children with high-frequency accelerometry monitoring: A methodological issue. *Preventive Medicine*, 44: 143–147.

Bellizzi, M.C. and Dietz, W.H. (1999) Workshop on childhood obesity: Summary of the discussion. *American Journal of Clinical Nutrition*, 70: 173–175.

Blair, S.N., Clark, D.G., Cureton, K.J. and Powell, K.E. (1989) Exercise and fitness in childhood: Implications for a lifetime of health. In: *Perspectives in Exercise Science and Sports Medicine, Vol. 2: Youth, Exercise and Sport* (Eds C.V. Gisolfi and D.R. Lamb), pp. 401–430. McGraw-Hill, New York.

Blair, S.N. and Cooper, K.H. (1997) Dose of exercise and health benefits. *Archives of Internal Medicine*, 157(2): 153–154.

Boreham, C. and Riddoch, C. (2001) The physical activity, fitness and health of children. *Journal of Sports Sciences*, 19: 915–929.

Brooks, F. and Magnusson, J. (2006) Taking part counts: Adolescents' experiences of the transition from inactivity to active participation in school-based physical education. *Health Education Research*, 21: 872–883.

Bundred, P., Kitchiner, D. and Buchan, I. (2001) Prevalence of overweight and obese children between 1989 and 1998: A population based series of cross sectional studies. *British Medical Journal*, 10(322): 326–328.

Cole, T.J., Bellizzi, M.C., Flegal, K.M. and Dietz, W.H. (2000) Establishing a standard definition for child overweight and obesity worldwide: International survey. *British Medical Journal*, 6(320): 1240–1243.

Davison, K.K. and Lawson, C.T. (2006) Do attributes in the physical environment influence children's physical activity? A review of the literature. *International Journal of Behavioural Nutrition and Physical Activity*, 27: 3–19.

Department for Transport (2005) National Transport Survey. www.dft.gov.uk/pgr/statistics/ (accessed 4/10/2007)

Department of Health (2004) *At Least Five a Week: Evidence on the Impact of Physical Activity and Its Relationship to Health*. A Report from the Chief Medical Officer. Department of Health, London.

Dugdill, L., Graham, R. and McNair, F. (2005) Exercise referral: The public health panacea for physical activity promotion? A critical perspective of exercise referral interventions; their development and evaluation. *Ergonomics*, 48: 1390–1410.

Dugdill, L. and Stratton, G. (2007) *Evaluating Sport and Physical Activity Interventions: A Guide for Practitioners*. University of Salford, UK.

Duncan, S.C., Duncan, T.E., Strycker, L.A. and Chaumeton, N.R. (2007) A cohort-sequential latent growth model of physical activity from ages 12 to 17 years. *Annals of Behavioral Medicine*, 33: 80–89.

Engstrom, I., Fallstrom, K., Karlberg, E., Sten, G. and Bjure, J. (1991) Psychological and respiratory physiological effects of a physical exercise programme on boys with severe asthma. *Acta Paediatrica Scandinavica*, 80: 1058–1065.

Epstein, L.H., Roemmich, J.N., Saad, F.G. and Handley, E.A. (2004). The value of sedentary alternatives influences child physical activity choice. *International Journal of Behavioural Medicine*, 11(4): 236–242.

Ferreira, I., van der Horst, K., Wendel-Vos, W., Kremers, S., van Lenthe, F. and Brug, J. (2007) Environmental correlates of physical activity in youth – A review and update. *Obesity Reviews*, 8(2): 129–154.

Foresight (2007) *Tackling Obesities: Future Choices Project*. Final report available from http://www.foresight.gov.uk/Obesity/Obesity_final/Index.html (accessed 25/11/07).

Gorely, T., Marshall, S.J. and Biddle, S.J. (2004) Couch kids: Correlates of television viewing among youth. *International Journal of Behavioral Medicine*, 11: 152–163.

Green, L.W. and Kreuter, M.W. (1999). *Health Promotion Planning. An Educational and Ecological Approach,* 3rd edn. Mayfield Publishing Company, Mountain View, California.

Gustafson, S.L. and Rhodes, R.E. (2006) Parental correlates of physical activity in children and early adolescents. *Sports Medicine*, 36: 79–97.

Hallal, P.C., Victora, C.G., Azevedo, M.R. and Wells, J.C. (2006) Adolescent physical activity and health: A systematic review. *Sports Medicine*, 36: 1019–1030.

Harter, S. (1985) *Manual for the Self-Perception Profile for Children*. University of Denver, Denver, CO.

Hills, A.P., King, N.A. and Armstrong, T.P. (2007) The contribution of physical activity and sedentary behaviours to the growth and development of children and adolescents. *Sports Medicine*, 37: 533–545.

Hume, C., Salmon, J. and Ball, K. (2005) Children's perceptions of their home and neighborhood environments, and their association with objectively measured physical activity: A qualitative and quantitative study. *Health Education Research*, 20(1): 1–13.

Janssen. I., Katzmarzyk, P.T., Boyce, W.F., Vereecken, C., Mulvihill, C., Roberts, C., Currie, C. and Pickett, W. (2005) Health Behaviour in School-Aged Children Obesity Working Group. Comparison of overweight and obesity prevalence in school-aged youth from 34 countries and their relationships with physical activity and dietary patterns. *Obesity Reviews*, 6: 123–132.

Jotangia, D., Moody, A., Stamatakis, E. and Wardle, H. (2005) *Obesity Among Children Under 11*. Publication commissioned by Department of Health, 2005. Available: http://www.dh.gov.uk (accessed 29/04/05).

Mackett, R.L., Lucas, L.L., Paskins, J. and Turbin, J. (2005) The therapeutic value of children's everyday travel. *Transportation Research*, 39: 205–219.

Malina, R.M. (1996) Tracking of physical activity and physical fitness across the lifespan. *Research Quarterly for Exercise and Sport*, 67(3): 48–57.

Marshall, S.J., Biddle, S.J.H., Sallis, J.F., McKenzie, T.L. and Conway, T.L. (2002) Clustering of sedentary behaviors and physical activity among youth: A cross-national study. *Pediatric Exercise Science*, 14: 401–417.

Marttila, J., Laitakari, J., Nupponen, R., Miilunpalo, S. and Paronen, O. (1998) The versatile nature of physical activity – on the psychological, behavioural and contextual characteristics of health-related physical activity. *Patient Education and Counseling*, 33(1): 29–38.

Medical Research Council (2000) A framework for development and evaluation of RCTs for complex interventions to improve health. Discussion document drafted by members of the MRC Health Services and Public Health Research Board.

NICE (National Institute of Health and Clinical Excellence) (2006) *Obesity: Guidance on the Prevention, Identification, Assessment and Management of Overweight and Obesity in Adults and Children (Clinical Guideline 43)*. Nice, London.

Nilsson, A., Ekelund, U., Yngve, A. and Sjostrom, M. (2002) Assessing physical activity among children with accelerometers using different time sampling intervals and placements. *Pediatric Exercise Science*, 14: 87–96.

Nowicka, P. and Flodmark, C.E. (2007) Physical activity – key issues in treatment of childhood obesity. *Acta Paediatrica*, 96: 39–45.

Pellegrini, A.D. and Bohn, C.M. (2005) The role of recess in children's cognitive performance and school adjustment. *Educational Researcher*, 34: 13–19.

Peterson, Y. (2005) Family therapy treatment: Working with obese children and their families with small steps and realistic goals. *Acta Paediatrica*, 94(448): 42–44.

Riddoch, C.J., Mattocks, C., Deere, K., Saunders, J., Kirkby, J., Tilling, K., Leary, S.D., Blair, S. and Ness, A. (2007) Objective measurement of levels and patterns of physical activity. *Archives of Disease in Childhood*, 92: 963–969.

Ridgers, N.D. (2007) *An Evaluation of a Playground Redesign on the Physical Activity and Behaviour of Children During Playtime*. PhD Thesis, Liverpool John Moores University.

Ridgers, N.D., Stratton, G., Fairclough, S.J. and Twisk J.W. (2007a). Children's physical activity levels during school recess: A quasi-experimental intervention study. *International Journal of Behavioral Nutrition and Physical Activity*, 21: 4–19.

Ridgers, N.D., Stratton, G., Fairclough, S.J. and Twisk, J.W. (2007b). Long-term effects of a playground markings and physical structures on children's recess physical activity levels. *Preventive Medicine*, 44: 393–397.

Sallis, J.F. and Patrick, K. (1994) Physical activity guidelines for adolescents: Consensus statement. *Pediatric Exercise Science*, 6: 302–314.

Sallis, J.F., Prochaska, J.J. and Taylor, W.C. (2000) A review of correlates of physical activity of children and adolescents. *Medicine and Science in Sports and Exercise*, 32: 963–975.

SIGN (Scottish Intercollegiate Guidelines Network) (2003) *Management of Obesity in Children and Young People: A National Clinical Guideline*. SIGN, Edinburgh. Available: www.sign.ac.uk (accessed 01/12/05).

Sproston, K. and Primatesta, P. (2002) *Health Survey for England*. Department of Health, London.

Stratton, G. (1996) Children's heart rates during physical activity lessons: A review. *Pediatric Exercise Science*, 8: 215–233.

Stratton, G. (2000) Promoting children's physical activity in primary school: An intervention study using playground markings. *Ergonomics*, 43(10): 1538–1546.

Stratton, G. and Mullan, E. (2005). The effect of multicolor playground markings on children's physical activity level during playtime. *Preventive Medicine*, 41: 828–833.

Stratton, G., Canoy, D., Boddy, L.M., Taylor, S.R., Hackett, A.F. and Buchan I.E. (2007) Cardiorespiratory fitness and body mass index of 9–11 year-old English children: A serial cross-sectional study from 1998 to 2004. *International Journal of Obesity*, 3(1): 1172–1178.

Strong, W.B., Malina, R.M., Blimkie, C.J., Daniels, S.R., Dishman, R.K., Gutin, B., Hergenroeder, A.C., Must, A., Nixon, P.A., Pivarnik, J.M., Rowland, T., Trost, S. and

Trudeau, F. (2005) Evidence based physical activity for school-age youth. *Pediatrics*, 146: 732–737.

Taylor, W.C., Baranowski, T. and Sallis, J.F. (1994) Family determinants of childhood physical activity: A social-cognitive model. In: *Advances In Exercise Adherence* (Ed R.K. Dishman), pp. 319–342. Human Kinetics, Champaign, IL.

Telama, R., Yang, X., Viikari, J., Välimäki, I., Wanne, O., and Raitakari, O. (2005) Physical activity from childhood to adulthood: A 21-year tracking study. *American Journal of Preventive Medicine*, 28: 267–273.

Tudor-Locke, C., Lee, S.M., Morgan, C.F., Beighle, A., and Pangrazi, R.P. (2006) Children's pedometer-determined physical activity during the segmented school day. *Medicine and Science in Sports and Exercise*, 38(10): 1732–1738.

Tomkinson, G.R. and Olds, T.S. (2007). Secular changes in aerobic fitness test performance of Australasian children and adolescents. In: *Pediatric Fitness: Secular Trends and Geographic Variability, Vol. 50, Medicine and Sport Science Series* (Eds G.R. Tomkinson and T.S. Olds), pp. 168–182. Basel, Karger.

Twisk, J.W., Kemper, H.C. and van Mechelen, W. (2000) Tracking of activity and fitness and the relationship with cardiovascular disease risk factors. *Medicine and Science in Sports and Exercise*, 32(8): 1455–1461.

van Sluijs, E.M., McMinn, A.M. and Griffin, S.J. (2007) Effectiveness of interventions to promote physical activity in children and adolescents: Systematic review of controlled trials.) *British Medical Journal*, 335(7622): 703.

Vertstraete, S.J.M., Cardon, G.M., De Clerq, D.L.R. and De Bourdeaudhuil, I.M.M. (2006) Increasing children's physical activity levels during recessin elementary schools: The effects of providing game equipment. *European Journal of Public Health*, 16: 415–419.

Welk, G.J. (1999) The Youth Physical Activity Promotion Model: A conceptual bridge between theory and practice. *Quest*, 51: 5–23.

9 Populations: older people and physical activity

Afroditi Stathi

Introduction

One of humanity's most important achievements and challenges is the improvement in life expectancy and the provision of the opportunity for more people to live longer lives. The number of people aged 60 and over, as a proportion of the global population, will double from 11% in 2006 to 22% by 2050 (World Health Organisation, 2006). By then, there will be more older people than children (aged 0–14 years) in the population for the first time in human history (United Nations, 2006). Furthermore, in the UK, the number of people aged over 65 has more than doubled since the early 1930s and is continuing to rise (Kinsella, 1996). In England in 2003, 16% of the national population were aged 65 and over; this is forecast to rise to 22% by 2028 (Office for National Statistics, 2006).

Although average life expectancy is increasing in the industrialised world, improvements in mortality may not necessarily be reflected by improvements in morbidity. By many, old age is seen as a period of decline and disengagement. In his editorial, Jeste (2005) challenges this notion and supports the view that instead of thinking of demographic ageing as the 'greying of the world' (p. 323), aging should be seen as the reason for 'the world becoming more golden' (p. 323). Current research evidence supports this optimism. Data from the Berlin Aging Study (Baltes and Mayer, 1999) demonstrate the ability of older people to show gains in mental and physical function, cognitive reserves, emotional intelligence, and wisdom. In a 9-year follow-up study of middle-age civil servants in the UK, Hillsdon *et al.* (2005) concluded that physical activity participation during mid-life could help in the maintenance of high physical function in later life.

Although decline of functional capacity is an inevitable part of the ageing process, the rate of this decline is largely determined by lifestyle factors as well as social, environmental and economic factors. Low levels of physical activity even in the absence of chronic conditions could lead to lower functional ability in later life. The rate of this decline could be reversible with the appropriate interventions at the intrapersonal, interpersonal and societal level.

Old age could be a period of continuing activity involvement, a necessary requirement for successful ageing (Rowe and Kahn, 1997). Active Ageing has been defined as 'the process of optimizing opportunities for health, participation and security in order to enhance quality of life as people age' (World Health Organization, 2002a, p. 12). Physical activity can contribute to the maintenance of physical and psycho-social health, and to the improvement of independence, competence and autonomy facilitating continuing participation in society and enhancing quality of life in later years.

This chapter provides an overview of the evidence regarding the role of physical activity on the enhancement and the maintenance of health, both physical and mental, in the later years of life. The effectiveness of interventions aimed at promoting physical activity among older people is discussed. A summary of key physical activity recommendations for older adults and recent public health initiatives demonstrates the importance of evidence-based approaches in physical activity. Stressing the need to translate evidence into practice, this chapter concludes with evidence-based advice on physical activity interventions for older adults over the age of 70.

Learning outcomes

This chapter aims to:

1. explain the scientific evidence underpinning the impact of physical activity on multiple dimensions of older adults' physical and mental health
2. analyse the effectiveness of physical activity interventions and the complexity of health behaviour change in later life
3. discuss the increasing public health importance of physical activity promotion for older people and explore new directions in physical activity and ageing research
4. interpret how evidence from research trials can be translated to recommendations for design and delivery of physical activity programmes targeting older adults living in the community

---

Physical activity and health: the evidence in older people

There is a substantial body of scientific evidence indicating that regular moderate-intensity physical activity can bring multi-dimensional health benefits to older adults (World Health Organisation, 2002b; Department of Health, 2004; Nelson *et al.*, 2007). These benefits are in the fields of both physical and mental health.

Reductions in risk arising from regular physical activity in older age are at least as strong as those found in middle age for all-cause mortality, cardiovascular disease, and type-2 diabetes (Lee and Skerrett, 2001; Knowler *et al.*, 2002; Thompson *et al.*, 2003). As a preventive tool, regular physical activity reduces the risk of falls and injuries from falls, which are major concerns for frail older people (Chang *et al.*, 2004). Structured exercise programmes could decrease the number of falls that are closely associated with functional impairment and disability (LaStayo *et al.*, 2003). Physical activity increases or preserves muscle strength and power, and maintains functional ability and independent living (Miller *et al.*, 2000; Department of Health, 2001; Fiatarone-Singh, 2002; Keysor, 2003; Taylor *et al.*, 2004; Young and Dinan, 2005). Brach *et al.* (2004) concluded that any type of physical activity is beneficial for protection against functional limitations. They stressed that participation in 20–30 minutes of moderate-intensity exercise on most days of the week seems to confer greater benefit for physical capacity.

Physical activity has an important therapeutic role in coronary heart disease, hypertension, obesity, osteoporosis, osteoarthritis, claudication and chronic obstructive pulmonary disease (American Geriatrics Society, 2001; Stewart *et al.*, 2002; Going *et al.*, 2003; American College of Sports Medicine, 2004). Physical activity also plays an important role in the management of pain, congestive heart failure and back pain (American Geriatrics Society Panel, 2002; Hagen *et al.*, 2002; Vignon *et al.*, 2006).

The beneficial effect of physical activity extends to frail people and people living in nursing homes (Fiatarone-Singh, 2002; Young and Dinan, 2005). Even frail older people with multiple co-morbidities and pre-existing functional impairment and disabilities can derive functional, mental and social benefits from exercise participation (Young and Dinan, 2005). Investigating the impact of a falls prevention exercise intervention on the quality of life of people living in nursing homes in England, Stathi and Simey (2007) found that exercise participation resulted in changes in a rather passive lifestyle. This lifestyle was characterised by dependence, and growing purposelessness and helplessness. Perceived improved mobility, decreased fear of falling, increased social interaction and feelings of achievement and competence contributed to an improvement in everyday life in the nursing home. This study provided a positive portrait of the human capacity for improvement, adaptation, and optimisation during the later years of life, which seems to remain intact even for institutionalised people.

Although the case for physical activity in older adults has largely been built on its impact on physical health and function, evidence is emerging for its positive effects on aspects of mental health. The Health

Survey for England (2005) showed that 28% of women and 22% of men aged 65 and over reported high levels of depression (Graig and Mindell, 2007). Depression scores increased with age with a prevalence of 40% of men and 43% of women aged 85 and older. The preventive effect of physical activity for mental disorders such as depression (Strawbridge et al., 2002), cognitive impairment, dementia and Alzheimer's disease in older adults (Laurin et al., 2001; Yaffe et al., 2001; Colcombe and Kramer, 2003; Abbott, 2004; Rovio et al., 2005) have been documented in large-scale prospective studies. Physical activity has been found to contribute to the management of dementia, depression and anxiety disorders (Blumenthal et al., 1999; Barbour and Blumenthal, 2005; Barnes et al., 2007) and improvement in sleep quality. Reviewing epidemiological observational studies, randomised human clinical trials and non-human animal studies, Kramer and Ericson (2007) concluded that physical activity is an inexpensive treatment with preventative and restorative properties for cognitive and brain function.

There is growing evidence of the positive impact of physical activity participation on various aspects of quality of later life (Rejeski and Mihalko, 2001; Biddle and Faulkner, 2002; Fox and Stathi, 2002; McAuley and Elavsky, 2006). Diener et al. (1999) suggested that the literature carries a bias towards negative mental states and therefore, more research documenting the positive dimensions of well-being and quality of life is required. Recently, there has been a greater recognition of the importance of the positive elements of well-being, such as self-esteem, self-confidence, positive mood, perceptions of health-related quality of life and life satisfaction (Biddle and Faulkner, 2002; Huppert et al., 2005). In a meta-analysis focusing on positive aspects of well-being, Netz et al. (2005) demonstrated that self-efficacy, self-perceptions and overall well-being levels of older people were significantly improved by physical activity participation.

These findings support the role of physical activity in providing mastery experiences and subsequently improved perceptions of functional ability and self-efficacy, in turn leading to improved well-being (McAuley et al., 2005a; McAuley et al., 2006). The ability of physical activity to alter self-efficacy is very important as self-efficacy is one of the most important determinants of future engagement in physical activities.

Participation in physical activity is linked with small but significant improvements in global self-esteem (Spence et al., 2005); however, it is thought to have the greatest influence on self-esteem at domain-specific levels (e.g., physical self-worth, physical competence; Fox, 2000). That is supported by evidence from Taylor and Fox (2005) who reported significant improvements in self-perceptions among 40- to 70-years-olds after a 10-week primary care exercise referral scheme and at a 6-month follow-up.

Findings from qualitative studies demonstrate that older people link successful ageing with a wide range of factors: positive attitude, realistic perspective in life, security and stability, social support, health and wellness, a sense of engagement, a sense of purpose in life and a sense of being useful to others and to society (Reichstadt *et al.*, 2007). Physical activity can contribute to successful ageing as it offers a multidimensional beneficial effect on personal development, independence, physical, mental and social aspects of well-being (Stathi *et al.*, 2002). In a recent European intervention, older participants stressed that the involvement in the trial made them feel useful and cited their contribution to science and society as one of the strongest motives for adherence to the programme (Fox *et al.*, 2007).

The beneficial effects of physical activity on both physical and psycho-social components of well-being are not independent from each other. Although not yet fully established, it is likely, that functional ability is particularly critical to mental well-being in older people as community mobility is required for the maintenance of independent living (Frank and Patla, 2003; Netz *et al.*, 2005).

Prevalence of physical activity in older adults

The wealth of evidence regarding the benefits of physical activity has not convinced older people to increase their physical activity levels. In the US, 91% of over-85-year-olds and 64% of 65- to 74-year-olds do not engage in any regular physical activity (Federal Interagency Forum on Aging-Related Statistics, 2004). Men and women over the age of 65 living in UK are the least physically active of any age group (Department of Health, 2004) and generate the highest expenditures for medical and social care (Department of Health, 2001). Eighty-two per cent of the over 75-year-olds and 61% of 65- to 74-year-olds achieve less than 30 minutes of weekly moderate intensity physical activity (Department of Health, 2004).

Adults over the age of 70 are the least likely to walk for more than 20 minutes in any one bout. Of this group, 26% make these trips three or more times a week, while 45% make such walks less than once a year or never (Office for National Statistics, 2005). According to the 2005 Health Survey for England (Graig and Mindell, 2007) 14% of men and 25% of women aged 65 and over are classified as 'walking impaired' (a walking speed of 0.5 metres per second or less). By the age of 85 and over, 36% of men and 56% of women were 'walking impaired'. Twenty-six per cent of men (25% of women) aged 65–69 to 57% of men (38% of women) aged 85 and over reported having at least one functional limitation (seeing, hearing, communication, walking, or using stairs). The most prevalent limitation among men was being unable to walk

200 yards or more unaided without stopping or discomfort (reported by 56% of men and 61% of women). More women than men had difficulty in walking up a flight of 12 stairs without resting (65% of women, 48% of men), and this was the most common limitation among women. Both these limitations showed age-related differences, with a higher proportion of those aged 85 or over reporting them than those aged 65–69 (Graig and Mindell, 2007). These data are in agreement with the findings of the English Longitudinal Study of Ageing (Banks *et al.*, 2006). In both surveys the general trends were that the ability to perform functional tests declined with age; this decline was sharper in the older age groups, and it started at a younger age for women than for men.

Measurement of physical activity in older people has primarily relied on self-report. Although attendance at organised exercise classes can be assessed with reasonable accuracy, identification of physical activity patterns and incidental activity that takes place throughout the day is more challenging for older adults to recall accurately with self-report questionnaires. New technologies such as accelerometry (see Chapter 4) can record minute-by-minute movement including physical activity intensity with precision. Therefore energy expenditure, volumes of light, sedentary and vigorous intensity activity and even volume of sedentary activities can be objectively measured (Washburn and Ficker, 1999; Craig *et al.*, 2003).

In the first study, undertaken in UK, France and Italy, to provide objective data on a large sample of adults aged 70 years and over, Davis and Fox (2007) used accelerometry to assess physical activity volume and intensity performed by older adults. Nearly half of the 161 participants who provided accelerometry data did not perform any sustained 10-minute moderate to vigorous physical activity bouts, and none met current physical activity recommendations. These low levels of daily movement are not likely to be adequate for optimal health benefits.

Effectiveness of interventions targeting older adults

Despite a significant evidence base about the benefits of physical activity, most older adults remain sceptical and resistant to adopting and maintaining active lifestyles. Survey data demonstrate a reduction in physical activity with ageing; however, reviews of adherence rates to intervention studies do not find a negative effect of age. In many trials, older adults have displayed higher levels of adherence (>75%) than younger persons (Martin and Sinden, 2001). In a systematic review of 38 randomised controlled trials, the participation rate was 90% in home-based interventions and 84% in group-based interventions (van der Bij *et al.*, 2002); these high adherence rates were not sustained in long-term interventions (≥ 1 year). In contrast, Fox *et al.* (2007) reported a 93% attendance for facility-based sessions and 85% for self-reported compliance with home-based sessions in a 1-year intervention. King *et al.* (1998) reviewing 29 studies reported a high short-term adherence (mean $\approx$ 75%). In a systematic review, Ashworth and colleagues (2005) comparing home- and centre-based interventions reported that home-based programmes demonstrated better adherence rates in the long-term. Taylor and colleagues (2004) concluded that the failure of long-term interventions to sustain high adherence rates identifies the need for more effective approaches for maintenance of exercise participation.

The combination of telephone supervision with home-based exercise programmes appears to be at least as effective in changing the level of physical activity in individuals in the short term as group-based approaches or face-to-face contact (King *et al.*, 1998; Marcus *et al.*, 2006). A meta-analysis of 43 endurance exercise interventions targeting adults over the age of 60 demonstrated that studies using centre-based exercise reported significantly larger effect sizes than studies using home-based exercise (Conn *et al.*, 2002). Conn *et al.* reported that interventions that promoted moderate and non-endurance physical activities (e.g. flexibility exercises) were associated with long-term changes in behaviour. Supporting these findings, Netz *et al.* (2005) reported that moderate exercise had a strong beneficial effect on older adults' psychological well-being. They concluded that high intensity physical activity is not needed to promote physical and mental health of older adults. Furthermore, Conn *et al.* (2002) showed that interventions focusing on moderate-intensity activity reported significantly larger effect sizes than interventions recommending low-intensity activity.

Although most interventions have targeted endurance-oriented activities taking place mainly in controlled facility-based environments, interventions which have targeted strength, flexibility and balance training also demonstrate promising outcomes (King *et al.*, 2000). Similarly, encouraging results have been reported for interventions targeting both physical activity and healthy eating (Kelley and Abraham, 2004; Aldana *et al.*, 2005). Although these initial findings indicate that multiple behaviour change interventions can be effective, more research is needed on whether, and how, to focus on more than one health behaviour in interventions with older adults.

Theoretical frameworks

In the meta-analysis by Conn *et al.* (2002) only 15 studies out of the 43 explicitly stated a theoretical framework which guided the development of the intervention. The most common framework was Social

Cognitive Theory (n = 6) followed by the Transtheoretical Model (n = 3) and Cognitive Behavioural Theory (n = 2). These data demonstrate that early interventions were largely atheoretical. However, in the last decade, most research designs have been informed by a combination of educational, behavioural and cognitive-behavioural strategies (Marcus *et al.*, 2006).

The use of cognitive-behavioural approaches has been the most effective whereas general health education approaches do not seem to motivate older people to increase their physical activity levels. In a series of studies, McAuley and colleagues have demonstrated the need for inclusion of social cognitive variables in models of exercise adherence stressing the pivotal role of self-efficacy in long-term maintenance of physical activity participation in older adults (McAuley *et al.*, 2005b). In the first study to examine the physical activity behaviour of older adults 5 years after their initial enrolment in a 6-month exercise trial, McAuley *et al.* (2007) identified self-efficacy and affect as key contributors to long-term maintenance of physical activity (McAuley & Blissmer, 2005).

Realistic goal setting, mastery experiences, positive feedback, and adaptation of exercise prescription to suit individual needs are all linked with enhanced self-efficacy and subsequent successful exercise involvement (McAuley *et al.*, 2000a, 2003). Positive perceptions about exercise benefits, positive feelings about exercise itself, and confidence in achieving valued health benefits, are important motivators for, and consistent predictors of, exercise adherence (Resnick *et al.*, 2000; Cohen-Mansfield *et al.*, 2003).

Support from family and friends has been shown to be a significant determinant of participation in physical activity (Booth *et al.*, 2000). Social opportunities and qualities associated with the exercise group (e.g. attachment, social integration, opportunity for nurturing and guidance, fun, perceptions of similarity and closeness) are important for increasing exercise adherence (Estabrooks and Carron 1999; McAuley *et al.*, 2000b, 2003). The communication and collaboration with health professionals and with exercise instructors each contribute to exercise adherence. Many people overcome the feeling of powerlessness by becoming more active as a consequence of a doctor's advice, which illustrates the power of some interpersonal factors (Booth *et al.*, 1997; Centers for Disease Control and Prevention, 2002). The exercise instructor's guidance, interest and the quality of their support are also important contributors to older people's exercise participation (Cohen-Mansfield *et al.*, 2004; Stathi *et al.*, 2004).

Changing behaviour and adopting a more active lifestyle is a complex task. The adoption of comprehensive multi-theoretical approach is needed in order to meet the challenge of understanding the motivational processes among older people and facilitating changes in activity behaviours (Schutzer and Graves, 2004; Standage and Duda, 2004; Grodesky *et al.*, 2006; see also Chapter 2 in this book).

A number of researchers have recently called for the incorporation of both individual-level and environmental-level factors in an integrated approach to physical activity research and practice in older adults. In a special issue of the *American Journal of Preventive Medicine*, Sallis (2003) called for a new thinking in physical activity research. This thinking is the base for a shift to the trans-disciplinary paradigm that combines concepts and methods from exercise science, behavioural science, urban planning, transportation, parks and recreation, and other scientific disciplines.

This paradigm follows, in large part, from the ecological model which emphasises multiple levels of influence on individual behaviour – intrapersonal, interpersonal and/or social, organisational, institutional, community and policy (Stokols *et al.*, 1996; Sallis *et al.*, 1998; Sallis and Owen, 1999). Building on previous ecological models of physical activity, Sallis *et al.* (2006) identified the need to focus on four active living domains (household activities, active recreation, active transport, occupational activities) and the characteristics of, and access to, places that physical activity can occur within these domains. The intrapersonal characteristics interact with the environment in many levels; the perceived environment, the social cultural environment, the natural environment, the information environment and the policy environment (Sallis *et al.*, 2006). Although there has been a call for the use of this multilevel approach to increase physical activity in persons across the lifespan (Doyle *et al.*, 1999), attempts to influence environmental and policy factors that may enhance physical activity participation in older adults are lacking (Li *et al.*, 2005a). That is evident when reviewing the effectiveness of interventions that mainly target a range of psycho-social variables aiming to change behaviours at the intrapersonal and interpersonal level.

Translating evidence to guidelines and practice

Based on the research evidence, physical activity guidelines have evolved through the decades and reflect the increasing importance of physical activity behaviour as a public health issue. The exercise guidelines in the 1970s, recommended vigorous exercise for 20 minutes at a time, three or more times a week. Based on the findings of a dose–response relationship between physical activity and various health outcomes, the mid-1990s saw the publication of the public health guidelines which recommended 30 minutes of moderate physical activity on most days of the week. Since then, specific recommendations have been developed for older adults (see Table 9.1 for a summary) that try to convey the message that older adults need to focus on multiple dimensions of physical activity. Cardiovascular training, strength training, flexibility and balance activities are all high priorities for older adults, because each dimension of physical activity is inversely linked to specific, serious medical conditions that contribute to reduced

Table 9.1 Summary of national and international physical activity recommendations for older adults 1997–2007.

1997 (Heidelberg guidelines for promoting physical activity among older people; World Health Organization, 1997)

These guidelines stressed the physical, psychological, social and societal benefits of physical activity. They introduced a health–fitness gradient and they stressed that older people have specific physical activity needs according to their position, moving from the physically fit–healthy to the physically unfit–unhealthy dependant

1998 (Exercise and physical activity for older adults: American College of Sports Medicine; Mazzeo *et al.*, 1998)

This position stand included recommendations for cardiovascular function, strength training, postural stability and flexibility, psychological function and included a section with recommendations for the frail and the very old adults

1999 (Guidelines: Promoting physical activity with older people. Active for life; Health Education Authority, 1999)

These guidelines aimed primarily at the statutory and voluntary sector and related agencies working with, or for, older people and highlighted ways in which these individuals or agencies can encourage the promotion of physical activity for people aged over 50

2002 (Keep fit for life. Meeting the nutritional needs of older persons; World Health Organisation, 2002b)

These guidelines suggested that older persons should build up to at least 30 minutes of aerobic exercise on most, if not all, days of the week. They also recommended strength training 2–3 days a week, with a day of rest between workouts and provided more specific recommendations for exercise in a fitness center or at home

2004 (At least five a week. A report from the Chief Medical Officer; UK Department of Health, 2004)

This report concluded that 'For general health benefit, adults should achieve a total of at least 30 minutes a day of at least moderate-intensity physical activity on five or more days of the week. Older adults should take particular care to keep moving and retain their mobility through daily activity. Additionally, specific activities that promote improved strength, coordination and balance are particularly beneficial for older people' (p. 3)

2007 (Guidelines for the promotion of physical activity with older people; British Heart Foundation, 2007)

These guidelines translate current recommendations into meaningful messages and offer extensive guidance on translating evidence on promoting physical activity with older people into practice

(Continued)

Table 9.1 (Continued).

2007 (Physical activity and public health in older adults: American College of Sports Medicine and American Heart Association; Nelson et al., 2007)

These recommendations stress that older adults should:

1. perform moderate-intensity aerobic physical activity for a minimum of 30 minutes on 5 days a week or vigorous-intensity aerobic activity for a minimum of 20 minutes on 3 days a week; in addition to routine activities of daily living if light- or moderate-intensity activities lasting less than 10 minutes in duration
2. at least twice a week perform muscle strengthening and twice a week flexibility activities
3. exceed the minimum recommended amount of physical activity when they wish to further improve their fitness, reduce their risk for chronic diseases and disabilities, or prevent unhealthy weight gain,
4. increase physical activity over time in a stepwise manner when not active at recommended levels, and
5. self-monitor their physical activity on a regular basis and re-evaluate plans as their abilities improve or as their health status changes

---

quality of life, morbidity and mortality. Recent randomised controlled trials have explored feasibility of exercise prescription that combines various components as suggested in the physical activity recommendations (Baker, 2007a,b).

These recommendations represent the goals older people must strive for. As the latest recommendations clearly present (Nelson et al., 2007; Table 9.1), due to health problems or low fitness levels, some individuals make require a lot of time to reach any of these recommended goals. The biggest challenge from a public health perspective is to help older people to adopt and adhere to regular physical activity. Any such effort needs to take into account the barriers older adults face in being active (Schutzer and Graves, 2004; Dawson et al., 2007), the complexity of physical activity behaviour and the complexity of lifestyle changes (Brawley et al., 2003; Cress et al., 2004).

Implications for public health policy

The need to meet the challenges of an ageing society has led to the development of policies which try to safeguard a good quality of life for older people (Department of Health, 2001; World Health Organization, 2002a). The current physical activity participation rates in older adults demonstrate that the target to get 70% of the population in England taking 30 minutes of moderate exercise, five times a week, by 2020 is over-optimistic (British Heart Foundation, 2007). Even a more realistic goal (1% increase year-on-year) would appear difficult to achieve and it will require political leadership and collaborations at all levels through the public and the private sector.

The high rates of sedentary lifestyles and the identification of the role of physical activity as an essential and viable lifestyle behaviour in later life has raised physical activity promotion up the public health agenda of many developed countries. In the US, a coalition of 46 national organisations released the National Blueprint: Increasing Physical Activity Among Adults Age 50 and Older – a major planning document designed to develop a national strategy for the promotion of physically active lifestyles among the mid-life and older adults (Chodzko-Zajko, 2001; Chodzko-Zajko et al., 2005). The Blueprint identified 18 strategies in five key areas: home and community, marketing and communication, medical systems, public policy and research. Furthermore, an overarching theme that crosses boundaries and require broad, comprehensive strategies was also identified (Sheppard et al., 2003).

In the UK, the National Coalition for Active Ageing (NCAA) was established in 2005 to bring together key agencies, voluntary organisations and stakeholders to act as a collective voice and to champion the promotion of physical activity among older people of all ages, interests and abilities. The British Heart Foundation, a founding member of the NCAA, published the Policy Blueprint for increasing physical activity levels in the over-50s (British Heart Foundation, 2007) to launch a nationwide public health campaign targeting older people. Translating the current physical activity recommendations (see Table 9.1) into practical action, this Policy Blueprint has identified five main themes reflecting the key phases that people go through when they decide to change health behaviours. These themes stress the need to: (a) raise awareness of the importance of physical activity for the over-50s, (b) increase the accessibility of physical activity opportunities focusing on the principles of active living, (c) involve health professionals who can promote and support older people trying to change their physical activity patterns, (d) involve the fitness industry to capitalise on the new market by providing appropriate facilities and opportunities, and (e) develop initiatives and partnerships across the country to promote physical activity in the over-50s.

New directions in physical activity and ageing research

A substantial body of scientific evidence stresses that the health benefits of regular physical activity extends over the entire life course. Good epidemiological data link physical activity and health status in older adults and they stress the need for large, prospective studies with chronic disease, disability and mental well-being as primary outcomes. Good experimental evidence has demonstrated the impact of physical activity on health. However, more rigorous data on the dose–response relationships between physical activity participation, physical fitness, and major chronic diseases and their risk factors is required. Furthermore, there is a need for more well conducted intervention studies focusing on the role of physical activity as a therapeutic tool for mental health disorders in later life and for the promotion of good mental and social well-being.

Research on quality of life in later life has over-relied on only health-related indicators, and there is need for more holistic approaches, as giving attention solely to physical activity is not sufficient for the promotion of older people's quality of life (Chodzko-Zajko, 2000). This new approach requires a transition from the positivist paradigm to more interpretive approaches that focus on the nature and the diversity of the ageing experience, the importance of different domains of quality of life for the individual and the complex realities of older people's lives.

Older people are the least physically active segment of the population. However, self-report data from a cross-sectional study in six European countries demonstrated that older people, even when they are not engaged in paid work, remain active and productive in individual activities outside the house, in community-centred activities and in home-based activities (Fortujin et al., 2006). Objective data from the Better Ageing project (which is discussed in more detail in the next section; Davis and Fox, 2007) indicated that the activity levels of people above 70 are very low. Detailed data on frequency, duration and location of activity involvement is needed in future studies. Objective ways of measuring older people's quantity, patterns (time and space) and modes of physical activity are also required. The use of new technologies (accelerometry and global positioning system, or GIS) will enable us to gather valuable information on when, where, and how older people accumulate their daily activities (see Chapter 4).

Recent intervention efforts have focused mainly on psychological factors that have only been successful in the short-term; they have not made a strong long-term impact. Therefore, longitudinal research which can inform the scientific community about the effectiveness of psycho-social strategies in attenuating the rate of declining levels of physical activity after the completion of intervention programmes are required (Brawley et al., 2003).

Targeting only a range of psycho-social variables aiming to change behaviours at the intrapersonal and interpersonal level to date has not brought the results needed to make changes at the population level. We need multi-level ecological approaches that will enable us to draw more complete pictures of how physical activity is embedded in older adults' lives, and what the determinants and the constraints are for the adoption and maintenance of an active lifestyle. Contemporary research and policy focus on how communities and neighbourhoods could facilitate the promotion of physical activity and healthy living (Fisher *et al.*, 2004; Li *et al.*, 2005b; World Health Organisation, 2006; Edwards and Tsouros, 2006). Furthermore, most interventions have focused on age-specific groups losing the potential opportunities to capitalise on the interaction of different generations in intergenerational physical activity experiences (Marcus *et al.*, 2006). Promising new interventions in the neighbourhood, the local community and in residential care stress the need for design and evaluation of more innovative approaches targeting community settings where different generations meet naturally. Even among age specific groups there is need for more research with older people, older than 70 years, and frail people, living either in the community or in residential care.

Case study: the Better Ageing Project

Outline of project: One of the key policy proposals of the Active Ageing Project (World Health Organisation, 2002a) is the development of 'culturally appropriate, population based information and guidelines on physical activity for older men and women' (p. 48). These recommendations have been incorporated into recent research. The Better Ageing Project – a European Commission-funded research project (2002–2005) investigated the causes of frailty and the effects of a 12-month standardised exercise intervention, in people aged over 70 years, on aspects of motor control, strength, functionality, steadiness, physical activity patterns and well-being. The standardised exercise programme used in this research was initially developed and widely used as part of a falls prevention project (Skelton and Dinan, 1999). It was modified to fit local conditions but had the following general features:

- two instructor-led group exercise sessions/week, lasting 60–80 minutes
- one home-based exercise session lasting 40–60 minutes
- diary monitoring of all exercise
- home-based exercise substituted for group sessions during holidays

The research offered the opportunity to objectively document the daily physical activity patterns, functionality and psychological well-being of samples of healthy older people in England, France and Italy. This produced the largest objective data set currently existing in Europe with over 200 subjects contributing to the project.

The following section will provide a translation of these research findings (Davis and Fox, 2007; Fox *et al.*, 2007) into implications and guidelines for the design and delivery of exercise programmes for people aged 70 and older.

Evaluation outcomes: Quantitative evidence from this study showed a 93% attendance to facility-based sessions. The self-reported compliance to home-based sessions was 85%. Among this healthy group of volunteers, few people (about 30% men and 20% women) met current recommendations for adults to accumulate 30 minutes or more of moderate physical activity per day, through continuous bouts of 10 minutes or more. The activity levels steadily declined with age within the 70–85+ age groups. Very few older people took part in activities more demanding than walking at 6 kilometres per hour and that was a rare event across weekly records.

There is a serious deterioration in the muscular and motor function of older people with age. As older people have very limited physical activity, there is great scope to increase physical activity in older people, particularly at levels of moderate intensity where greatest health benefits will be experienced. In summary, despite much impairment affecting the performance of the motor system as a whole, older individuals retain a remarkable adaptability to physical activity. After engaging in a comprehensive 12-month exercise programme there was a significant reversal of muscle wasting and weakness combined with improvements in neuromuscular control, exercise tolerance and performance of daily activities.

In support of the physical benefits found, semi-structured individual interviews discovered that many participants experienced improvements in strength and functional ability. Participants felt that these positive changes were evident in the performance of their daily activities. They also reported that the engagement in the programme prevented them regressing to an unfit and inactive state.

Active older people were more likely to report higher levels of psychological well-being. Time spent sitting was negatively related to most well-being indicators. Older people who move more often and more intensively might experience better mental health. Participants in this study reported feeling better about themselves, their confidence in their abilities and their bodies as a result of their exercise achievements. Some participants reported increased social interaction within and outside the scheduled classes and some reported changing other health behaviours such as dietary intake. These positive changes were reflected in the exercising women in some small but significant improvement in mental well-being indicators as measured by standardised questionnaires (Fox et al., 2007). The exercising men maintained high levels of well-being as compared with a significant deterioration in the men in the non-exercising control group. It is possible that only small changes were recorded due to a ceiling effect because participants were healthy, reasonably active volunteers, and quite high in well-being at baseline.

Application to practice: Based on the findings from the Better Ageing Project, an effective exercise programme that optimises physical, mental and social well-being and facilitates adherence for older people over the age of 70 should have the following features:

- specialist-led group exercise sessions supported by home-based physical activity
- multiple components including warm-up, aerobic, resistance, co-ordination, balance and flexibility/mobility exercises
- the strength component should focus on all main muscle groups building from two to three sets of 8–10 repetitions and from 60% to 80% of 1 repetition maximum
- aerobic exercise conducted at 60–80% of predicted maximum heart rate
- steady and careful individually based progression, particularly in the early stages
- provision of regular individual attention in order to reassure, build confidence, and make participants feel wanted
- feedback key to adherence and confidence building – strength training feedback is intrinsic and overt
- establishment of intergenerational rapport (instructor/participant)
- a strong information/educational element, particularly in the early stages
- an enjoyable, social and welcoming atmosphere
- a strong group allegiance and sense of ownership
- proximity to residences in a conducive, accessible, well-lit facility

Conclusion and implications for practice

Regular moderate intensity physical activity can bring multi-dimensional health benefits to older adults. Interventions targeting a range of psycho-social variables aiming to change behaviours at the intrapersonal and interpersonal level have been effective in the short term. Implementing evidence-based interventions is both challenging and unpredictable when the programmes are delivered in the community. This chapter has highlighted the need for evidence-based approaches in physical activity promotion with older adults. Promoting physically active lifestyles requires more than establishing isolated programmes and facilities. Targeting at one-level does not seem to be sufficient. Multi-level ecological approaches focusing on active living are needed. Within these approaches, innovative programmes that recognise the broad range of capacities among older people, meet their needs and respect their lifestyle choices could contribute to a more active older adult population with multiple benefits for the individual and the society.

References

Abbott, R.D. (2004) Walking and dementia in physically capable elderly men. *Journal of American Medical Association*, 292: 1447–1453.

Aldana, S.G., Greenlaw, R.L., Diehl, H.A., Salberg, A., Merrill, R.M. and Ohmine, S. (2005) Effects of an intensive diet and physical activity modification program on the health risks of adults. *Journal of the American Diet Association*, 105: 371–381.

American College of Sports Medicine (2004) Position stand: Exercise and hypertension. *Medicine and Science in Sports and Exercise*, 36: 533–553.

American Geriatrics Society (2001) Exercise prescription for older adults with osteoarthritis pain: Consensus practice recommendations. A supplement to the AGS Clinical Practice Guidelines on the Quality Standards Subcommittee of the American Academy of Neurology. *Neurology*, 56: 1154–1166.

American Geriatrics Society Panel on Persistent Pain in Older Persons (2002) The management of persistent pain in older persons. *Journal of American Geriatrics Society*, 50(6): 205–224.

Ashworth, N.L., Chad, K.E., Harrison, E.L., Reeder, B.A. and Marshall, S.C. (2005) Home versus center based physical activity programs in older adults. *Cochrane Database of Systematic Reviews*, 1: CD004017.

Baker, M., Atlantis, E. and Singh, M.A.F. (2007a) Multi-modal exercise programs for older adults. *Age and Ageing*, 36(4): 375–381.

Baker, M.K., Kennedy, D.J., Bohle, P. L., Campbell, D.S., Knapman, L., Grady, J., Wiltshire, J., McNamara, M., Evans, W., Atlantis, E. and Fiatarone-Singh, M. (2007b) Efficacy and feasibility of a novel tri-modal robust exercise prescription in a retirement community: A randomized, controlled trial. *Journal of the American Geriatrics Society* 55(1): 1–10.

Baltes, P.B. and Mayer, K.U. (1999) *The Berlin Aging Study: Aging from 70 to 100.* Cambridge University Press, New York.

Banks, J., Breeze, W., Lessof, C. and Nazroo, J. (2006) *Retirement, Health and Relationships of the Older Population in England. The 2004 English Longitudinal Study of Ageing.* Institute for Fiscal Studies, London.

Barbour, K.A. and Blumenthal, J.A. (2005) Exercise training and depression in older adults. *Neurobiology Aging,* 26: 119–123.

Barnes, D.E., Whitmer, R.A. and Yaffe, K. (2007) Physical activity and dementia: The need for prevention trials. *Exercise and Sports Sciences Reviews,* 35(1): 24–29.

Biddle S.J.H. and Faulkner, G.E. (2002) Psychological and social benefits of physical activity. In: *Active Aging* (Eds K.M. Chan, W. Chodzko-Zajko, W. Frontera and A. Parker), pp. 89–164. Lippincott, Williams and Wilkins, Hong Kong.

Blumenthal, J.A., Babyak, M.A., Moore, K.A., Craighead, E., Herman, S., Khatri, P., Waugh, R., Napolitano, M.A., Forman, L.M., Appelbaum, M., Murali Doraiswamy, P. and Ranga Krishnan, K. (1999) Effects of exercise training on older patients with major depression. *Archives of Internal Medicine,* 159: 2349–2356.

Booth, M.L., Bauman, A., Owen, N. and Gore, C.J. (1997) Physical activity preferences, preferred sources of assistance, and perceived barriers to increased activity among physically inactive Australians. *Preventive Medicine,* 26(1): 131–137.

Booth, M.L., Owen, N., Bauman, A., Clavisi, O. and Leslie, E. (2000) Social-cognitive and perceived environment influences associated with physical activity in older Australians. *Preventive Medicine,* 31(1): 15–22.

Brach, J.S., Simonsick, E.M., Kritchevsky, S., Yaffe, K., Newman, A.B. for the Health, Aging and Body Composition Study Research Group (2004) The association between physical function and lifestyle activity and exercise in the health, aging and body composition study. *Journal of the American Geriatrics Society,* 52(4): 502–509.

Brawley, L.R., Rejeski, W. J., and King, A.C. (2003) Promoting physical activity for older adults: The challenge for changing behavior. *American Journal of Preventive Medicine,* 25: 172–183.

British Heart Foundation (2007) *30 Minutes a Day: Policy Blueprint for Increasing Physical Activity Levels in the over 50s.* British Heart Foundation, London.

Centers for Disease Control and Prevention (2002) Prevalence of health-care providers asking older adults about their physical activity levels-US, 1998. *Morbidity and Mortality Weekly Report,* 51(19): 412–414.

Chang, T.J., Morton, C.S., Rubenstein, Z.L., Mojica, M.A., Maglione, M., Suttorp, J.M., Roth, E.A. and Shekelle, P.G. (2004) Interventions for the prevention of falls in older adults: Systematic review and meta-analysis of randomised clinical trials. *British Medical Journal,* 328: 680–687.

Chodzko-Zajko, W. (2000) Successful aging in the new millennium: The role of regular physical activity. *Quest,* 52: 333–343.

Chodzko-Zajko, W. (2001) National Blueprint: Increasing physical activity among adults age 50 and older. *Journal of Aging and Physical Activity*, 9: 1–28.

Chodzko-Zajko, W., Sheppard, L., Senior, J., Park, C.H., Mockenhaupt, R. and Bazarre, T. (2005) The national blueprint for promoting physical activity in the mid-life and older adult population. *Quest*, 57(1): 2–11.

Cohen-Mansfield, J., Marx, M.S. and Guralnik, J. (2003) Motivators and barriers to exercise in an older community-dwelling population. *Journal of Aging and Physical Activity*, 11: 242–253.

Cohen-Mansfield, J., Marx, M.S., Biddison, J.R. and Guralnik, J.M. (2004) Socio-environmental exercise preferences among older adults. *Preventive Medicine*, 38: 804–811.

Colcombe, S. and Kramer, A.F. (2003) Fitness effects on the cognitive function of older adults: A meta-analytic study. *Psychological Science*, 14: 125–130.

Conn, S.V., Valentine, C.J. and Cooper, M.H. (2002) Interventions to increase physical activity among aging adults: A meta-analysis. *Annals of Behavioral Medicine*, 24(3): 190–200.

Craig, C., Marshall, A., Sjostrom, M., Bauman, A., Booth, M., Ainsworth, B., Pratt, M., Ekelund, U., Yngve, A., Sallis, J. and Oja, P. (2003) International physical activity questionnaire: 12-country reliability and validity. *Medicine and Science in Sport and Exercise*, 35: 1381–1395.

Cress, M.E., Buchner, D.M., Prohaska, T., Rimmer, J., Brown, M., Macera, C., DePietro, L. and Chodzko-Zajko, W. (2004) Physical activity programs and behavior counseling in older adult populations. *Medicine and Science in Sports and Exercise*, 36(11): 1997–2003.

Davis, M. and Fox, K. (2007) Physical activity patterns assessed by accelerometry in older people. *European Journal of Applied Physiology*, 100(5): 581–589.

Dawson, J., Hillsdon, M., Boller, I. and Foster, C. (2007) Perceived barriers to walking in the neighbourhood environment and change in physical activity levels over 12 months. *British Journal of Sports Medicine*, 41 (9): 562–568.

Department of Health (2001) *National Service Framework for Older People: Modern Standards and Service Models*. Department of Health, London.

Department of Health (2004) *At least five a week: Evidence on the impact of physical activity and its relationship to health*. A report from the Chief Medical Officer. Department of Health, London.

Diener, E., Suh, E.H., Lucas, R.E. and Smith, H.L. (1999) Subjective well-being: Three decades of progress. *Psychological Bulletin*, 125(2): 276–302.

Doyle, S., Kelly-Schwartz, A., Schlossberg, M. and Stockard, J. (1996) Active community environments and health – The relationship of walkable and safe communities to individual health. *Journal of the American Planning Association*, 72(1): 19–31.

Edwards, P. and Tsouros, A. (2006) *Promoting Physical Activity and Active Living in Urban Environments: The Role of Local Governments*. World Health Organization, Regional Office for Europe, Denmark.

Estabrooks, P. and Carron, A.V. (1999) Group cohesion in older adult exercisers: Prediction and intervention effects. *Journal of Behavioral Medicine*, 22: 575–588.

Federal Interagency Forum on Aging-Related Statistics (2004) *Older Americans 2004: Key Indicators of Well-Being*. Federal Interagency Forum on Aging-Related Statistics. Government Printing Office, Washington, DC.

Fiatarone-Singh, M.A. (2002) Exercise comes of age: Rationale and recommendations for a geriatric exercise prescription. *Journals of Gerontology Series A – Biological Sciences and Medical Sciences*, 57: 262–282.

Fisher, K.J., Li, F.Z., Michael, Y. and Cleveland, M. (2004) Neighborhood-level influences on physical activity among older adults: A multilevel analysis. *Journal of Aging and Physical Activity*, 12(1): 45–63.

Fortuijn, J.D., van der Meer, M., Burholt, V., Ferring, D., Quattrini, S., Hallberg, I.R., Weber, G. and Wenger, G.C. (2006) The activity patterns of older adults: A cross-sectional study in six European countries. *Population, Space and Place*, 12(5): 353–369.

Fox, K.R. (2000). Self-esteem, self-perceptions and exercise. *International Journal of Sport Psychology*, 31(2): 228–240.

Fox, K.R. and Stathi, A. (2002) Physical activity and mental health in older adults: Current evidence and future perspectives. *Psychology: Journal of Greek Psychological Society*, 9: 563–580.

Fox, K.R., Stathi, A., McKenna, J. and Davis, M. (2007) Physical activity and mental well-being in older people participating in the Better Ageing Project. *European Journal of Applied Physiology*, 100(5): 591–602.

Frank, J.S. and Patla, A.E. (2003) Balance and mobility challenges in older adults: Implications for preserving community mobility. *American Journal of Preventive Medicine*, 25: 157–163.

Going, S., Lohman, T., Houtkopper, L., Metcalfe, L., Flint-Wagner, H., Blew, R., Stanford, V., Cussler, E., Martin, J., Teixeira, P., Harris, M., Milliken, L., Figueroa-Galvez, A. and Weber, J. (2003) Effects of exercise on bone mineral density in calcium-replete post-menopausal women with and without hormone replacement therapy. *Osteoporosis International*, 14(8): 637–643.

Graig, R. and Mindell, J. (2007) *The Health of Older People-Key Findings*. The Information Centre, London.

Grodesky, J.M., Kosma, M. and Solmon, M.A. (2006) Understanding older adults' physical activity behavior: A multi-theoretical approach. *Quest*, 58(3): 310–324.

Hagen, K., Hilde, G., Jamtvedt, G. and Winnem, J. (2002) The Cochrane review of advice to stay active as a single treatment for low back pain and sciatica. *Spine*, 27: 1736–1741.

Health Education Authority (1999) *Guidelines: Promoting Physical Activity with Older People*. Health Education Authority, London.

Hillsdon, M.M., Brunner, E.J., Guralnik, J.M. and Marmot, M.G. (2005) Prospective study of physical activity and physical function in early old age. *American Journal of Preventive Medicine*, 28(3): 245–250.

Huppert, F., Baylis, N. and Keverne, B. (2005) *The Science of Well-Being*. Oxford University Press, Oxford.

Jeste, D.V. (2005) Feeling fine at a hundred and three: Secrets of successful aging. *American Journal of Preventive Medicine*, 28(3): 323–324.

Kelley, K. and Abraham, C. (2004) Randomised Control Trial of a theory-based intervention promoting healthy eating and physical activity amongst out-patients older than 65 years. *Social Science and Medicine*, 59: 787–797.

Keysor, L.J. (2003) Does late-life physical activity or exercise prevent or minimise disablement? *American Journal of Preventive Medicine*, 25: 129–136.

King, A.C., Pruitt, L.A., Phillips, W., Oka, R., Rodenburg, A. and Haskell, W.L. (2000) Comparative effects of two physical activity programmes on measured and perceived physical functioning and other health-related quality of life outcomes in older adults. *Journal of Gerontology*, 55(2): M74–M83.

King, A.C., Rejeski, W.J. and Buchner, D.M. (1998) Physical activity interventions targeting older adults: A critical review and recommendations. *American Journal of Preventive Medicine*, 15(4): 316–333.

Kinsella, K. (1996) Demographic aspects. In: *Epidemiology in Old Age* (Eds S. Ebrahim and A. Kalache), pp. 32–40. BMJ Publishing, London.

Kramer, A.F. and Erickson, K.I. (2007) Capitalizing on cortical plasticity: Influence of physical activity on cognition and brain function. *Trends in Cognitive Sciences*, 11(8): 342–348.

Knowler, W.C., Barrett-Connor, E., Fowler, S.E., Hamman, R.F., Lachin, J.M., Walker, E.A. and Nathan, D.M. (2002) Reduction in the incidence of type 2 diabetes with lifestyle intervention of metformin. *New England Journal of Medicine*, 346: 393–403.

LaStayo, P.C., Ewy, G.A., Pierotti, D.D., Johns, R.K. and Lidstedt, S. (2003) The positive effects of negative work: Increased muscle strength and decreased fall risk in a frail elderly population. *Journal of Gerontology: Medical Sciences*, 58(A): 419–424.

Laurin, D., Verreault, R., Lindsay, J., MacPherson, K. and Rockwood, K. (2001) Physical activity and risk of cognitive impairment and dementia in elderly persons. *Archive Neurology*, 58: 498–504.

Lee, I.M. and Skerrett, P.J. (2001) Physical activity and all-cause mortality: What is the dose–response relation? *Medicine and Science in Sports and Exercise*, 33: 459–471.

Li, F.Z., Fisher, K.J., Bauman, A., Ory, M.G., Chodzko-Zajko, W., Harmer, P., Bosworth, M. and Cleveland, M. (2005a) Neighborhood influences on physical activity in middle-aged and older adults: A multilevel perspective. *Journal of Aging and Physical Activity*, 13(1): 87–114.

Li, F.Z., Fisher, K.J. and Brownson, R.C. (2005b) A multilevel analysis of change in neighborhood walking activity in older adults. *Journal of Aging and Physical Activity*, 13(2): 145–159.

Marcus, B.H., Williams, D.M., Dubbert, P.M., Sallis, J.F., King, A.C., Yancey, A.K., Franklin, B.A., Buchner, D., Daniels, S.R. and Claytor, R.P (2006) Physical activity intervention studies – What we know and what we need to know – A scientific statement from the American Heart Association Council on Nutrition, Physical Activity, and Metabolism (Subcommittee on Physical Activity); Council on Cardiovascular Disease in the Young; and the Interdisciplinary Working Group on Quality of Care and Outcomes Research. *Circulation*, 114(24): 2739–2752.

Martin, K.A. and Sinden, A.R. (2001) Who will stay and who will go? A review of older adults' adherence to randomized controlled trials of exercise. *Journal of Aging and Physical Activity,* 9(2): 91–114.

Mazzeo, R.S., Cavanagh, P., Evans, W.J., Fiatarone, M., Hagberg, J., McAuley, E. and Startzell, J. (1998) Exercise and physical activity for older adults. *Medicine and Science in Sports and Exercise*, 30(6): 992–1008.

McAuley, E. and Blissmer, B. (2000) Self-efficacy determinants and consequences. *Exercise and Sport Science Reviews*, 28: 85–88.

McAuley, E. and Elavsky, S. (2006) Physical activity, aging, and quality of life. implications for measurement. In: *Measurement Issues in Aging and Physical Activity* (Eds W. Zhu and W. Chodzko-Zajko), pp. 57–68. Human Kinetics, Urbana- Champaign, IL.

McAuley, E., Blissmer, B., Katula, J., Duncan, T.E. and Mihalko, S.L. (2000a) Physical activity, self-esteem, and self-efficacy relationships in older adults: A randomized controlled trial. *Annals of Behavioral Medicine*, 22(2): 131–139.

McAuley, E., Blissmer, S., Marquez, D.X., Jerome, G.J., Kramer, A.F. and Katula, J. (2000b) Social relations, physical activity, and well-being in older adults. *Preventive Medicine*, 31(5): 608–617.

McAuley, E., Elavsky, S., Jerome, G.J., Konopack, J.F. and Marquez, D.X. (2005a) Physical activity-related well-being in older adults: Social cognitive influences. *Psychology and Aging*, 20(2): 295–302.

McAuley, E., Elavsky, S., Motl, R., Konopack, J., Hu, L. and Marquez, D. (2005b) Physical activity, self-efficacy, and self-esteem: Longitudinal relationships in older adults. *Journal of Gerontology. Series B-Psychological Sciences and Social Sciences*, 60(5): 268–275.

McAuley, E., Jerome, G.J., Elavsky, S., Marquez, D.X. and Ramsey, S.N. (2003) Predicting long-term maintenance of physical activity in older adults. *Preventive Medicine,* 37: 110–118.

McAuley, E., Konopack, J.F., Motl, R.W., Morris, K.S., Doerksen, S.E. and Rosengren, K.R. (2006) Physical activity and quality of life in older adults: Influence of health status and self-efficacy. *Annals of Behavioural Medicine*, 31(1): 99–103.

McAuley, E., Morris, K.S., Motl, R.W., Hu, L., Konopack, J.F., and Elavsky, S. (2007). Long-term follow-up of physical activity behaviour in older adults. *Health Psychology*, 26(3): 375–380.

Miller, M., Rejeski, W.J., Reboussin, B.A., TenHave, T. and Ettinger, W. (2000) Physical activity, functional limitations, and disability in older adults. *Journal of the American Geriatrics Society*, 48: 1264–1272.

Nelson, M.E., Rejeski, W.J., Blair, S.N., Duncan, P.W., Judge, J.O., King, A.C., Macera, C.A. and Castaneda-Sceppa, C. (2007) Physical activity and public health in older adults – Recommendation from the American College of Sports Medicine and the American Heart Association. *Circulation*, 116(9): 1094–1105.

Netz, Y., Wu, M.J., Becker, B.J. and Tenenbaum, G. (2005) Physical activity and psychological well-being in advanced age: A meta-analysis of intervention studies. *Psychology and Aging,* 20(2): 272–284.

Office for National Statistics (2006) http://www.statistics.gov.uk/downloads/theme_population/InteractivePDF_March2006.pdf (accessed 21/8/2007).

Office for National Statistics (2005) *National Travel Survey*. The Department for Transport, London.

Reichstadt, J., Depp, C.A., Palinkas, L.A., Folsom, D.P. and Jeste, D.V. (2007) Building blocks of successful aging: A focus group study of older adults' perceived contributors to successful aging. *American Journal of Geriatric Psychiatry*, 15(3): 194–201.

Rejeski, W.J. and Mihalko, S.L. (2001) Physical activity and quality of life in older adults. *Journal of Gerontology: Medical Sciences*, 56(A): 23–35.

Resnick, B., Palmer, H., Jenkins, L.S. and Spellbring, A.M. (2000) Path analysis of efficacy expectations and exercise behaviour in older adults. *Journal of Advanced Nursing*, 31(6): 1309–1315.

Rovio, S., Kareholt, L., Helkala, E.L., Viitanen, M., Winblad, B., Tuomilehto, J., Soininen, H., Nissinen, A. and Kivipelto, M. (2005) Leisure-time physical activity at midlife and the risk of dementia and Alzheimer's disease. *Lancet Neurology*, 4: 705–711.

Rowe, J.W. and Kahn, R.L. (1997) Successful aging. *Geronologist*, 37(4): 433–440.

Sallis, J.F. (2003) New thinking on older adults' physical activity. *American Journal of Preventive Medicine*, 25(3): 110–111.

Sallis, J.F., Bauman, A., and Pratt, M. (1998) Environmental and policy – Interventions to promote physical activity. *American Journal of Preventive Medicine*, 15(4): 379–397.

Sallis, J.E., Cervero, R.B., Ascher, W., Henderson, K.A., Kraft, M.K. and Kerr, J. (2006) An ecological approach to creating active living communities. *Annual Review of Public Health*, 27: 297–322.

Sallis, J.F. and Owen, N. (1999) *Physical Activity and Behavioral Medicine*. Sage, Beverley Hills, CA.

Schutzer, K.A. and Graves, B.S. (2004) Barriers and motivations to exercise in older adults. *Preventive Medicine*, 39: 1056–1061.

Sheppard, L., Senior, J. Park, C.H., Mockenhaupt, R., Chodzko-Zajko, W. and Bazzarre, T. (2003) The National Blueprint Consensus Conference Summary Report. Strategic priorities for increasing physical activity among adults aged >50. *American Journal of Preventive Medicine*, 25: 209–213.

Skelton, D. and Dinan, S. (1999) Exercise for falls management: Rationale for an exercise programme aimed at reducing postural instability. *Physiotherapy, Theory and Practice*, 15: 105–120.

Spence, J.C., McGannon, K.R. and Poon, P. (2005) The effect of exercise on global self-esteem: A quantitative review. *Journal of Sport and Exercise Psychology*, 27(3): 311–333.

Standage, M. and Duda, J.L. (2004) Motivational processes among older adults in sport and exercise settings. In: *Developmental Sport and Exercise Psychology: A Lifespan Perspective* (Ed M.R. Weiss), pp. 357–381. Fitness Press, Morgan Town, VW.

Stathi, A. and Simey, P. (2007) Quality of life in the fourth age: Exercise experiences of nursing home residents. *Journal of Aging and Physical Activity*, 15: 272–286.

Stathi, A., Fox, K.R. and McKenna, J. (2002) Physical activity and dimensions of subjective well-being in older adults. *Journal of Aging and Physical Activity*, 10: 76–92.

Stathi, A., McKenna, J. and Fox, K.R. (2004) The experiences of older people participating in exercise referral schemes. *The Royal Journal for the Promotion of Health*, 124(1): 18–23.

Stewart, K., Hiatt, W., Regensteiner, J. and Hirsch, A. (2002) Exercise training for claudication. *New England Journal of Medicine*, 347: 1941–1951.

Stokols, D., Allen, J. and Bellingham, R.L. (1996) Translating social ecological theory into guidelines for community health promotion. *American Journal of Health Promotion*, 10: 282–298.

Strawbridge, W.J., Deleger, S., Roberts, R.E. and Kaplan, G.A. (2002) Physical activity reduces the risk of subsequent depression for older adults. *American Journal of Epidemiology*, 156: 328–334.

Taylor, A.H., Cable, N.T., Faulkner, G.E., Hillsdon, M., Narici, M. and Van der Bij, A.K. (2004) Physical activity and older adults: A review of health benefits and the effectiveness of interventions. *Journal of Sports Sciences*, 22: 703–725.

Taylor, A.H. and Fox, K.R. (2005) Effectiveness of a primary care exercise referral intervention for changing physical self-perceptions over 9 months. *Health Psychology*, 24(1): 11–21.

Thompson, P.D., Buchner, D., Pina, I.L., Balady, G.J., Williams, M.A., Marcus, B.H., Berra, K., Blair, S.N., Costa, F., Franklin, B., Fletcher, G.F., Gordon, N.F., Pate, R.R., Rodriguez, B.L., Yancey, A.K. and Wenger, N.K. (2003) Exercise and physical activity in the prevention and treatment of atherosclerotic cardiovascular disease – A statement from the Council on Clinical Cardiology (Subcommittee on Exercise, Rehabilitation, and Prevention) and the Council on Nutrition, Physical Activity, and Metabolism (Subcommittee on Physical Activity). *Circulation*, 107(24): 3109–3116.

United Nations (2006) Population Ageing 2006. United Nations Department of Economic and Social Affairs, Population Division, New York. http://www.un.org/esa/population/publications/ageing/ageing2006.htm (accessed 20/10/07).

Van der Bij, A.K., Laurant, M.G.H. and Wensing, M. (2002) Effectiveness of physical activity interventions for older adults. *American Journal of Preventive Medicine*, 22(2): 120–133.

Vignon, E., Valat, J.P., Rossignol, M., Avouac, B., Rozenberg, S., Thoumie P., Avouac, J., Nordin, M. and Hilliquin, P. (2006) Osteoarthritis of the knee and hip and activity: A systematic international review and synthesis (OASIS). *Joint Bone Spine*, 73(4): 442–455.

Washburn, R.A. and Ficker, J.L. (1999) Physical Activity Scale for the Elderly (PASE): The relationship with activity measured by a portable accelerometer. *Journal of Sports Medicine and Physical Fitness*, 39(4): 336–340.

World Health Organisation (1997) The Heidelberg guidelines for promoting physical activity among older persons. *Journal of Aging and Physical Activity*, 5: 2–8.

World Health Organization (2002a) Active ageing: A policy framework. Department of Health Promotion, Noncommunicable Disease Prevention and Surveillance, Geneva.

World Health Organization (2002b) *Keep Fit for Life. Meeting the Nutritional Needs of Older Persons*. World Health Organization, Geneva.

World Health Organization (2006) *Global Age-Friendly Cities: A Guide*. World Health Organisation, Geneva.

Yaffe, K., Barnes, D., Nevitt, M., Lui, L.Y. and Covinsky, K. (2001) A prospective study of physical activity and cognitive decline in elderly women: Women who walk. *Archives of International Medicine,* 161: 1703–1708.

Young, A. and Dinan, S. (2005) Activity in later life. *British Medical Journal*, 330: 189–191.

10 Physical activity and mental health

Diane Crone, Linda Heaney and Christopher S. Owens

Introduction

Mental health problems are increasingly common in society, with approximately 1 in 6 adults likely to experience a mental health problem/disorder at any one time (Department of Health, 2004a). During the past decade there has been an increasing interest in the role that physical activity can play in the treatment and maintenance of mental health problems, and in mental health promotion. This chapter reviews the evidence underpinning the use of physical activity for people with mental health problems and outlines the policy context for practice in this area. It concludes with a case study from practice which centres on the development of an evidence base which can directly lead into the enhancement of services in the area of physical activity and well-being promotion in a mental health trust.

Learning outcomes

The chapter aims to provide:

1. an appreciation of mental health problems and understanding of the structure and function of mental health services in the treatment and care of people with mental health problems
2. an understanding of the position of physical activity promotion with the current mental health policy and services
3. an understanding of the evidence base underpinning the use of physical activity as an adjunct to treatment for people with mental health problems
4. an appreciation of the holistic role physical activity can have for people with mental health problems, particularly those with severe mental illness
5. an appreciation of how a partnership between a university and a local mental health trust can be used to develop an evidence base developed by those that are involved with the receipt and delivery of services that can feed directly into the enhancement of local practice

Types of mental health problems

Mental illness is defined by the American Psychiatric Association (APA) as 'a clinically significant behavioural or psychological syndrome or pattern that occurs in an individual and that is associated with present distress, or disability, or with significantly increased risk of suffering death, pain, disability, or an important loss of freedom' (1994, p. 21). There are a number of illnesses within this classification, but for the purpose of this chapter, we shall explain the more common disorders of depression and anxiety, and the term severe mental illness (SMI).

Depressive disorders are characterised by low mood, lack of enjoyment, lethargy, lack of motivation and feelings of hopelessness and worthlessness. Often there are accompanying changes in sleep and appetite (Biddle and Mutrie, 2001). These symptoms may continue for many months, leading to increasing social isolation and withdrawal. Anxiety disorders can manifest in a number of different ways. Of particular relevance are the phobic disorders, which prevent social interactions as a person becomes overwhelmingly anxious and excessively self-conscious in everyday social situations (National Institute of Mental Health, 2006). In particular, social anxiety is a common mental disorder on a lifetime basis, ranging from 12% to 14% (Stein, 2006).

The more severe mental illnesses, such as schizophrenia, potentially have the greatest impact on a person's ability to pursue physical activity independently. SMI is commonly defined as people who have a diagnosis of schizophrenia, organic mental illness or bipolar disorder (Gask, 2004). Carless and Sparkes (2008) explain that research with people with SMI, for example schizophrenia, is uncommon and that, given the impact of the illness on lives of people who experience it, the use of physical activity may not lead to remission. However, they conclude that as a part of a holistic treatment plan for people with SMI, findings from the limited research that is available suggests that it has much to give to the quality of life of a person with SMI. Symptoms of schizophrenia can include disturbances in psychological processes such as language, communication, sense of self, mood, affect and relationship to the external world (Gask, 2004). It is not surprising, therefore, that physical activity levels are known to be low in this population group; in addition, when they do attempt to attend and participate in physical activity sessions, their lack of social skills and the stigmatisation by society may also be inhibiting factors. The use of medication is particularly long term for SMI, and often has side effects of drowsiness and weight gain, commonly leading to obesity (Marder et al., 2004). Generally, people with schizophrenia die prematurely; the illness itself, its treatment with medication and lifestyle choices all contribute to the excess morbidity and mortality (Allebeck, 1989; Baxter, 1996; Brown *et al.*, 2000). Excessive body weight increases the morbidity and mortality and is the biggest risk factor for type II diabetes in schizophrenia. However, much of the increased mortality of schizophrenia may be preventable through lifestyle and risk factor modification, e.g. the uptake of physical activity, healthy eating and so on, which supports the calls for further research to support the development of practice in this area.

Overview of mental health services in England

Mental health services in England are provided at both a primary and secondary care level. Primary care mental health services can be provided by general practitioners, practice nurses, specialised primary care mental health professionals, health visitors, counsellors and social workers. The majority of people who attend health care with a mental health problem receive a primary care response (Kendrick *et al.*, 1994). A primary care response is where people who have common mental disorder (mainly anxiety and/or depression) seek advice and treatment from a general practitioner (Boardman and Parsonage, 2007). The remaining individuals (approximately 10–15%) receive care from secondary mental health services (Boardman and Parsonage, 2007).

Secondary health care mental health services are provided by both acute and specialised mental health services. During the past 20 years, there have been many changes to mental health services, especially in secondary services (Boardman and Parsonage, 2007). In this period, community services have developed and asylums have closed (Boardman, 2005). Specialised mental health services are provided by mental health trusts, which care for those with more complex and/or enduring mental health problems. In comparison to services in primary care, specialist mental health services are more clearly prescribed in the National Health Service (NHS) Plan (Department of Health, 2000) and Implementation Guides (Department of Health, 2001a, 2002a,b,c,d, 2003a,b,c,d, 2004b,c). They cover three broad areas: community-based teams, in-patient services (including aftercare accommodation) and day services. In addition, these specialist services are complemented by forensic services, rehabilitation services and other sub-specialist services such as perinatal and eating disorder services (Boardman and Parsonage, 2007).

Services for working-age adults are primarily focused around community mental health teams. Community mental health teams are viewed as the mainstay of the system and the core around which newer services are developed (Department of Health, 2002a). These teams consist of psychiatrists, community psychiatric nurses, occupational therapists, social workers, community care workers, psychologists and other therapists. They are required to focus on people with severe and complex problems through the Care Programme Approach (CPA) (Department of Health, 1990a,b). Under this framework, each patient has a 'care co-ordinator' who is responsible for co-ordinating the care that the person receives. Regular meetings, called care-planning meetings are held whereby the patient's care is reviewed and plans are made for the future (Department of Health, 1990a,b). In some trusts, the patient or service user can have the inclusion of a physical activity programme in their programme. However, although a recent audit in the South West region of England found an extensive array of physical activity opportunities for people with mental health problems (Crone and Stembridge, 2007) the provision is not a statutory requirement and it is still considered to be an underutilised adjunct to standard treatment (Callaghan, 2004).

In addition, there are also more intensive community teams who can provide around-the-clock support for patients experiencing an exacerbation of their mental health problems such as assertive outreach teams, crisis resolution teams and early intervention in psychosis teams. In-patient beds are also available, although there has been a steady decline in these over the past 50 years (Simpson *et al.*, 1993). Furthermore, non-statutory services such as charitable groups (e.g. Rethink and Mental Health Foundation) also provide valuable services for people with mental health problems in conjunction with statutory services.

The place of physical activity in mental health policy and services

The National Service Framework for Mental Health (Department of Health, 1999) emphasises the use of physical activity as an opportunity for relaxation and purposefulness. Since the publication of this document, and with the increasing profile of physical activity research regarding its relationship with mental health, there have been numerous publications with references to the role that physical activity can play for general well-being and in the specific treatment, prevention and maintenance of mental health problems, for example Choosing Health: Making healthier choices easier (Department of Health, 2004d). Additionally, with the acknowledgement of other health concerns of this group, for example levels of obesity (Cormac *et al.*, 2005; Department of Health, 2006a), this has further provided a rationale for the use of physical activity in the care plans of people with mental health problems (see Table 10.1).

Subsequently, there has been a surge in the opportunities for physical activity in mental health services. In Crone and Stembridge's (2007) review, over 100 physical activity opportunities were identified across the region, ranging from walking groups to football projects.

Table 10.1 Review of national documents and references to mental health, well-being and physical activity.

Title	Relevance of physical activity
National Quality Assurance Framework: Exercise Referral Schemes (Department of Health, 2001b)	Recognised the importance of well-being as a fundamental outcome of those attending exercise referral schemes in the UK
Schizophrenia: Full national clinical guideline on core interventions in primary and secondary care [National Institute for Clinical Excellence (NICE), 2003]	States that primary care is best placed to monitor the physical health of those with schizophrenia and should do so regularly, through practice care registers. This should include screening for diabetes/endocrine disorders, cardiovascular system disorders, and lifestyle factors. Secondary services should undertake regular and full assessments of the physical health of their service users, addressing all the issues relevant to a person's quality of life and well-being. If service users choose not to see a general practitioner, then physical care should be monitored by secondary services. In addition, higher physical morbidity of those with schizophrenia should be considered in all assessments, including secondary. This should be done through the CPA
At least five a week (Department of Health, 2004e)	Acknowledged role of exercise for general well-being and for the treatment of mental health problems
Choosing Health: Making healthier choices easier (Department of Health, 2004d)	This landmark public health White Paper acknowledges the beneficial role of physical activity for reducing the risk of depression and having positive benefits for mental health including reduced anxiety, enhanced mood and self-esteem. Reference is also made to extending the models of physical healthcare for those with mental health problems across all primary care trusts
Depression: Management of depression in primary and secondary care (NICE, 2004)	Support is expressed in the guidelines for using exercise as a treatment for depression. In addition, recommends from a clinical viewpoint that patients of all ages with mild depression should be advised of the benefits of following a structured and supervised exercise programme
Healthy Body and Mind: Promoting Healthy Living for People Who Experience Mental Distress [National Institute for Mental Health in England (NIMHE)/ Mentality, 2004]	It addresses higher mortality and morbidity of those with severe mental illness saying that specialist care is an inappropriate service setting for attending to the physical health needs of this group, and acknowledges social exclusion. Primary care trusts should commission mental health services to be more integrated with primary care and social care. Primary care trusts also need to make strategic links with health promotion. A need for effective communication between primary and secondary care should be the responsibility of both of these. Community mental health teams have a role in educating primary care staff in mental health issues. A good practice point made is that joint community psychiatric nurses and practice nurse led weight management groups exist

Mental Health and Social Exclusion: Social Exclusion Unit Report (Social Exclusion Unit, 2004)	Focused on inequalities in access to services and tackling poor physical health. There is a section on secondary services and also on exercise. The section on secondary services states that secondary services should offer strengthened advice and support the use of the CPA. This should be done through the CPA process. The primary care trusts and secondary services have the lead responsibility for drawing up a local action plan to address the issues in this report
The General Medical Services Contract (Department of Health, 2004f)	States that general practitioner's should be encouraged to be more proactive in addressing the physical health needs of those with severe mental illness, which could include for example the referral of patients to physical activity programmes, such as exercise referral schemes
Making it possible: Improving Mental Health and Well-being in England (NIMHE, 2005)	Emphasises that local priorities for action to improve mental health and well-being will be determined by local needs assessment informed by evidence of effectiveness. Greater access to sporting activities and action to reduce isolation and exclusion also play a part. Positive steps to well-being include keeping physically active, eating well and moderate drinking
Health, work and well-being – Caring for our future: A strategy for the health and well-being of working-age people (Department of Health, 2005)	Sets out to identify ways to improve the provision of and access to management of common mental health problems in order to enhance well-being. The aim of the strategy is to reduce relapse rates and prolonged periods of treatment for those with a severe mental illness. There is a role for physical activity in this strategy
Choosing health: Supporting the physical health needs of people with severe mental illness (Department of Health, 2006a)	Recognises the importance of managing physical ill health among people with mental illness through the implementation of the 'Well-Being Support Programme' piloted by Lilly. This programme involves specialist teams working in partnership with primary and social care providers in order to help support people with severe mental illness who are vulnerable to physical ill health. The use of physical health consultations with a nurse lead is mentioned in which those with a mental illness are provided with relevant health and health promotion information, particularly relating to physical activity

(Continued)

Table 10.1 (Continued).

Title	Relevance of physical activity
From values to action: The Chief Nursing Officer's review of mental health nursing (Department of Health, 2006b)	Highlights the importance of mental health nurses encouraging physical exercise through developing physical healthcare assessment skills and actively engaging in health promotion strategies with service users as recommended by the public health White Paper Choosing Health: Making healthier choices easier (Department of Health, 2004d)
Our health, our care, our say: a new direction for community services (Department of Health, 2006c) Our health, our care, our say: making it happen (Department of Health, 2006d)	States that public bodies should do more to support individuals and give everyone an equal chance to become and stay healthy, active and independent. It is in this particular paper that the NHS 'Life check' is introduced, which consists of an initial self assessment, followed by a discussion with a health trainer about what can be done to improve health. This paper also states that the UK Government will take steps to make the 'positive steps' more widely known. This includes being physically active, eating well and a moderate alcohol intake
From segregation to inclusion: Commissioning guidance on day services for people with mental health problems [NIMHE/ Care Services Improvement Partnership (CSIP), 2006]	Provides guidance on day services for people with mental health problems. The main principles include improving cross sector worker including with sports and leisure providers. Secondary care services should be involved in this cross sector working. Day services should also be available in every primary care trust area, as determined by local need. The functions of day services include providing opportunities for social contact and support, supporting people to retain existing social and leisure activities, and supporting people to access mainstream social/leisure opportunities of their choosing. Performance indicators include initial assessments in primary and secondary care that should include activities and care plans which should include targets (i.e. activities). It is stressed in this act that the majority of activities provided should be based in mainstream integrated settings

These opportunities were found to be largely embedded within mental health services, and were partnership projects with funding from a range of sources including local government, mental health services and charitable groups (Crone and Stembridge, 2007). It would appear from the survey that this popularity in physical activity for people with mental health problems is prevalent within the community and the existence of these projects supports the continued calls for the use of physical activity for mental health benefits (Department of Health, 2006a).

Physical activity and mental health – the evidence

The positive alliance between exercise and mental health has long been acknowledged, recognised nearly 100 years ago, with exercise being used as a component of recreational therapy for psychiatric patients (Dishman, 2000). From the 1970s onwards, there has been a surge of papers consistently demonstrating a positive relationship between physical activity and mental health which has culminated in a substantial body of evidence and various reviews (e.g. Biddle *et al.*, 2000; Fontaine, 2000; Biddle and Mutrie, 2001; Lawlor and Hopker, 2001; Daley, 2002; Phillips *et al.*, 2003; Dunn *et al.*, 2005; Penedo and Dahn, 2005; Saxena *et al.*, 2005; Stathopoulou *et al.*, 2006).

Depression

Research investigating the link between depression and physical activity has been conducted in both clinical and non clinical settings, using a range of scales including the Beck Depression Inventory (Beck *et al.*, 1961), the Hospital Anxiety and Depression Scale (Zigmond and Snaith, 1983) and the General Health Questionnaire (Goldberg *et al.*, 1980). The range of measures used to define depression makes the comparison between studies problematic but despite this there is a consensus that there is a positive link between physical activity and depression (Mutrie, 2000). Despite their being some concern regarding the use of physical activity as a clinical intervention (e.g. Burbach, 1997) reviews generally conclude that physical activity has a beneficial effect on mild to moderate depression (Lawlor and Hopker, 2001; Phillips *et al.*, 2003; Faulkner and Biddle, 2004; Craft, 2005), and in terms of a dose response, public health recommendations for aerobic exercise have been found to be an effective treatment for mild to moderate major depressive disorder (Dunn *et al.*, 2005).

Anxiety-related disorders

Research on the effect of physical activity on anxiety includes a series of meta-analysis (McDonald and Hodgdon, 1991; Long and van Stavel, 1995) and reviews of reviews (such as Paluska and Schwenk, 2000;

Taylor, 2000; Biddle and Mutrie, 2001). This summary will focus on research which has investigated the effect of chronic or acute exercise on anxiety disorders (such as generalised anxiety disorder, obsessive compulsive disorder, specific phobias, social anxiety disorder, panic disorder and post-traumatic stress disorder).

Meta-analyses (e.g. McDonald and Hodgdon, 1991; Petruzzello et al., 1991; Long and van Stavel, 1995) have found a significant effect for anxiety and exercise. In summarising these meta-analyses, Biddle and Mutrie (2001) concluded that aerobic exercise was found to produce greater effects than non aerobic exercise, but no difference was found for different types of aerobic activity. Duration of the exercise session was significant when exercise lasted between 21 and 30 minutes, in comparison to durations of up to 20 minutes (Petruzzello et al., 1991). However, when the findings from the studies with durations of fewer than 20 minutes were compared to other anxiety reducing treatments, there was no significant difference between the two lengths of session time compared to other treatments. Intensity was, however, found to be of influence, with both moderate and high-intensity exercise found to be beneficial for anxiety reduction. The links between exercise and anxiety were supported by Leith's (1994) review of experimental studies, with moderate-intensity rather than high-intensity exercise, reducing anxiety during and after exercise. Stephens' (1988) population study also included evidence on anxiety and exercise. Once again findings support the meta-analyses that symptoms of anxiety were less likely to be reported in more active individuals.

In terms of acute exercise and anxiety reduction, research demonstrates a positive relationship between the two with findings often reported together with psychological measures such as blood pressure (Taylor, 2000). Other research has investigated environmental factors such as the exercise environment and time of day (McAuley et al., 1995; Trine and Morgan, 1997). Environments were found to effect the reduction but time of day had no influence. The emergence of this work, once again reflects the developing interest in the environment and other factors complementary to the exercise intervention on mental health changes.

In summary, the empirical evidence regarding anxiety and exercise suggests that meta analyses, experimental and epidemiological studies support an anxiety reducing effect for exercise (Biddle and Mutrie, 2001), that exercise is as effective as other medication free anxiety treatments and that trait anxiety reductions have the greatest effect when chronic exercise is over 10 weeks in duration but is not dependent on physiological fitness changes (Taylor, 2000). Qualitative research supports this positive relationship (Morrissey, 1997), but despite this consensus, Taylor (2000) concludes that given the diversity of research designs and interventions used, it is difficult to draw specific conclusions.

Severe mental illness

There has been limited research into SMI and physical activity (Carless and Sparkes, 2008). Nevertheless, in a critical review of the role of exercise in psychosis (Ellis *et al.*, 2007), research findings demonstrated a positive trend towards improved mental health for those participants taking part in supervised exercise programmes. However, the review was hindered by the available research and the consistency of research design. Ellis *et al.* (2007) concluded that although a positive effect for exercise can be assumed the lack of consistency with research design hindered the ability to determine the size of effects and the most successful type of physical activity intervention.

The research that is available suggests that as a part of a holistic care plan it can have a positive effect and participation can result in decreased auditory hallucinations (Faulkner and Sparkes, 1999), a sense of achievement and social interaction (Carless and Douglas, 2004; Fogarty and Happell, 2005), which are important aspects of holistic well-being.

There has also been some qualitative research in this area that has demonstrated a relationship between physical activity and the management of symptoms, for people with psychotic illnesses. For example, Faulkner and Sparkes's (1999) ethnographic study of people with schizophrenia reported that distraction and social interaction experienced by participants was influential in providing increases in self esteem, a reduction in auditory hallucinations, improved sleep patterns and general behaviour. Qualitative research has also concluded that positive involvement in physical activity programmes, such as walking, can develop positive emotional experiences, a sense of achievement, social interaction and mental health benefits (Carless and Douglas, 2004; Fogarty and Happell, 2005; Crone, 2007) and an opportunity to return to 'normal' previously enjoyed activities, such as running (Carless, in press). This qualitative research provides support for the use of physical activity for people with mental health problems from a holistic perspective in that it can help them to derive many aspects of positive mental well-being.

How does physical activity affect mental health problems?

Unfortunately researchers and mental health professionals are not yet able to definitely provide an answer to this question. Despite numerous mechanisms being suggested for the relationship, to date no consensus has been agreed upon (Crone *et al.*, 2005b, 2006). This lack of consensus is largely due to the methodological and ethical difficulties of researching specific mechanisms and as such, no single mechanism has been substantiated as responsible (Morrissey, 1997; Daley, 2002; Carless and Faulkner, 2003). The mechanism is likely to be a combination of physiological, biochemical and psycho-social aspects (Biddle and Mutrie, 2001); however, there is also growing evidence that the actual process of exercising, rather than the exercise itself, is influential in eliciting various mental health benefits (Faulkner and Sparkes, 1999). Morrissey (1997), Crone *et al.* (2005b) and Crone (2007) support this finding, and also highlight the importance of social interaction opportunities that participants report whilst exercising, as influential to mental health benefits. The lack of consensus over the mechanism responsible for this relationship may be the cause of some of the scepticism amongst mental health professionals of the use of physical activity as an effective adjunct to treatment (Faulkner and Biddle, 2001).

Holistic benefits of physical activity

Although there is evidence linking physical activity to mental health problems, there is criticism of this, for example because of the variability of measurement tools used and small subject sizes, and perhaps because of a lack of consensus on the mechanism responsible for the relationship. However, despite these concerns the call from policy and research for the inclusion of physical activity into mental health services for the treatment of people with mental health problems is important because of the holistic worth of physical activity for this group of individuals.

Engagement in physical activity, as detailed above, can have many other benefits for these population groups, for example psycho-social aspects such as positive emotional experiences, a sense of achievement, social interaction and mental health benefits (Carless and Douglas, 2004; Fogarty and Happell, 2005; Crone, 2007; Crone and Guy, 2008) and an opportunity to return to 'normal' previously enjoyed activities, such as running (Carless, in press). It can also address health concerns within this population group, including higher rates of physical inactivity, obesity and smoking prevalence (Kendrick, 1996; McCreadie, 2003; Crone *et al.*, 2005a). These health concerns are known to result in higher levels of morbidity and premature mortality in people with mental health problems, when compared with the general population (Brugha *et al.*, 1989; Brown *et al.*, 1999). The inclusion, therefore, of exercise within mental health services is evidence based, contemporary, and in line with the government's public health agenda to increase physical activity levels within the population (Department for Culture, Media and Sport/Strategy Unit, 2002; Department of Health, 2004a,d, 2005) and specifically for people with mental health problems (Mental Health Foundation, 2005; Department of Health, 2006a).

Practical guidelines to date

The substantial evidence linking physical activity to mental health has resulted in recommendations for exercise to be used as an adjunct to other forms of treatment in mental illness (Burbach, 1997; Biddle *et al.*, 2000; Daley, 2002). As a consequence, the publication of UK practitioner guidelines for people working in mental health services (Grant, 2000) has resulted in an abundant range of physical activities being developed within mental health services and with local leisure partners, within the UK (Crone and Stembridge, 2007). However, the current guidelines for practice are solely based upon positivist evidence and would benefit from the inclusion of findings from research from interpretivist paradigms. For example, research that examines service users' perspectives of the role and function of exercise could feed into developing Grant's (2000) practitioner guidelines further. The inclusion of research with service users' perspectives would go some way to developing a more eclectic nursing based evidence base, which according to Geanellos (2004), has a critical contribution to the development of effective mental health services. The development of both an eclectic evidence base and the practitioner guidelines may enable people with mental health problems participating in exercise programmes to have positive, worthwhile, and meaningful experiences that can be influential to their treatment and to their quality of life.

Case study: Research in mental health services

Since 2000, a research partnership between the University of Gloucestershire and the NHS Foundation Trust (formerly Gloucestershire Partnership NHS Trust) has resulted in a series of research projects that have led to understanding more about the lives of people with mental health problems and the place of physical activity and well-being within their lives. This has assisted with the development of practice and has reinforced the important role of promoting well-being and a healthy lifestyle for this group of individuals.

Prior to the development of any interventions or service enhancement an audit of the lifestyle behaviour of people with severe mental illness was conducted within the city of Gloucester. The aim of the study was to compare the lifestyle behaviour of people with severe mental illness with the general population of Gloucestershire. The rationale underpinning the study had evolved from previous research identifying that this group were likely to have less healthy lifestyles than the general population, were less likely to be offered health promotion advice and interventions, and that physical health needs of service users were frequently neglected (Cohen and Hove, 2001; Dean *et al.*, 2001). Establishing the lifestyle behaviour of this group helped to identify specific local evidence regarding service users of the trust. These findings assisted in developing specific practice and enhancement of current practice in the area of lifestyle, a known risk factor for other common diseases and premature death in people with mental health problems (Brown *et al.*, 1999).

Findings of the lifestyle audit research (Crone *et al.*, 2005b) included that the severe mental health population in the study had lower perceptions of health when compared with data from the general population of Gloucestershire. Furthermore, there were higher reported body mass index scores, a higher percentage of smokers and lower levels of self-reported physical activity. There were, however, lower reported levels of alcohol consumption. Although the findings lacked statistical significance, due to the sample size, the research concluded with recommendations for practice. These have since informed discussions regarding service development and enhancement, and reinforced the existence of sports therapy and weight management groups that were already in existence.

Gloucestershire Partnership NHS Trust have had a commitment to addressing lifestyle issues since the early 1990s with the appointment of an exercise scientist to work as a 'sports therapist'. Currently there are now five 'sport therapists' in existence in the county who have the responsibility for leading and delivering sport and physical activity sessions within the trust, as part of service users treatment plans. This physical activity is deemed an integral part of service.

Geonellos (2004) proposed that research investigating service users' perspectives is central to the development of an effective mental health service. Service users' perspectives on the role of physical activity is an under researched topic. However, as physical activity is an established form of therapy, it is important to explore and understand the perspectives of service users who take part in it, especially given that it is a recommended adjunct to their treatment. As a consequence, a study undertaken by Crone and Guy (2008) investigated the perceived role of sports therapy from the perspectives of service users in the trust. They concluded that, for the people who participate in sport therapy in mental health services, it has a role to play in their quality of life and is an integral part of their health care. However, the research concluded that although there are many perceived benefits to be gained from participation, according to these participants, to achieve these there are many factors to overcome. These include, for example motivation and anxiety, and increasing general knowledge within mental health services regarding the role of physical activity in the treatment of mental health problems.

As a result of this research the profile of sport therapy has increased within the trust. It has also assisted with reinforcing the strategic role of physical activity in treatment, and of the need to ensure service users are informed and understand the evidence and rationale for its use in their treatment plans. The findings from Crone and Guy (2008) highlighted that although healthy lifestyle activities were actively provided in the trust there seemed, at times, a lack of strategic inclusion of these, within the workings of the trust. The promotion of lifestyle behaviour within mental health services centres on the treatment of individuals and fundamentally the enhancement of their quality of life. In light if this, and as a consequence of the previous research in this area (i.e. Crone et al., 2005b; Crone and Guy, 2008), the question arose regarding how embedded the promotion and concept of well-being was, within the trust.

As a consequence, a qualitative investigation was undertaken to explore, examine and enquire into service users' and mental health professionals' understandings, experiences and opinions of well-being and its promotion within the trust. This qualitative investigation involved focus groups and interviews with service users and a range of mental health professionals including mental health nurses, sports therapists and psychiatrists (Owens, 2007). Findings concluded that well-being promotion and provision of services that promote well-being existed within the trust, for example sports therapy and weight management groups, but there were concerns regarding service provision for the future, due to the reforms, reorganisation and financial cuts that had taken place due to national mental health service reform. Detailed earlier in this chapter is evidence that well-being is evident in national mental health policy, and although there was ample evidence of well-being promotion within the trust, there was found to be limited reference to this in local trust policy. To place these findings into some kind of context, it is probable that these findings would at least be no different to any other investigation of this kind, in other trusts within England. In fact, given that this particular trust has had a commitment to promoting lifestyle issues for many years, it is possible that these findings suggest a more conducive environment for well-being promotion than actually exists elsewhere. However, with respect to this geographical area, these findings highlight the importance of investigating the perspectives of mental health professionals and service users to appreciate what is known and understood by them, in respect to well-being promotion within their trust. These findings, coupled with the conclusions from the previous research projects, assist in the further development and enhancement of evidence based practice within the trust, which is reinforced and supported by current national policy.

Case study summary

These research projects represent a partnership between the University and the trust that also involves student placements (see Crone *et al.*, 2005c, for a review), the sharing of leisure facilities, and professional development opportunities for sports therapy staff in the trust. Through this research the use of sports therapy and the promotion of well-being within the trust, has been examined and results have highlighted that it is evident and a valued aspect of treatment. It has also suggested where further developments and increases in profile could be enhanced. Furthermore, the partnership between the University and the local mental health trust has led to a 'local' evidence base which has both relevance and ownership by those involved in receiving, delivering and designing services within a mental health trust. It also ensures that these issues have a continuous profile, highlighting their importance in an ever changing National Health Service. Future developments are likely to be guided by these findings and the symbiotic partnership that has evolved over the past decade.

Summary and implications for practice

Physical activity has an important role in the enhancement of quality of life for people with mental health problems, and for some it can act as an adjunct to treatment for their condition. Opportunities exist within mental health services and the local community for people with mental health problems to engage in physical activity, but these may not always be embedded strategically within the care plans of service users. This chapter has attempted to present a case for the use of physical activity within a health policy context and based on the available evidence from both positivist and interpretivist paradigms. The importance of recognising the value of the development of an eclectic evidence base derived from complementary paradigms is important if we are to fully comprehend the value, role and effectiveness of the use of physical activity for people with mental health problems within our society.

References

Allebeck, P. (1989) Schizophrenia: A life shortening disease. *Schizophrenia Bulletin*, 15 (1): 81–89.

American Psychiatric Association (1994) *Diagnostic and Statistical Manual of Mental Disorders*. American Psychiatric Association, Washington.

Baxter, D.N. (1996) The mortality experience of individuals on the Salford Psychiatric care register: I All cause mortality. *British Journal of Psychiatry*, 168: 772–779.

Beck, A.T., Ward, C.H., Mendelsohn, M., Mock, J. and Erbaugh, H. (1961) An inventory for measuring depression. *Archives of General Psychiatry*, 4: 561–571.

Biddle, S.J.H. and Mutrie, N. (2001) *Psychology of Physical Activity: Determinants, Well-being and Interventions*. Routledge, London.

Biddle, S.J.H., Fox, K.R. and Boucher, S.H. (2000) *Physical Activity and Psychological Well-Being*. Routledge, London.

Brugha, T.S., Wing, J.K. and Smith, B.L. (1989) Physical health of the long term mentally ill in the community. Is there unmet need? *British Journal of Psychiatry*, 155: 777–781.

Boardman, J. (2005) New services for old – An overview of mental health policy. In: *Beyond the Water Towers: The Unfinished Revolution in Mental Health Services 1985–2005* (Eds A. Bell and P. Lindley), pp. 27–36. Sainsbury Centre for Mental Health, London.

Boardman, J. and Parsonage, M. (2007) *Delivering The Government's Mental Health Policies – Services, Staffing and Costs*. Sainsbury Centre for Mental Health, London.

Brown, S., Birtwhistle, J., Roe, L. and Thompson, C. (1999) The unhealthy lifestyles of people with schizophrenia. *Psychological Medicine*, 29: 697–701.

Brown, S., Barraclough, B. and Inskip, H. (2000) Causes of the excess mortality of schizophrenia. *British Journal of Psychiatry*, 177: 212–217.

Brugha, T.S, Wing, J.K. and Smith, B.L. (1989) Physical health of the long term mentally ill in the community: Is there unmet need? *British Journal of Psychiatry*, 155: 777–781.

Burbach, F.R. (1997) The efficacy of physical activity interventions within mental health services: Anxiety and depressive disorders. *Journal of Mental Health*, 6: 543–566.

Callaghan, P. (2004) Exercise: A neglected intervention in mental health care? *Journal of Psychiatric and Mental Health Nursing*, 11(4): 476–483.

Carless, D. and Douglas, K. (2004) A golf programme for people with severe and enduring mental health problems. *Journal of Mental Health Promotion*, 3(4): 26–39.

Carless, D. and Faulkner, G. (2003) Physical activity and mental health. In: *Perspectives On Health and Exercise* (Eds J. McKenna and C. Riddoch), pp. 61–82. Palgrave MacMillan, Houndsmead.

Carless, D. and Sparkes, A. (2008) The physical activity experiences of men with serious mental illness: Three short stories. *Psychology of Sport and Exercise*, 9(2) 191–210.

Carless, D. (in press) Narrative, identity and recovery from serious mental illness: A life history of a runner. *Qualitative Research in Psychology*.

Cohen, A. and Hove, M. (2001) *Physical Health of the Severe and Enduing Mentally Ill – A Training Pack for GP Educators*. Sainsbury Centre for Mental Health & Department of Health, London.

Cormac, I., Ferriter, M., Benning, R. and Saul, C. (2005) Physical health and health risk factors in a population of long-stay psychiatric patients. *Psychiatric Bulletin*, 29: 18–20.

Craft, L. (2005). Exercise and clinical depression: Examining two psychological mechanisms. *Psychology of Sport and Exercise*, 6 (2): 151–171.

Crone, D. (2007) Walking back to health: A qualitative investigation into Service user's experiences of a walking project. *Issues in Mental Health Nursing*, 28(2): 167–183.

Crone, D. and Guy, H. (2008) 'I know it is only exercise, but to me it is something that keeps me going': A qualitative approach to understanding mental health service users' experiences of sports therapy. *International Journal of Mental Health Nursing*, 17: 197–207.

Crone, D. and Stembridge, L. (2007) Physical activity for people with mental health problems: An audit of provision within the south west of England. *Mental Health Today*, April: 30–32.

Crone, D., Heaney, L., Herbert, R., Morgan, J., Johnston, L. and MacPherson, R. (2005a) A comparison of lifestyle behaviour and health perceptions of people with severe mental illness and the general population. *Journal of Mental Health Promotion*, 3(4): 19–25.

Crone, D., Smith, A. and Gough, B. (2005b) 'I feel totally at one, totally alive and totally happy': A psycho-social explanation of the physical activity and mental health relationship. *Health Education Research*, 20(5): 600–611.

Crone, D., Smith, A. and Gough, B. (2006) The physical activity and mental health relationship – A contemporary perspective from qualitative research. *Gymnica,* 36(3), 29–36.

Crone, D., Meek, L., Edwards, D., Price, L. and Webber, E. (2005c) Creative partnerships for promoting physical activity. *A Life in the Day*, 9 (1): 21–23.

Daley, A. (2002) Exercise therapy and mental health in clinical populations: Is exercise therapy a worthwhile intervention. *Advances in Psychiatric Treatment*, 8: 262–270.

Dean, J., Todd, G., Morrow, H. and Sheldon, K. (2001) 'Mum, I used to be good looking… look at me now': the physical health needs of adults with mental health problems: The perspectives of users, carers and front-line staff. *International Journal of Mental Health Promotion,* 3(4): 16–24.

Department of Culture, Media and Sport/Strategy Unit (2002) *Game Plan: A Strategy for Delivering Government's Sport and Physical Activity Targets*. Cabinet Office, London.

Department of Health (1990a) *The Care Programme Approach. Circular: HC(90)23/ LASSL(90)11*. Department of Health, London.

Department of Health (1990b) *The Care Programme Approach for People with a Mental Illness Referred to the Specialist Psychiatric Services*. Department of Health, London.

Department of Health (1999) *The National Service Framework for Mental Health*. Department of Health, London.

Department of Health (2000) *The NHS Plan: A Plan for Investment, a Plan for Reform*. Department of Health, London.

Department of Health (2001a) *Mental Health Policy Implementation Guide*. Department of Health, London.

Department of Health (2001b) *National Quality Assurance Framework: Exercise Referral Schemes*. Department of Health, London.

Department of Health (2002a) *Community Mental Health Teams: Policy Implementation Guide*. Department of Health, London.

Department of Health (2002b) *Mental Health Policy Implementation Guide: Adult Acute Inpatient Care Provision*. Department of Health, London.

Department of Health (2002c) *Mental Health Policy Implementation Guide: Dual Diagnosis Good Practice Guide*. Department of Health, London.

Department of Health (2002d) *Mental Health Policy Implementation Guide: National Minimum Standards for General Adult Services in Psychiatric Intensive Care Units (Picu) and Low Secure Environments*. Department of Health, London.

Department of Health (2003a) *Mental Health Policy Implementation Guide: Support, Time and Recovery (Str) Workers*. Department of Health, London.

Department of Health (2003b) *Mainstreaming Gender and Women's Mental Health: Implementation Guidance*. Department of Health, London.

Department of Health (2003c) *Fast Forwarding Primary Care Mental Health, Graduate Primary Care Mental Health Workers: Best Practice Guidance*. Department of Health, London.

Department of Health (2003d) *Fast Forwarding Primary Care Mental Health, 'Gateway' Workers: Guidance*. Department of Health, London.

Department of Health (2004a) *Choosing Health? a Consultation on Improving People's Health – Resource Pack*. Department of Health, London.

Department of Health (2004b) *Policy Implementation Guide. Community Development Workers for Black and Minority Ethnic Communities. Interim Guidance*. Department of Health, London.

Department of Health (2004c) *Developing Positive Practice to Support the Safe and Therapeutic Management of Aggression and Violence in Mental Health Inpatient Settings: Mental Health Policy Implementation Guide*. Department of Health, London.

Department of Health (2004d) *Choosing Health: Making Healthier Choices Easier*. Department of Health, London.

Department of Health (2004e) *At Least Five a Week*. Department of Health, London.

Department of Health (2004f) *The New General Medical Services Contract*. Department of Health, London.

Department of Health (2005) *Health, Work and Well-Being – Caring for Our Future: A Strategy for the Health and Well-Being of Working Age People*. Department of Health, London.

Department of Health (2006a) *Choosing Health: Supporting the Physical Health Needs of People with Severe Mental Illness*. Department of Health, London.

Department of Health (2006b) *From Values to Action: The Chief Nursing Officer's Review of Mental Health Nursing*. Department of Health, London.

Department of Health (2006c) *Our Health, Our Care, Our Say: A New Direction for Community Services*. Department of Health, London.

Department of Health (2006d) *Our Health, Our Care, Our Say: Making It Happen*. Department of Health, London.

Dishman, R.K. (2000) Introduction. *International Journal of Sport Psychology*, 31: 103–109.

Dunn, A., Trivedi, M., Kampert, J., Clark, C. and Chambliss, H. (2005) Exercise treatment for depression efficacy and dose response. *American Journal of Preventative Medicine*, 28(1): 1–8.

Ellis, N., Crone, D., Davey, R. and Grogan, S. (2007) Exercise interventions as a therapy for psychosis: A critical review. *British Journal of Psychiatry*, 46(1): 95–111.

Faulkner, G. and Biddle, S. (2004) Exercise and depression: Considering variability and contextuality. *Journal of Sport and Exercise Psychology*, 26(1): 3–18.

Faulkner, G. and Biddle, S.J.H. (2001) Exercise as therapy: It's just not psychology! *Journal of Sports Sciences*, 19: 433–444.

Faulkner, G. and Sparkes, A. (1999) Exercise as therapy for schizophrenia: An ethnographic study. *Journal of Sport and Exercise Psychology*, 21(1): 52–69.

Fogarty, M. and Happell, B. (2005) Exploring the benefits of an exercise program for people with schizophrenia: A qualitative study. *Issues in Mental Health Nursing*, 26: 341–351.

Fontaine, K.R. (2000) Physical activity improves mental health. *The Physician and Sports Medicine*, 28(10): 83–84.

Gask, L. (2004) *A Short Introduction to Psychiatry*. Sage, London.

Geanellos, R. (2004) Nursing based evidence: Moving beyond evidenced based practice in mental health nursing. *Journal of Evaluation in Clinical Practice*, 10(2): 177–186.

Goldberg, D.P., Steele, J.J., Smik, C. and Spivey, L. (1980) Training family doctors to recognize psychiatric illness with increased accuracy. *Lancet*, 6:2(8193): 521–523.

Grant, T. (Ed) (2000) *Physical Activity and Mental Health – National Consensus Statements and Guidelines for Practitioners*. Health Education Authority, London.

Kendrick, T. (1996) Cardiovascular and respiratory risk factors and symptoms among general practice patients with long-term mental illness. *British Journal of Psychiatry*, 169: 733–739.

Kendrick, T., Burns, T., Freeling, P. and Sibbald, B. (1994) Provision of care to general practice patients with long-term mental illness: A survey in 16 practices. *British Journal of General Practice*, 44: 301–305.

Lawlor, D.A. and Hopker, S.W. (2001) The effectiveness of exercise as an intervention in the management of depression: Systematic review and meta-regression analysis of randomized controlled trials. *British Medical Journal*, 322: 1–8.

Leith, L. (1994) *Foundations of Exercise and Mental Health*. Fitness Information Technology Inc, USA.

Long, B.C. and van Stavel, R. (1995) Effects of exercise training on anxiety: A meta-analysis. *Journal of Applied Sports Psychology*, 7: 167–189.

McAuley, E., Bane, S.M., Ruddolph, D.L. and Lox, C.L. (1995) Physique anxiety and exercise in middle aged adults. *Journal of Gerontology*, 50B: 229–235.

McCreadie, R.G. (2003) Diet, smoking and cardiovascular risk in people with schizophrenia: Descriptive study. *British Journal of Psychiatry*, 183: 534–539.

McDonald, D.G. and Hodgdon, J.A. (1991) *Psychological Effects of Aerobic Fitness Training: Research and Theory*. Springer-Verlag, New York.

Marder, S.R., Essock, S.M., Miller, A.L., Buchanan, R.W., Casey, D.E., Davis, J.M., Kane, J.M., Lieberman, J.A., Schooler, N.R., Covell, N., Stroup, S., Weissman, E.M., Wirshing, D.A., Hall, C.S., Pogach, L., Pi-Sunyer, X., Bigger, J.T., Friedman, A., Kleinberg, D., Yevich, S.J., Davis, B. and Shon, S. (2004) Physical health monitoring of patients with schizophrenia. *American Journal of Psychiatry*, 161: 1334–1349.

Mental Health Foundation (2005) *Up and Running?* Mental Health Foundation, London.

Morrissey, M. (1997) Exercise and mental health: A qualitative study. *Mental Health Nursing*, 17: 6–8.

Mutrie, N. (2000) The relationship between physical activity and clinically defined depression. In: *Physical Activity and Psychological Well-Being* (Eds S.J.H. Biddle, K.R. Fox and S.H. Boutcher), pp. 46–62. Routledge, London.

National Institute for Clinical Excellence (2003) *Schizophrenia: Full National Clinical Guideline on Core Interventions in Primary and Secondary Care*. National Institute for Clinical Excellence, London.

National Institute for Clinical Excellence (2004) *Depression: Management of Depression in Primary and Secondary Care*. National Institute for Clinical Excellence, London.

National Institute for Mental Health in England (2005) *Making It Possible: Improving Mental Health and Well-Being in England*. National Institute for Mental Health in England, Leeds.

National Institute for Mental Health in England/ Care Services Improvement Partnership (2006) *From Segregation to Inclusion: Commissioning Guidance on Day Services for People with Mental Health Problems*. National Institute for Mental Health in England/ Care Services Improvement Partnership, London.

National Institute for Mental Health in England/Mentality (2004) *Healthy Body and Mind: Promoting Healthy Living for People Who Experience Mental Distress*. NIMHE/ Mentality, London.

National Institute of Mental Health (2006) *Anxiety Disorders*. National Institute of Mental Health. http://www.nimh.nih.gov/publicat/NIMHanxiety.pdf (accessed 22/05/07).

Owens, C. (2007) *A Qualitative Investigation into the Place and Promotion of Wellbeing for Service Users Within Mental Health Services: A Case Study of Gloucestershire Partnership NHS Trust*. Unpublished MSc (Research) thesis, University of Gloucestershire.

Paluska, S.A. and Schwenk, T.L. (2000) Physical activity and mental health – Current concepts. *Sports Medicine*, 29(3): 167–180.

Penedo, F.J. and Dahn, J.R. (2005) Exercise and well-being: A review of mental and physical health benefits associated with physical activity. *Current Opinion in Psychiatry*, 18(2): 189–193.

Petruzzello, S.J., Landers, D.M., Hatfield, B.D., Kubitz, K.A. and Salazar, W. (1991) A meta-analysis on the anxiety reducing effects of acute and chronic exercise: Outcomes and mechanisms. *Sports Medicine*, 11: 143–182.

Phillips, W.T., Kiernan, M. and King, A.C. (2003) Physical activity as a non-pharmacological treatment for depression: A review. *Complementary Health Practice Review*, 8(2): 139–152.

Saxena, S., Van Ommeren, M., Tang, K. and Armstrong, T. (2005) Mental health benefits of physical activity. *Journal of Mental Health*, 14(5): 445–451.

Simpson, C.J., Seager, C.P. and Robertson, J.A. (1993) Home-based care and standard hospital care for patients with severe mental illness: A randomised controlled trial. *British Journal of Psychiatry*, 162: 239–243.

Social Exclusion Unit (2004) *Mental Health and Social Exclusion: Social Exclusion Unit Report*. Stationery Office, London.

Stein, M.B. (2006) An epidemiologic perspective on social anxiety disorder. *Journal of Clinical Psychiatry*, 67 (12): 3–8.

Stephens, T. (1988) Physical activity and mental health in the United States and Canada: Evidence from four population studies. *Preventative Medicine*, 17: 35–47.

Stathopoulou, G., Powers, M.B., Berry, A.C., Smits, J.A.J. and Otto, M.W. (2006) Exercise interventions for mental health: A quantitative and qualitative review. *Clinical Psychology: Science and Practice*, 13(2): 179–193.

Taylor, A. (2000) Physical activity, anxiety and stress. In: *Physical Activity and Psychological Well-Being* (Eds S.J.H. Biddle, K.R. Fox and S.H. Boutcher), pp. 10–45. Routledge, London.

Trine, M.R. and Morgan, W.P. (1997) Influence of time of day on the anxiolytic effects of exercise. *International Journal of Sports Medicine*, 18: 161–168.

Zigmond, A.D. and Snaith, R.P. (1983) The hospital anxiety and depression scale. *Acta Scandinavia*, 67(6): 361–370.

11 International developments in physical activity promotion

Jim McKenna

Introduction

This chapter aims to explore international developments within the field of physical activity and its promotion. The content is premised upon the idea that new approaches, or revisions of old ones, provide directions for physical activity promotion and for determining the key outcomes of trials. Examples are provided under the thinking of 'if it exists internationally, why not here? [in the UK]'. International data are also useful in that they generate opportunities to make comparisons with other familiar and unfamiliar countries. Often these comparisons may be unfavourable for the UK, such as the recent UNICEF (2007) review of well-being of young people, in 18 developed countries. However, taking a positive view on such comparisons can catalyse change. For example, in the UNICEF report UK children were in the bottom third of the rankings for five of the six categories including family and peer relationships, health and safety and sense of well-being. Part of the impact of such reports is that they compel practitioners and researchers to investigate and learn from causes and effects in the most and least successful examples.

Learning outcomes

The aims of the chapter are to:

1. identify a wide range of perspectives and evidence underpinning the promotion of physical activity internationally
2. describe levels of physical activity in different countries
3. discuss new recommendations for fitness and/or physical activity and consider their relevance to the UK
4. explain new international evidence regarding the role of physical activity in weight control, diabetes and a range of non-medical outcomes
5. identify perspectives on physical activity promotion for children and adolescents

---

6. consider how physical activity is promoted in medicalised settings and in the workplace
7. assess the different ways in which cost-effectiveness is identified in a range of international settings

Physical activity levels

Physical activity and physical fitness continues to be a cause for concern among public health advocates (Department of Health, 2004). Rising rates of sedentary-related health problems co-exist (Booth *et al.*, 2000). Globally, physical inactivity is estimated to cause 10–16% of cases of breast cancer, colon and rectal cancers and diabetes mellitus (WHO, 2003, 2004). For ischaemic heart disease the figure is approximately 22%, with almost 2 million deaths per annum being attributable to physical inactivity. Data from six EU countries (and based on a liberal definition of physical activity (*'Do you do any gymnastics, physical activity or sports?'*: Yes = 1, No = 0) showed that almost 7 in 10 respondents reported being 'active'. However, this figures hides considerable variability; 88% Finnish respondents (n = 400); 64.1% from Saxony, eastern Germany(n = 913), 63.2% from Flanders, Belgium (n = 389), and 37.4% from Catalonia, Spain (n = 380) (Stähl *et al.*, 2001) considered themselves 'active'. Although the study was not established to identify prevalence, the figures suggest wide variability, even between countries separated by small distances and travelling times. This appears to justify intervening and evaluating outcomes at a community level, e.g. the Australian Rockhampton walking project (Brown *et al.*, 2006) and the sister 10,000 Steps Ghent project from the Netherlands (De Cocker *et al.*, 2007).

Eurobarometer data (Sjöströem *et al.*, 2002) based on standardised questionnaire responses also indicate wide variability of physical activity across EU countries. The World Health Organisation (Cavill *et al.*, 2006) also report countries where age-group physical activity is at higher and lower levels than in the UK, for example in Ireland 51% of girls and 61% of boys were active versus 11% and 25% for their French counterparts. Even though recent analyses of nationally representative data contends that adult physical activity has declined from 1991 to 2004 (Stamatakis *et al.*, 2007), the broad sweep of evidence consistently suggests that fewer than 1 in 2 UK adults achieve even weak adherence to current recommendations. This has given rise to a longer-term concern that we may be creating an environment wherein children are growing up and adopting sedentary norms of parents. Further, qualitative evidence from UK adults suggests that walking is not yet an accepted form of exercise (O'Donovan and Shave, 2007). It remains a cause for concern that walking does not count towards health either for men or women (Darker *et al.*, 2007) despite the growth of walking-specific promotions and the evidence that the walking speeds typifying walking in a park will often create the stimulus equivalent to moderate intensity exercise for most middle-aged adults (Murtagh *et al.*, 2002).

International comparisons of levels of involvement in physical activity are always challenging, although there are indications of change in some countries. In the Western Pacific there may have been some national increases in adult physical activity in New Zealand, achieved through a national awareness raising campaign ('Push play') which encouraged 30+ minutes of daily physical activity. Singapore also has promising preliminary changes in physical activity associated with the 'Trim and fit' campaign as for Canada's 'Canada on the Move' campaign (Craig *et al.*, 2007). In contrast, there are suggestions of declining physical activity in Australia (WHO, 2003) which might recast our image of Australia as a land of healthy, active outdoor living. There are always unusual examples from which we might take inspiration. For example, as part of their 'Move for Health' programme the Thai Ministry of Public Health organised the world's largest health festival called The Power of Exercise, in Bangkok, November, 2002 (http://www.who.int/mediacentre/news/releases/pr88/en/index.html). Further, an attempt was made to break the Guinness World Record, by bringing more than 70 000 people together in a mass aerobics routine, led by the Prime Minister. In Tonga, spurred by concerns for his own inactivity-related well-being the king decreed a national programme of physical activity! The ubiquity of campaigns across the globe can be compared to our most recent genuinely nationwide campaign, which was Active for Life in 1996–1999 (Hillsdon *et al.*, 2002).

New recommendations: fitness and/or physical activity?

One recent development for physical activity promotion is that fitness (*aka* 'exercise capacity') is now firmly back on the public health agenda (see Chapter 3). Recent US studies show how, even in the presence of hypertension [and high body mass index (BMI), high cholesterol and diabetes], risks for death are reduced in a graded response to increased fitness in both men (Myers *et al.*, 2002) and women (Gulati *et al.*, 2003). Indeed, these findings suggest that risks return to normal population values when exercise capacity exceeds 8 METs [MET = standard metabolic equivalent; 1 MET = the energy (oxygen) used by the body whilst sitting quietly; any activity that burns >6 METs is considered vigorous intensity physical activity].

These data, based on the selective samples with access to maximal treadmill testing, may help to revitalise services providing independent prognostic fitness testing (Mark and Lauer, 2003). Graded responses within these data suggest that even relatively low levels of physical activity can increase metabolic fitness, producing beneficial adaptations in the many physiological and biochemical indices linked to coronary heart disease (Booth *et al.*, 2000). Further, growing evidence is now linking physical activity to various positive outcomes among cancer patients (Knols *et al.*, 2005) including children (Brouwer *et al.*, 2007) and women (Stevinson *et al.*, 2007).

As a consequence of these data, new US recommendations for physical activity promotion were released in August 2007 (see Chapter 1). These are intended to provide more comprehensive and explicit public health recommendations (Haskell *et al.*, 2007). Importantly, the recommendations refocus attention on exercise intensity, where all healthy adults, up to 65 years, need moderate intensity, aerobic physical activity for a minimum of 30 minutes on 5 days each week or vigorous intensity aerobic activity for a minimum of 20 minutes on 3 days each week. The relevance of this new recommendation for over 65-year-olds can be seen more fully in Chapter 9. As well as clarifying the frequency of moderate intensity exercise and revaluing vigorous intensity exercise, these new guidelines specify the complementarity of moderate and vigorous intensity exercise. However, they separate the 'blur' that may exist around promoting 'moderate-to-vigorous physical activity' (MVPA) as a single entity. One further development is that muscle-strengthening is added to these new guidelines, with implications for bone health and ability to prevent falls in over-65s, which again, is more fully explored in Chapter 9.

Although these recommendations may appear to refute the lifestyle activity message, they emphasise that short bouts of activity (10 minutes or more) can be combined to meet the 30 minute daily goal. For older adults (65+ years) the guidelines include several important differences including combining the development of moderate intensity aerobic activity, muscle-strengthening activity, reducing sedentary behaviour and risk management (Nelson *et al.*, 2007). A further consideration is that these recommendations represent a considerably more complicated (and tailored) physical activity message. On the one hand, this may present a problem to enshrine the message within catchy slogans or maxims. On the other hand, they more faithfully represent the evidence and more fully inform individuals about how they can meet personal needs.

In something of a paradigm shift, a growing number of researchers worldwide are now focusing their attention on the effects of sedentary living. It is likely that this development will offer interesting opportunities for converting findings into effective intervention approaches. It remains to be seen how the STRRIDE (Studies of Targeted Risk Reduction Interventions through Defined Exercise) findings regarding the impact of inactivity, derived from control group participants, can be adapted within interventions (Slentz et al., 2005). Indeed, a growing body of research is emerging about the factors that promote sedentary living (e.g. Biddle, 2007) and on the 'Non Exercise Activity Thermogenesis' (NEAT) consequences of sitting, rather than standing in both children and adults (Lanningham-Foster et al., 2005). These have implications for classroom design, and in adult employees (Levine and Miller, 2007), these have implications for workstation design. These findings may offer important opportunities to develop interventions that aim to reduce prolonged sitting time either in the workplace or in leisure time.

Physical activity, weight control and diabetes

Weight control is of major importance in treating adult-onset diabetes, which is so commonly associated with levels of weight gain that compromise well-being. In a range of recent important randomised controlled trial studies, including STRRIDE (USA), the Finnish Diabetes Prevention Study (Lindström et al., 2006) and the Diabetes Prevention Programme (Knowler et al., 2002), walking that exceeded the equivalent of 10–12 miles per week, of moderate intensity, consistently suspended further weight gain. Other studies suggest that a minimum of 40 minutes physical activity per day, on every day of the week, can maintain weight loss, which is important given contemporary rises in obesity and associated diabetes. The detail of STRRIDE provides useful information for exercise promoters, highlighting not only the beneficial effects of regular physical activity but also the deleterious effects of remaining inactive (through assessing important markers of cardiovascular well-being over 18 months). STRRIDE data are especially important since they are based on a long-term randomised controlled trial design, meaning that participants have an even chance of being allocated to either the treatment or control groups. In this way, data are thought to be representative of the samples recruited at baseline.

The details of STRRIDE are also important for exercise promoters and for public health more generally. After drawing a mixed sample of 175 sedentary adults with mild-to-moderate dyslipidaemia, each was randomly allocated to either 6 months in a control group or ~8 months in one of three exercise groups. In the first group physical activity was low in volume and of moderate intensity, equivalent to walking 12 miles a week (19.2 kilometres) at 40–55% of peak oxygen consumption. In the second group the same volume of activity was completed more vigorously, equivalent to jogging 12 miles a week at 65–80% of peak oxygen consumption. In the third group vigorous intensity activity, equivalent to jogging 20 miles a week was prescribed.

Computed tomography scans were analysed for abdominal fat pre-post intervention. Controls gained visceral fat (8.6%). At the equivalent of 11 miles of exercise per week, at either intensity, accumulation of visceral fat was prevented, while the highest volume of exercise resulted in decreased visceral (–6.9%), subcutaneous (–7.0%) and abdominal fat. STRRIDE emphasised how a range of associated adaptations, including adipose fat and high-density lipoprotein (HDL) density were all responsive to this level of activity. However, despite these important findings, Kruger et al. (2006) showed that the positive role of physical activity is often under-appreciated by individuals attempting to lose weight, which underlines the need for regular reminders within consultations with clients.

In the Finnish Diabetes Prevention Study (Laaksonen et al., 2005; Lindström et al., 2006) one further set of findings is important. Based on intention-to-treat analysis (which integrates participants who comply with those who do not), rates of new cases of diabetes were assessed according to tertiles for physical activity change (highest versus lowest tertile). The highest physical activity tertile were 74% less likely to develop diabetes; this was only reduced to 71% after accounting for dietary changes, meaning that physical activity was the most potent of these behavioural changes, which included fat reduction, increased fruit/vegetables and fibre intake. In a similar vein, more recent work from the EPIC-Norfolk Prospective Population Study has shown that four behaviours, including regular physical activity, not smoking, regularly consuming five or more fruits and vegetables per day and moderate alcohol intake can lead to an average of 14 years of extra life compared to people undertaking none of these behaviours (Khaw et al., 2008).

Pedometers have become increasingly important in the promotion of walking, although the evidence of effectiveness has not been confirmed in adults. One recent systematic literature review (Bravata et al., 2007) found that pedometer use, particularly with a daily step goal, was associated with significant increases in physical activity (averaging an extra 2491 steps per day over controls) and significant decreases in body mass index and blood pressure. Analyses were based upon eight randomised controlled trails and 18 observational studies ($n = 2767$ participants). There is also moderate evidence that pedometers can positively influence physical activity in workplace settings as has been evidenced by the recent NICE (National Institute of Health and Clinical Excellence) review (Dugdill et al., 2007).

Non-medical outcomes resulting from physical activity

While adaptations that directly impact on markers of disease are important (including blood vessel inflammation), another body of evidence is increasingly addressing how physical activity contributes to subjective perspectives, such as quality of life, which are predictors of longevity and subsequent well-being (Sullivan, 2003). One recent meta-analysis (Netz et al., 2005) emphasised physical activity impact on well-being among older adults. Findings were based on 36 studies (only 22 of which included both control and treatment groups), and a wide range of outcome measures. Analyses were also consistent with the outcomes from a range of qualitative studies, in this case highlighting that mean-change effects for any physical activity intervention ($d^c = 0.24$) were three times greater than for control groups ($d^c = 0.09$). Within interventions behavioural change mechanisms were most strongly linked to subjective estimates of changes in self-efficacy, overall sense of well-being and sense of self. These data were limited to older people without clinical disorders and while the effects sizes were small, they were statistically significant.

Social support is widely understood as important for establishing and then maintaining good health (Eng et al., 2002). Researchers increasingly show how positive emotions linked to relationships enhance our capacity to heal or fight disease (Dickens et al., 2004). However, new data are reporting that it is also important to consider the negative effects associated with family, friends, colleagues and neighbours. Recent, challenging findings from the field of medical sociology have highlighted some negative effects for becoming obese (Christakis and Fowler, 2006). Using data drawn from over 12 000 adults enrolled in the US' Framingham Study, collected in 1971 and again in 2003, analysis showed that the risk for becoming obese dramatically increased when a friend, sibling or spouse gained weight.

More specifically, the chances of becoming obese increased by 57% if a friend had became obese in a given interval. When a sibling became obese, the chance increased by 40%, if a spouse became obese, the chance increase was 37%. Among same-sex friendships, the probability of obesity increased by 71% if the friend became obese. For sisters, the risk was 67%, compared to 44% for brothers. However, neither opposite-sex friends nor siblings had any effect on increasing risk, suggesting the influence of hitherto unknown factors within the relationship. It remains to be seen whether, or how, this 'network medicine' can be used to foster positive behaviours like physical activity, exercise or sport.

Cross-cultural competence describes the developed abilities of individuals from one cultural to operate effectively with individuals and/or groups from another culture. This is a relatively new theme that is playing a part in refining existing physical activity promotion. One recent set of studies, conducted on older adults in Taiwan, have shown how there may be culturally distinctive understandings of physical activity and the role that it can play within any cultural groupings. For example, in Taiwan, with its strong collectivist Chinese influence, communal physical activity (think of large groups doing Tai Chi in public spaces) is not only seen as good activity but also as a signal of community spirit and integration (Ku *et al.*, 2006, 2007). Interviews also confirmed that family loyalty is such a driving force that it provides an important incentive for older people not to impose on their children (even though they may still be living in the same house and the 'carers' may be over 60 years of age themselves!). These features have much to say about how cross-cultural competence might be enhanced for black and minority ethnic groups in the UK. Importantly, they remind us that individuals from a 'majority' can quickly, but wrongly, make assumptions about the lives of 'minorities'. These assumptions may not only compromise attempts to become more active, but also underline cultural separation rather than unity.

Health literacy is another emergent theme that has exorcised health promoters in recent years. Based on an assumption that low health literacy is linked to a low capacity to understand and then respond to health-related messages, recent English data are important. Over 2 years Blank *et al.* (2007) drew data to identify the effects of physical activity and diet change on standardised measures of mental health from 39 low-socio-economic districts ($n = 10419$). Comparable data were collected from neighbourhood districts with similar demographic characteristics. These data are important not only because they represent communities rarely studied in close detail, but also because the key study outcomes are internationally comparable, especially in Europe. Further, the neighbourhoods contributing to this study were also those who were the target of substantial government in investment to improve health and well-being (New Deal for Communities, 2001–2005), in the assumption that low health literacy predominated in these communities.

Baseline data indicated that both the assumption of low health literacy and the need for investment may have been justified. Participating communities were characterised by a poorer mental health profile than indicated in two samples drawn from the EU in 2005–2006, particularly for 'happiness' and 'peacefulness'. Although there were no European Union comparisons for this variable, fewer than 4 in 10 self-rated their health as 'good'.

Results over 2 years showed that even though levels of physical activity were low, increases were reported over 2 years [based on responses to an interviewer-administered question about the numbers of bouts (0–13) of exercise lasting 'for 20 minutes at a time']. However, these changes were associated with important positive improvements in mental health. Further, an improvement in mental health indices was identified after comparing outcomes for contrasting neighbourhoods and despite no changes in either diet or physical activity. The authors speculate that a further effect of providing exercise classes is to improve the local sense of community. In effect, having these classes and such opportunities may be an important way of signalling an upturn in quality of life in areas of widespread social deprivation. Extending this idea further, health professionals may consider the value of intensifying efforts to promote new exercise opportunities in such communities, irrespective of attendance.

Physical activity promotion for children and adolescents

Key issues relating to physical activity levels and methods by which these levels are identified have recently been reported (Armstrong and Welsman, 2007; see also Chapter 4). Notwithstanding these limitations, evidence consistently suggests that across the EU, boys tend to be more active than girls, especially in vigorous forms of activity. The availability of sensitive, but cheaper, motion sensor technology has allowed large-scale studies to be undertaken with methods that overcome the limitations of self-report questionnaires and diaries. The newest devices have the capacity to record patterns of physical activity in very fine detail (measures can be taken and stored every 2 seconds with the newer devices) and for up to 14 days. Researchers continue to seek ways to more fully represent the detail that can often be lost in the types of analysis being conducted in most contemporary studies. Combining minute-by-minute scores are useful for describing overall activity, but there is more to be done to explore such data for patterns and styles of physical activity in a range of populations.

However, even allowing for the limitations of these analytical approaches, accelerometer-based studies are yielding important data. For example, very recent UK data has produced challenging figures regarding the numbers of children meeting recommended levels of physical activity. These data emerged from a major birth cohort study in the UK, Avon Longitudinal Study of Parents and Children. Among over 5000 11-year-olds, all born in the Avon region in 1995, motion sensors were worn for seven continuous days between 2003 and 2005. In boys (who were more active than girls) 40% undertook continuous moderate-to-vigorous physical activity (MVPA) for 5 minutes, whereas the equivalent figure for girls was 22%. Only 2% of respondents met the criterion for continuous MVPA of at least 20 minutes duration, instead undertaking most activity at a lower intensity (Riddoch et al., 2007). While the authors have acknowledged that their criterion for MVPA may be higher than that adopted elsewhere, if these findings are both accurate and generalisable, they emphasise the scale of the need for more effective physical activity promotion among young people in the UK.

A range of school-based interventions have been reported, although caution should be exercised when considering the transfer of findings across nations. For example, public school studies from the US (Luepker *et al.*, 1996) often reflect differently resourced systems and are based on a unique ethnic mix of pupils and teacher practices that have no parallel in Europe. Further, the acceptability of the developments must reflect the distinctive traditions and aspirations of teacher groups. However, their achievements should be noted, and under the idea that 'if it exists, it is possible', they certainly deserve our consideration for example SPARK (Sports, Play and Active Recreation for Kids; Sallis *et al.*, 1998), CATCH Kid's Club (Kelder *et al.*, 2005). Other studies are currently underway and may have greater relevance for the UK setting, for example Ireland's impending Take PART study.

Much of what influences children's activity beyond the school reflects different aspirations for young people. For example, parental aspirations often provide a strong, and perhaps limiting, context for younger children's activity in the home and at weekends. Care of children may be an area for attention and one recent meta-analysis, conducted in the Netherlands (van Sluijs *et al.*, 2007), highlights the importance of multi-component interventions, although there were doubts that blending family/home, school and community approaches will help all children and young people to meet current physical activity recommendations. Effects were strongest for adolescents in this review, with conclusions based on data drawn from 57 studies from Australia, Belgium, Canada, Ireland, Greece, France, Finland, Netherlands, Spain, Taiwan and UK. However, this evidence base was dominated by US studies.

Notwithstanding these outcomes, UK data appear to reflect trends toward restricted physical activity at home and in movement to and from the home, presumably due to adults' perspectives on the relative safety of the outside world. Hillman *et al.* (1991) showed that the level of parental licence offered to UK 9-year-olds in 1979, for playing outside the home, by 1991 was only available to 13-year-olds. In the same period, 80% of 7- to 8-year-olds went to school on their own in the 1970s, falling to fewer than 1 in 10 in 1990. These findings have clear relevance for the promotion of active commuting; in the UK, and between 1991 and 2002 the proportion of children walking or cycling to school declined from 60% to 51% in primary and from 46% to 38% in secondary children (Department for Transport, 2004).

Data drawn from Derby, UK, in June 2006 (Smith *et al.*, 2007), suggests that among over 5000 year 4 (aged 8–9), year 8 (ages 12–13) and year 10 pupils (ages 15–16), 3422 actively commuted (walked/cycled) on 4 or more occasions per week, whereas 1235 reported no time in active commuting. Importantly, active commuting was associated with more pupils meeting weekly physical activity recommendations of 1 hour a day (73.9% of regular commuters, 47.9% of irregularly active commuters and 37.5% of non-active commuters), even though average daily commuting MVPA was 18.4 ± 16.4 minutes and represented just 15% of average weekday values. Even after removing the contribution from active commuting, daily active commuters achieved an average extra 34 minutes of MVPA. These data not only highlight the value of this form of activity for meeting recommendations but also suggest that there may be different audiences for active commuting interventions and distinctive ways to be an active commuter (e.g., walking plus using public transport). Active commuting has been the focus of extensive attention in many countries, including Australia (Merom et al., 2006), Canada (Pabayo and Gauvin, 2007), Denmark (Cooper et al., 2003, 2005), Russia (Tudor-Locke et al., 2002), Scotland (Alexander et al., 2005), Switzerland (Bringolf-Isler et al., 2007) and the US (Sirard et al., 2005a,b). The distinctive levels of active commuting among young people reported in the different studies reflect distinctive definitions of what constitutes active commuting (e.g. allowing for more than just walking or not) and ways of measuring commuting behaviour (e.g. self-reporting, parental or teacher observations, accelerometry).

Academic performance

Once children get to school, concerns focus on how to improve their academic performance. Researchers continue to investigate the link between academic performance and physical activity, presumably in the hope of identifying learning-related effects of active living. One recent 16-month randomised controlled trial conducted in British Columbia, Canada, achieved a daily average increase of 47 minutes physical activity per day and was associated with no negative impact on academic performance (Ahamed et al., 2007). Eight schools completed the study and were randomized either to intervention (INT) or usual practice (UP). Children (n = 143 boys; 144 girls) in grades 4 and 5 (ages) were recruited for the study.

At older ages (15 and 16 years), 590 pupils (292 females, 49.2%) in year 10 (ages 15 and 16) across four schools in the Bristol area (England, UK) who were undertaking important public examinations, completed Baecke's physical activity diaries (Baecke et al., 1982) immediately prior to entering their examination period (McKenna and Bennett, 2005). In a prospective design, physical activity levels were identified and then used to address examination outcomes identified three months later. Examinations results matched national profiles and showed that physical activity behaviour neither advantaged nor disadvantaged examination outcomes, based on grades provided by the examination boards and by teachers' predicted grades (recorded in May of the same year). Although 411 students felt that being active during the examinations would positively influence their results, 75.8% reported at least one source of pressure to reduce their physical activity (personal pressure 47.3%, parents 43.0%, teachers 40.6% and friends 8.7%). Uniquely, students who personally decided to restrict leisure time (n = 276), rather than reduce physical activity, achieved grades closest to teachers' predictions ($P < 0.05$) and more A to C passes [7.02 (3.80) versus 5.26 (3.79), $P < 0.01$]. In the context of growing pressures on school playtimes (or recess periods) evidence for 'no harm' may be a first step in stabilising the activity of more young people during the school day.

One interesting recent Canadian study (Pabayo et al., 2006) focused on the impact of after-school sports programmes. Specifically, the study was based on 10 schools to identify the impact of a 1 year (1999–2000) teacher ban on extracurricular sports on secondary school children's physical activity. Effects measured in 979 grade 7 pupils (mean age 12.7 years) indicated children in the 'ban' schools were more responsive to extracurricular-based physical activity once it was reinstated. These data are both encouraging and perplexing; should teachers intentionally remove opportunities only to reinstate them more fully later? However, the data may also have relevance to (re)introducing after-school activities following staff turnover or protracted absence, which reflects the reality of daily life in schools.

Physical activity promotion in health care systems

In the US, in October 2007, with the backing of the American Medical Association, the 'Exercise is Medicine' campaign (http://www.exerciseis-medicine.org/taskforce) was launched. This was based on the understanding that health care professionals (doctors, nurses and the other professions allied to medicine) can deliver effective exercise promotion by automatically including this as a topic of conversation at every meeting. In this way, successes are likely to be followed up, which has been a running issue in convincing staff to undertake physical activity promotion (McKenna and Vernon, 2004).

In Scotland, during 2004, both practice nurses ($n = 149$) and health visitors ($n = 186$) reported high involvement (9 out of 10 respondents) in the promoting of physical activity (Douglas et al., 2006). The authors of this study highlighted a problem within their findings; that both groups thought that physical activity behaviour was increasing in Scotland. An alternative interpretation is that it is this attitude which supports continued involvement in physical activity promotion. These data contrast with the recurrent finding among doctors that lack of skill or evidence of demonstrable effectiveness each undermine efforts to offer systematic physical activity support for patients. It is important to note that the sample was predominantly comprised of female respondents, contrasting strongly with many studies based on family doctors.

Aittasalo et al. (2006), based on sampling all family doctors in Finland, highlighted the problems of substantially altering behaviours within individual consultations with patients. Despite being able to change some features of local promotion, over 4 years national-level change was not reported in the proportions of doctors asking patients about their physical activity, or for frequency of using pre-prepared resources.

Recent Australian data (Eakin *et al.*, 2007) suggest that family doctors have patients who they consider more preferentially for receiving physical activity promotion. This may encourage the adoption of more refined targets for interventions focused on promotional behaviour. Physical activity advice from doctors was reported by 24.2% of 2478 Rockhampton respondents during a walking promotion (2001–2003), where doctors' advice was a central tenet of the community-wide intervention. This contrasted with a rate of 1-in-5 in a comparison control community and with national estimates for physical activity counselling in 1.5% of consultations, suggesting responsiveness of doctors to participating in community-based initiatives. In Rockhampton, advice was more likely to be given to males, overweight/obese people, those with chronic conditions, and those most frequently visiting their doctors. In US longitudinal data (Ma *et al.*, 2004), physical activity was reported in ≤30% of visits with adults with known hyperlidemia, diabetes, hypertension or obesity. Like the Australian data, this figure appears to have risen over the study period 1992–2000, although these US data also suggest doctor's preferences for promoting physical activity promotion to clinically unwell patients.

For post-coronary US patients physical activity promotion 'within the past 12 months' was reported by 53.2% of respondents (Wofford *et al.*, 2007) although multivariate analyses indicated that the 33.2% who met the recommendations did so independently of being advised in this way, which brings into question the effectiveness of interventions that doctors make. Among diabetic patients, nationally representative data suggests that over twice as many diabetics (73% of 26 878) were 'ever' advised about physical activity by any health professional than were adults without diabetes (Morrato *et al.*, 2006). In multivariate analysis doctors' preferences for secondary prevention were again confirmed; the strongest correlates of promoting physical activity were BMI and accompanying cardiovascular risk factors.

Other nations, with distinctive medical systems, and stages of development in relation to physical activity promotion through general practice, are beginning to better understand the issues they face in establishing this as routine practice. In Switzerland (Jimmy and Martin, 2004) 90% of inactive patients agreed to participate in a general practice-based physical activity intervention. Following the trend among adolescents in Spain (Ortega-Sanchez *et al.*, 2004), effectiveness in the Swiss participants increased over time with one-third reported as active at 7 weeks and nearly half at 14 months. It remains to be seen how any such lag effects might be optimised by follow-up interventions. Following-up patients was a characteristic of UK doctors who systematically promoted physical activity (McKenna and Vernon, 2004).

In another study in Barcelona in the Catalan region of Spain (Puig Ribera *et al.*, 2006a,b), where rates of sedentary-related health problems are rising, mixed methods were used to better understand the context of physical activity promotion. Attention will be paid to this study as it replicates many of the issues found in other countries, even those with differently oriented health care systems. The consistency of these findings to others suggests the centrality of system orientation for establishing more consistent physical activity promotion within public health care.

In a first stage of the work, surveys were distributed to family doctors and nurses. Subsequently, interviews were conducted with doctors, nurses, representatives from medical organisations, academics and physical activity promoters. Focusing on important barriers to undertaking more regular physical activity promotion, respondents highlighted a strong sense that the political climate was wrong for physical activity promotion to become widely accepted among doctors, nurses and patients. Further, doctors sensed that they were continually reminded of the value of drug therapy by the recurrent calling of pharmaceutical representatives (while they also noted the absence of similar advocacy for physical activity). Others noted that the lack of time in consultations was a problem.

Consistent with studies (excluding Jimmy and Martin, 2004) from around the world, doctors also felt that patients were reluctant to discuss physical activity since they were attending consultations to seek immediate remediation for health problems. There were other factors that limited public health promotion of physical activity and these included lack of training, although this was occasionally resolved by having a personal interest in being physically active. Physical activity promotion was also considered to be something of a burden and only to be considered if a 'cure' pathway could be identified. However, there was a general concern that doctors had limited understanding of the health (or disease) effects of physical activity (Graham *et al.*, 2005). Collectively, these data underline the need for more detailed training and for making time available to promote physical activity more effectively. This limited secondary prevention and largely precluded primary prevention opportunities.

Further, few practitioners trusted their knowledge of local facilities (e.g. exercise specialists, centres, clubs). In this way, staff members were unable to provide examples of local places to go for further help or people who could provide more detailed information. Indeed, doctors were broadly suspicious of people who were not medical doctors and this mistrust only intensified when discussion focused on voluntary groups. Clearly in this context, this limited the capacity of doctors to engage patients with community-based services, which further added to the over-burdened perspective that predominated among study contributors.

Workplace physical activity promotion

It is no surprise that, consistent with setting-based approaches (Whitelaw et al., 2001) toward physical activity, the workplace continues to attract the attention of physical activity promoters (Gilson et al., 2007, 2008; see Chapter 7). As an essential part of the working day, journeys to and from work (active commuting) are increasingly thought to increase total physical activity. Recent attempts have focused on changing office furniture to include treadmills and cycle ergometers in place of seating to increase daily energy expenditure under the notion of walking while working (Levine and Miller, 2007). These authors calculated that replacing time spent sitting at the computer with walking computer time by 2–3 hours per day, allowing for other factors (diet, etc.) being held constant, weight loss of 20–30 kg per year may result. In related work (Thompson et al., 2007) walking workstations increased daily step counts by 2000, which equates to an increase of 100 kcal per day. Of course, there are considerable costs associated with replacing/duplicating and also maintaining active-office equipment and cost-effectiveness analysis will need to support these interventions however it emphasises the importance of not sitting at a desk for too long!

Other approaches have focused on showing the health impact of active commuting. Australian data (Ming Wen and Rissel, 2007) based on 6810 respondents showed that men who cycled to work (odds ratio 0.49, 95% CI 0.31–0.76) as well as those who used public transport (odds ratio 0.65, 95% CI 0.53–0.81) – which involves more walking to and from stops – reduced the likely of being overweight and obese compared to men who drove to work. Over 5 years, regular walking or cycling to work was also associated with reduced adiposity and reduced weight gain (Wagner et al., 2001).

Epidemiological evidence for 1 hour (or for 25 miles) of weekly cycling was associated with a 50% reduction in risk of dying from all causes over 10 years (Morris et al., 1990). Further, in adults, a cycling to work intervention was associated with a 30% lower risk of mortality in both sexes (Vuori et al., 1994; Andersen et al., 2000), perhaps because cycling involves higher exercise intensities than say, walking. A recent meta-analysis of the general effect of active commuting showed an 11% reduction in cardiovascular risk, with stronger effects in women than men (Hamer and Chidi, 2007). Recent work has also shown how the promotion of commuting by public transport also contributes to increased physical activity (Zheng, 2008), presumably through walking to and from the various termini. Although there are clear lines of evidence underlining the health value of active commuting it remains frustrating to health promoters that it is best achieved, albeit with short-term effects, through public transport strikes and fuel shortages.

A growing body of literature is now highlighting that physical activity, as part of wider programme of provision within the workplace, is being seen as having a wide morale-building effect. While physical and medical outcomes are valued, a growing trend among employers recognises that the 'well' employee has a better chance of being a more effective employee when management is also 'well'. Collectively, and using the language of 'wellness', this creates a 'well' organisation (Chartered Management Institute, 2007). Central to this understanding is that physical activity during the working day, or in the employee's lifestyle, reduces health care costs and absenteeism as well as improving performance. Recent data from UK white collar employees (Coulson *et al.*, in press) compared self-assessed work performance in people who exercised on one day but not on another in a randomised controlled trail design with cross-over. Effects, measured using the Work Limitations Questionnaire, showed recurrent differences in performance estimates favouring the exercise day.

Other work (van Vegchel *et al.*, 2005) is refining the notion of work to reflect subjective estimates of the nature of the workplace, conceptualised within the Effort-Reward Imbalance (ERI) model, and their link to employee well-being and health. ERI is characterised by conceptualising the employee experience of work in relation to two constructs; effort required to compete daily tasks and rewards provided while undertaking those tasks. In a review of 45 empirical studies, employees who characterise their workplace as high effort, low reward, risks for health were increased. These risks were accentuated by the additional factor of a culture of over-commitment. It may be that such environments have most to gain from, but are least likely to integrate, physical activity interventions.

In this context, it is worthwhile considering the research that focuses on the beneficial 'spill-over' of physical activity into other realms of life. This work can be profound in helping individual to redress lost work-life balance (McKenna and Thew, 2008). For example, in an Australian randomised controlled trial with regular exercise has recently been shown to benefit by being preceded by a short period of self-regulation training (Oaten and Cheng, 2006). Further, a host of further adaptive behaviours were reported by participants, suggesting the value of such salutogenic preparations before undertaking physical activity. Many of these newly adopted behaviours, which include reduced TV watching, improved emotional control and reduced stress and alcohol intake, all making further contributions to well-being. The US PREMIER study (Svetkey *et al.*, 2003; Elmer *et al.*, 2006) suggests that concurrent promotion of multiple behavioural changes is as effective, or better than, sequential counselling (i.e. one behaviour change at a time), and sustains improved health for up to 18 months. Combining the findings from Oaten and Cheng (2006) and those from STRRIDE, suggests that a new range of physical activity interventions should be undertaken to address inactivity and/or sustain the already active segments of the population.

Cost-effectiveness of physical activity

Cost-effectiveness analysis is increasingly being required as an integral part of intervention research. As health care systems nudge toward rationing care, attention is focusing on those interventions which deliver clinically meaningful outcomes with best financial value. Despite the problems of comparing currencies, ways of calculating health care costs and the preliminary nature of the existing data, there are interesting examples of cost-effectiveness estimates for different diseases and of physical activity for moderating these costs. For comparison, costs per head (assuming 60 million inhabitants) average approximately £2000 in the NHS.

One 6-year prospective observation of National Health Insurance beneficiaries in rural Japan highlighted how sedentary-related factors contributed to national medical costs (Ohmori-Matsuda *et al.*, 2007). Between 1996 and 2001, medical costs were collated for a sample of 12,340 participants (n = 7034 women) who were asymptomatic for cardiovascular disease or cancer at baseline and who made a claim during the study period. At baseline, participants were identified as overweight/obese (BMI $\geq$ 25.0 kg/m^2), hypertensive ($\geq$ 140/90 mm Hg or self-reported medication) or hyperglycaemic (blood glucose $\geq$ 150 mg/dl or self-reported history of diabetes) and annual costs were identified for each year of the study. For the three conditions where physical activity could have a strongly moderating effect, total mean monthly medical costs were equivalent to USD 12.7 million, with individuals identified with none of the three risks making average monthly claims of $193.4. Hypertension alone increased this figure by 33%, whereas hyperglycaemia increased costs by 48.3%. Where overweight/obesity, hypertension and hyperglycaemia combined, average annual medical costs increased by 91%. These figures highlight the scale of cost saving that physical activity might help to produce.

In a second study within the same insurance system, the role of physical activity (in this case walking) was identified for cost saving impact. Estimates of physical activity were based on 26 110 men and women aged 40–79 years. Analyses excluded people who were simply unable to walk and showed that self-reported walking for ≥ 1 hour a day reduced health care charges by 8%, compared to people who walked less than this (Kuriyama et al., 2004). This compared with increases of 8.3% for ever having smoked (versus never having smoked) and 7.1% for BMI ≥ 25.0 kg/m² (versus < 25.0 kg/m²). Combining factors showed a graded rise in costs, while the presence of all three harmful factors increases averaged 42.6%. These data are especially interesting for a number of reasons; first the costs relate directly to the claims made against medical insurance and in this care system this service covers almost all available medical care services. Thus, the data are more valuable than projections of cost saving and they relate to a country demonstrating consistently greater longevity than in the UK. Second, they are based on self-reported behaviour and status; a process which has often been subject to major criticism.

In worksite health promotion terms, each dollar invested among 6246 employees in Nevada, USA, over 2 years was associated with approximately $15 savings when absenteeism and lost productivity was included in the calculations for 'loss' (Aldana et al., 2005). The intervention associated with this intervention was characterised by 11 different elements of content (including dental care, reducing TV watching, fitness challenges and car safety) and delivered to a wide range of locations, so was available electronically as well as face-to-face.

The aim of STRRIDE, conducted in the US, was to identify the most effective of the two intervention options, versus the control, in promoting change in physical activity, measured using 7-day physical activity recall diaries. The intervention was motivationally tailored to 224 healthy but sedentary participants (aged 18–65 years) randomly allocated to either phone, print or control conditions. Intervention cost-effectiveness was assessed using prospectively assessed costs (Sevick et al., 2007). Analysis indicated that the print intervention was the most cost-effective intervention for engaging participants in physical activity. Compared to previous research, the cost associated with print intervention ($480 at 12 months) was greater than the $117 identified by Stevens et al. (1998) and by Elley et al. (2003) ($120) in general practices. The cost of successfully engaging one participant in a more active lifestyle in these same studies also favour the STRRIDE print group ($955), versus $1240 (Elley et al., 2004) and $1153 (Stevens et al., 1998).

Although it seems automatic that once sufficient cost-effectiveness figures are established then physical activity promotion will also follow. However, this is not the case and data from Leipzig (Hambrecht et al., 2004) highlight this resistance to change among cardiologists. After randomising men with stable and documented coronary artery disease either to exercise (20 minutes daily cycle ergometry) or to angioplasty, event-free survival was higher in the exercise group (80%) than in the angioplasty group (70%) over 1 year. Further, the costs attributable to angioplasty were almost double that of exercise, mostly being attributable to reduced re-hospitalizations and repeat revascularizations. Yet, such is the challenge facing physical activity promoters that despite the obvious advantages of physical activity, even today angioplasty remains the favoured option for surgeons and male patients. These data underline that showing cost-effectiveness alone does not initiate and then sustain change in professional practice.

Conclusion: implications for practice

Using data from different countries highlights that there are new reasons and ways to promote physical activity. For the UK, the evidence suggests that key areas to focus on are on more effective delivery across the life course and for different population groups. Many of these issues have a direct bearing on how physical activity specialists interact with respective professional groups and in different settings. Client groups are becoming increasingly refined and the future for physical activity promotion appears to rely on getting the right messages to the right people in the right ways. The challenges in establishing measures that ensure international equivalence in terms of intervention outcome are likely to remain for some time, but should not be used to resist change. Exercise professionals need to use such data to extract the catalysing factors that enrich and nourish their physical activity promotion practice. In particular, researchers, especially those working in community settings, need to move away from reliance on self-reported physical activity, towards more objective measures such as pedometers or motion sensors (see Chapter 4).

England (not Scotland, Wales or Northern Ireland, who each have their own health concerns) is lacking in population based campaigns, national statistics and interventions when compared to other countries. New NHS policy announcements, made in January 2008, offer considerable potential not only to address local issues, but also to generate new practices that include the socially disadvantaged and excluded. In this way, provision will meet the growing needs of public health, which increasingly addresses softer notions of quality of life, emotional well-being and performance.

References

Ahamed, Y., Macdonald, H., Reed, K., Naylor, P-J., Liu-Ambrose, T. and McKay, H. (2007) School-based physical activity does not compromise children's academic performance. *Medicine and Science in Sports and Exercise*, 39: 371–376.

Aittasalo, M., Miilunpalom S., Stähl, T. and Kukkonen-Harjula, K. (2006) From innovation to practice; initiation, implementation and evaluation of a physician-based physical activity promotion programme in Finland. *Health Promotion International*, 22: 19–27.

Aldana, S.G., Merrill, R.M., Price, K., Hardy, A. and Hager, R. (2005) Financial impact of a comprehensive workplace health promotion program. *Preventive Medicine*, 40: 131–137.

Alexander, L.M., Inchley, J.T., Currie, D., Cooper, A.R. and Currie, C. (2005) The broader impact of walking to school among adolescents: Seven day accelerometry based study. *British Medical Journal*, 331: 1061–1062.

Andersen, L.B., Schnohr, P., Schroll, M. and Hein, H.O. (2000) All-cause mortality associated with physical activity during leisure-time, work, sports, and cycling to work. *Archives of Internal Medicine*, 160: 1621–1628.

Armstrong, N. and Welsman, J.R. (2007) Physical activity patterns of European youth with reference to methods of assessment. *Sports Medicine*, 36: 1067–1086.

Baecke, J.A., Burema, J. and Frijters, J.E. (1982) A short questionnaire for the measurement of habitual physical activity in epidemiological studies. *American Journal of Clinical Nutrition*, 36: 936–942.

Biddle, S.J.H. (2007) Sedentary behaviour. *American Journal of Preventive Medicine*, 33: 502–504.

Blank, L., Grimsley, E., Ellis, E. and Peters, J. (2007) Community-based lifestyle interventions: Changing behaviour and improving health. *Journal of Public Health*, 29: 236–245.

Booth, F., Gordon, S., Carlson, C. and Hamilton, M. (2000) Waging war on modern chronic diseases: Primary prevention through exercise biology. *Journal of Applied Physiology*, 88: 774–787.

Bravata, D.M., Smith-Spangler, C., Sundaram, V., Gienger, A.L., Lin, N., Lewis, R., Stave, C.D., Olkin, I. and Sirard, J.R. (2007) Using pedometers to increase physical activity and improve health: A systematic review. *Journal of the American Medical Association*, 298: 2296–2304.

Bringolf-Isler, G., Mäder, U., Ruch, N., Sennhauser, F.H. and Fahrländer, C. SCARPLOL team. (2007) Personal and environmental factors associated with active commuting to school in Switzerland. *Preventive Medicine*, 46(1): 67–73.

Brouwer, C.A.J., Gietema, J.A., Kamps, W.A., de Vries, E.G.E. and Postma, A. (2007) Changes in body composition after childhood cancer treatment: Impact on future health status – A review. *Critical Reviews in Oncology/Haematology*, 63: 32–46.

Brown, W.J., Mummery, W.K., Eakin, E.G. and Schofield, G. (2006) 10,000 Steps Rockhampton: Evaluation of a whole community approach to improving population levels of physical activity. *Journal of Physical Activity and Health*, 1: 1–14.

Cavill, N., Kahlmeier, S. and Racioppi, F. (Eds) (2006) *Physical Activity and HEALTH in Europe*. WHO, Geneva.

Chartered Management Institute (2007) *Healthy Workplace, Healthy Workforce; A Guide for Managers*. Chartered Management Institute, London.

Christakis, N.A. and Fowler, J.H. (2006) The spread of obesity in a large social network over 32 years. *New England Journal of Medicine*, 357: 370–379.

Cooper, A.R., Bo Anderson, L., Wedderkopp, N., Page, A.S. and Froberg, K. (2005) Physical activity levels of children who walk, cycle, or are driven to school. *American Journal of Preventive Medicine*, 29: 179–184.

Cooper, A.R., Page, A.S., Foster, L.J. and Qahwaji, D. (2003) Commuting to school: Are children who walk more physically active? *American Journal of Preventive Medicine*, 25: 273–276.

Coulson, J., McKenna, J. and Field, M. (in press) Exercise at work and work performance. *International Journal of Workplace Health Management*.

Craig, C.L., Tudor-Locke, C. and Bauman, A. (2007) Twelve-month effects of Canada on the Move: A population-wide campaign to promote pedometer use and walking. *Health Education Research*, 22: 406–413.

Darker, C.D., Larkin, M. and French, D.P. (2007) An exploration of walking behaviour – An interpretive phenomenological approach. *Social Science and Medicine*, 65: 2172–2183.

De Cocker, K.A., Boureaudhuij, I.M., Brown, W.J. and Cardon, G.M. (2007) Effects of '10000 Steps Ghent': A whole community intervention. *American Journal of Preventive Medicine*, 33: 455–463.

Department of Health (2004) *At Least Five a Week. Evidence on the Impact of Physical Activity and its Relationship to Health*. A Report from the Chief Medical Officer. Department of Health, London.

Department of Transport (2004) *National Travel Survey, 2004*. Department of Transport, London

Dickens, C.M., McGowan, L., Percival, C., Douglas, J., Tomenson, B., Cotter, L., Heagerty, A. and Creed, F.H. (2004) Lack of a close confidant, but not depression, predicts further cardiac events after myocardial infarction. *Heart*, 90: 518–522.

Douglas, F., van Teijlingen, E., Torrance, N., Fearn, P., Kerr, A. and Meloni, S. (2006) Promoting physical activity in primary care settings: Health visitors' and practice nurses' views and experiences. *Journal of Advanced Nursing*, 55: 159–168.

Dugdill, L., Brettle, A., Hulme, C., McCluskey, S. and Long, A.F. (2007) Intervention guidance on workplace health promotion with reference to physical activity and what works in motivating and changing employees' health behaviour. Systematic Review for the National Institute of Health and Clinical Excellence, University of Salford, Salford.

Eakin, E., Brown, W., Schofield, G., Mummery, K. and Reeves, M. (2007) General Practitioner advice on physical activity – who gets it? *American Journal of Health Promotion*, 21: 225–228.

Elley, C.R., Kerse, N.M. and Arroll, B. (2003) Effectiveness of counselling patients on physical activity in general practice: Cluster randomised controlled trial. *British Medical Journal*, 326: 793–798.

Elmer, P.J., Obarzanek, E., Vollmer, W.M., Simons-Morton, D., Stevens, V.J., Young, D.R., Lin, P-H., Champagne, C., Harsha, D.W., Svetkey, L.P., Ard, J., Brantley, P.J., Proschan, M.A., Erlinger, T.P. and Appel, L.J. for the PREMIER Collaborative Research

Group (2006) Effects of comprehensive lifestyle modification on diet, weight physical fitness and blood pressure control: 18-month results of a randomized trail. *Annals of Internal Medicine*, 144: 485–495.

Eng, P.M., Rimm, E.B., Fitzmaurice, G. and Kawachi, I. (2002) Social ties and changes in social ties in relation to subsequent total and cause-specific mortality and coronary heart disease in men. *American Journal of Epidemiology*, 155: 700–709.

Gilson, N., McKenna, J. and Cooke, C. (2007) Walking towards wellbeing and productivity: A randomised controlled trial in university employees. *Preventive Medicine*, 44: 167–169.

Gilson, N., McKenna, J. and Cooke, C. (2008) Experiences of route and task-based walking in a university community: Qualitative perspectives in a randomised control trial. *Journal of Physical Activity and Health*, 5(1): 172–178.

Graham, R.C., Dugdill, L. and Cable, N.T. (2005) Health professionals' perspectives in exercise referral: Implications for the referral process. *Ergonomics*, 48: 1411–1422.

Gulati, M., Dilip, M.S., Pandey, K., Arnsdorf, D.K., Lauderdale, M.F., Thisted, D.S., Wicklund, R.H., Al-Hani, A.J. and Black, H.R. (2003) The St James Women Take Heart Project. *Circulation*, 108: 1554–1559.

Hambrecht, R., Walther, C., Möbius-Winkler, S. and Hambrecht, R. (2004) Percutaneous coronary angioplasty compared with exercise training in patients with stable coronary artery disease: A randomized trial. *Circulation*, 109: 1371–1378.

Hamer, M. and Chidi, Y. (2007) Active commuting and cardiovascular risk; A meta analytic review. *Preventive Medicine*, 46(1): 9–13.

Haskell, W.L., Lee, I.M., Pate, R.R., Powell, K.E., Brassington, S.N., Bliwise, D. and Haskell, W. (2007) Physical activity and public health. Updated recommendation for adults from the American College of Sports Medicine and the American Heart Association. *Circulation*, 116, 1081–1093.

Hillman, M., Adams, J. and Whitelegg, J. (1991) *One False Move: A Study of Children's Independent Mobility*. Policy Studies Institute, London.

Hillsdon, M., Thorogood, M. and White, I. (2002) Advising people to take more exercise is ineffective: A randomised controlled trial of physical activity promotion in primary care. *International Journal of Epidemiology*, 31: 8–15.

Jimmy, G. and Martin, B.W. (2004) Implementation and effectiveness of a primary care based physical activity counselling scheme. *Patient Education and Counseling*, 56: 323–331.

Kelder, S., Hoelscher, D. M., Barroso, C.S., Walker, J.L., Cribb, P. and Hu, S. (2005) The CATCH Kids Club: A pilot after-school study for improving elementary students' nutrition and physical activity. *Public Health Nutrition*, 8: 133–140.

Khaw, K.T., Wareham, N., Bingham, S., Welch, A., Luben, R. and Day, N. (2008) Combined impact of health behaviours and mortality in men and women: The EPIC-Norfolk Prospective Population Study. *PLoS Med,* 5(1): e12.

Knols, R., Aaronson, N.K., Uebelhart, D., Fransen, J. and Aufdemkampe, G. (2005) Physical exercise in cancer patients during and after medical treatment: A systematic review of randomized and controlled clinical trials. *Journal of Clinical Oncology*, 23: 3830–3842.

Knowler, W.C., Barrett-Connor, E., Fowler, S.E., Hamman, R.F., Lachin, J.M., Walker, E.A. and Nathan, D.M. (2002) Reduction in the incidence of type 2 diabetes with lifestyle intervention or metformin. *New England Journal of Medicine*, 346: 393–403.

Kruger, J., Galuska, D.A., Serdula, M.K. and Kohl, H.W. (2005) Physical activity profiles of US adults trying to lose weight. *Medicine and Science in Sport and Exercise*, 37: 364–368.

Ku, P.-W., McKenna, J., Fox, K.R. and Hong, L.-Y. (2006) Prevalence of leisure-time physical activity in Taiwanese adults: Results of four national surveys, 2000–2004. *Preventive Medicine*, 43: 454–457.

Ku, P.-W., McKenna, J. and Fox, K.F. (2007) Physical activity and ageing well in Taiwan. *Journal of Ageing and Physical Activity*, 15: 382–397.

Kuriyama, S., Hozawa, A., Ohmori, K., Suzuki, Y., Nishino, Y., Fujita, K., Tsubono, Y. and Tsuji, I. (2004) Joint impact of health risks on health care charges; 7-year follow-up of National Health Insurance beneficiaries in Japan (the Ohsaki Study). *Preventive Medicine*, 39: 1194–1199.

Laaksonen, D.E., Lindstrom, J., Lakka, T.A., Eriksson, J.G., Niskanen, L., Wikstrom, K. Aunola, S., Keinänen-Kiukaanniemi, S., Laakso, M., Valle, T.T., Ilanne-Parikka, P., Louheranta, A., Hämäläinen, H., Rastas, M., Salminen, V., Cepaitis, Z., Hakumäki, M., Kaikkonen, H., Härkönen, P., Sundvall, J., Tuomilehto, J. and Uusitupa, M., for the Finnish Diabetes Prevention Study Group (2005) Physical activity in the prevention of type 2 diabetes. The Finnish Diabetes Prevention Study. *Diabetes*, 54: 158–165.

Lanningham-Foster, L.M., Jensen, T.B., McCrady, S.K., Nyse, L.J., Foster, R.C. and Levine, J.A. (2005) Laboratory measurement of posture allocation and physical activity in children. *Medicine and Science in Sports and Exercise*, 37: 1800–1805.

Levine, J.A. and Miller, J.M. (2007) The energy expenditure of using a 'walk-and-work' desk for office workers with obesity. *British Journal of Sports Medicine*, 41: 558–561.

Lindström, J., Ilanne-Parikka, P., Peltonen, M., Aunola, S., Eriksson, J.G., Hemiö, K. Hämäläinen, H., Härkönen, P., Keinänen-Kiukaanniemi, S., Laakso, M., Louheranta, A., Mannelin, M., Paturi, M., Sundvall, J., Valle, T.T., Uusitupa, M., Tuomilehto, J., on behalf of the Finnish Diabetes Prevention Study Group (2006) Sustained reduction in the incidence of type 2 diabetes by lifestyle intervention: Follow-up of the Finnish Diabetes Prevention Study. *Lancet*, 368: 1673–1679.

Luepker, R.V., Perry, C.L., McKinlay, S.M., Nader, P.R., Parcel, G.S., Stone, E.J., Webber, L.S., Elder, J.P., Feldman, H.A. and Johnson, C.C. (1996) Outcomes of a field trial to improve children's dietary patterns and physical activity. The Child and Adolescent Trial for Cardiovascular Health. CATCH collaborative group. *Journal of the American Medical Association*, 275: 768–776.

Ma, J., Urizar, G.G., Alehegn, T. and Stafford, R.S. (2004) Diet and physical activity counseling during ambulatory care visits in the United States. *Preventive Medicine*, 39: 815–822.

Mark, D.B. and Lauer, M.S. (2003) Exercise capacity: The prognostic variable that doesn't get enough respect. *Circulation*, 108: 1534–1536.

McKenna, J. and Bennett, C. (2005) Physical activity behaviour during preparation for public examinations. *Journal of Sports Sciences*, 24: 1262.

McKenna, J. and Coulson, J. (2005) How does exercising at work influence work performance? A randomised cross-over trial. *Medicine and Science in Sports and Exercise*, 37(5): S323.

McKenna, J. and Thew, M. (2008) Getting the balance right: Managing work-home conflict. In: *Lifestyle Management in Health and Social Care* (Eds M. Thew and J. McKenna), pp. 57–84, Blackwell, Chichester.

McKenna, J. and Vernon, M. (2004) How GPs promote lifestyle activity. *Patient Education & Counseling*, 54: 101–106.

Merom, D., Tudor-Locke, C., Bauman, A. and Rissel, C. (2006) Active commuting to school among NSW primary school children: Implications for public health. *Health and Place*, 12: 678–687.

Ming Wen, L. and Rissel, C. (2007) Inverse associations between cycling to work, public transport, and overweight and obesity; Findings from a population based study in Australia. *Preventive Medicine*, 46(1): 29–32.

Morrato, E.H., Hill, J.O., Wyatt, H.R., Ghushchyan, V. and Sullivan, P.W. (2006) Are health care professionals advising patients with diabetes or at risk of developing diabetes to exercise more? *Diabetes Care*, 29: 543–548.

Morris, J.N., Clayton, D.G., Everitt, M.G., Semmence, A.M. and Burgess, E.H. (1990) Exercise in leisure time: Coronary attack and death rates. *British Heart Journal*, 63: 325–334.

Murtagh, E.M., Boreham, C.A.G. and Murphy, P.H. (2002) Speed and exercise intensity of recreational walkers. *Preventive Medicine*, 35: 397–400.

Myers, J., Prakesh, M., Froelicher, V., Do, D., Partington, S. and Atwood, J.E. (2002) Exercise capacity and mortality among men referred for exercise testing. *New England Journal of Medicine*, 346: 793–801.

Nelson, M.E., Rejeski, W.J., Blair, S.N., Duncan, P.W., Judge, J.O., King, A.C., Macera, C.A. and Castaneda-Sceppa, C. (2007) Physical activity and public health in older adults. *Circulation*, 116 (9): 1094–1105.

Netz, Y., Becker, B.J., Tenenbaum, G. and Wu, M.-J. (2005) Physical activity and psychological well-being in advanced age: A meta-analysis of intervention studies. *Psychology and Aging*, 20: 272–284.

New Deal for Communities (2006) Research Report 17: An Interim Evaluation. Office of the Deputy Prime Minister, CRESR, Sheffield Hallam University.

Oaten, M. and Cheng, K. (2006) Longitudinal gains in self-regulation from regular physical exercise. *British Journal of Health Psychology*, 11: 717–733.

O'Donovan, G. and Shave, R. (2007). British adults' views on the health benefits of moderate and vigorous activity. *Preventive Medicine*, 45: 432–435.

Ohmori-Matsuda, K., Kuriyama, S., Hozawa, A., Nakaya, N., Shimazu, T. and Tsuji, I. (2007) The joint impact of cardiovascular risk factors upon medical costs. *Preventive Medicine*, 44: 349–355.

Ortega-Sanchez, R., Jimenez-Mena, C. and Cordoba-Garcia, R. (2004) The effect of office-based physician's advice on adolescent exercise behaviour. *Preventive Medicine*, 38: 219–226.

Pabayo, R., O'Loughlin, J., Gauvin, L., Paradis, G. and Gray-Donald, K. (2006) Effect of a ban on extracurricular sport activities by secondary school teachers on physical activity levels of adolescents: A multilevel analysis. *Health Education and Behaviour*, 33: 690–702.

Pabayo, R. and Gauvin, L. (2007) Proportions of students who use various modes of transport to and from school in a representative population-based sample of children and adolescents. *Preventive Medicine*, 46(1), 63–66.

Puig Ribera, A., McKenna, J. and Riddoch, C. (2006a) Attitudes and practices of physicians and nurses regarding physical activity promotion in the Catalan primary health care system. *European Journal of Public Health*, 15: 569–575.

Puig Ribera, A., McKenna, J. and Riddoch, C. (2006b) Physical activity promotion in general practices of Barcelona: A case study. *Health Education Research*, 21, 538–548.

Riddoch, C.J., Mattocks, C., Deere, K. Saunders, J., Kirkby, J., Tilling, K., Leary, S.D., Blair, S.N. and Ness, A.R. (2007) Objective measurement of levels and patterns of physical activity. *Archives of Disease in Childhood*, 92: 963–969.

Sallis, J.F., McKenzie, T.L., Alcaraz, J.E., Kolody, B., Faucette, N. and Hovell, M.F. (1998) The effects of a 2-year physical education program (SPARK) on physical activity and fitness in elementary school students. Sports, Play and Active Recreation for Kids. *American Journal of Public Health*, 87: 1328–1334.

Sevick, M.A., Napolitano, M.A., Papandonatos, G.D., Gordon, A.J., Reiser, L.M. and Marcus, B.H. (2007) Cost-effectiveness of alternative approaches for motivating activity in sedentary adults: Result of project STRRIDE. *Preventive Medicine*, 45: 54–61.

Sirard, J.R., Riner, J.R., McIver, K.L. and Pate, R.P. (2005a) Physical activity and active commuting to elementary school. *Medicine and Science in Sport and Exercise*, 37: 2062–2069.

Sirard, J.R., Ainsworth, B.E., McIver, K.L. and Pate, R.R. (2005b) Prevalence of active commuting at urban and suburban elementary schools in Columbia, SC. *American Journal of Public Health*, 95: 236–237.

Sjöströem, M., Oja, P., Hagströmer, M., Smith, B. and Bauman, A. (2002) Health-enhancing physical activity across European Union countries: The Eurobarometer study. *Journal of Public Health*, 14: 291–300.

Slentz, C.A., Aitken, L.B., Houmard, J.A., Bales, C.W., Johnson, J.L., Tanner, C.J., McCartney, J.S., Duscha, B.D. and Kraus, W.E. (2005) Inactivity, exercise and visceral fat. STRRIDE: A randomized controlled study of exercise intensity and amount. *Journal of Applied Physiology*, 99: 1613–1618.

Smith, A., McKenna, J. and Radley, D. (2007). The impact of regular active commuting to school on achieving 60 minutes of physical activity on weekdays in children. *Journal of Sports Sciences*, 25: S23–S24.

Stähl, T., Rütten, A., Nutbeam, D., Bauman, A., Kannas, L., Abel, T., Lüschen, G., Rodriquez, D.J.A., Vinck, J. and van der Zee, J. (2001) The importance of the social environment for physically active lifestyle – Results from an international study. *Social Science and Medicine*, 52: 1–10.

Stamatakis, E., Ekelund, U. and Wareham, N.J. (2007) Temporal trends in physical activity in England: The Health Survey for England 1991 to 2004. *Preventive Medicine*, 45: 416–423.

Stevens, W., Hillsdon, M., Thorogood, M. and McArdle, D. (1998) Cost effectiveness of a primary care based physical activity intervention in 45–74 year old men and women: A randomized controlled trial. *British Journal of Sports Medicine*, 32: 236–241.

Stevinson, C., Faught, W., Steed, H., Tonkin, K., Ladha, A.B., Vallance, J.K., Capstick, V., Schepansky, A. and Courneya, K.S. (2007) Associations between physical activity and quality of life in ovarian cancer survivors. *Gynaecologic Oncology*, 106: 244–250.

Sullivan, M. (2003) The new subjective medicine; taking the patient's point of view on health and health care. *Social Science and Medicine*, 56: 1595–1604.

Svetkey, L.P., Harsha, D.W., Vollmer, W.M., Stevens, V.J., Obarzanek, E., Elmer, P.J., Lin, P-H., Champagne, C., Simons-Morton, D-G., Aickin, M., Proschan, M.A. and Appel, L.J. (2003) PREMIER: A clinical trial of comprehensive lifestyle modification for blood pressure control: Rationale, design and baseline characteristics. *Annals of Epidemiology*, 13: 462–471.

Thompson, W.G., Foster, R., Eide, D. and Levine, J.A. (2007) Feasibility of a walking work-station to increase daily walking. *British Journal of Sports Medicine*, 42: 225–228.

Tudor-Locke, C., Neff, L.J., Ainsworth, B.E., Addy, C.L. and Popkin, B.M. (2002) Omission of active commuting to school and the prevalence of children's health-related physical activity levels: The Russian longitudinal monitoring study. *Child: Care, Health and Development*, 28: 507–512.

UNICEF (2007) Child poverty in perspective: An overview of child well-being in rich countries. Innocenti Report Card 7, UNICEF Innocenti Research Centre, Florence.

van Sluijs, E.M.F., McMinn, A.M. and Griffin, S.J. (2007) Effectiveness of interventions to promote physical activity in children and adolescents: Systematic review of con-trolled trials. *British Medical Journal*, 335: 703–713.

van Vegchel, N., de Jonge, J., Bosma, H. and Schauefeli, W. (2005) Reviewing the effort-reward imbalance model; drawing up the balance of 45 empirical studies. *Social Science and Medicine*, 60: 1117–1131.

Vuori, I.M., Oja, P. and Paronen, O. (1994) Physically active commuting to work – Testing its potential for exercise promotion. *Medicine and Science in Sports and Exercise*, 26: 844–850.

Wagner, A., Simon, C., Ducimetiere, P., Montaye, M., Bongard, V., Yarnell, J., Bingham, A., Hedelin, G., Amouyel, P., Ferrières, J., Evans, A. and Arveiler, D. (2001) Leisure-time physical activity and regular walking or cycling to work are associated with adiposity and 5-year weight gain in middle-aged men: The PRIME Study. *International Journal of Obesity*, 25: 940–948.

Whitelaw, S., Baxendale, A., Bryce, C., MacHardy, L., Young, I. and Witney, E. (2001) 'Settings' based health promotion; A review. *Health Promotion International*, 16: 339–352.

WHO (World Health Organisation) (2003) WHO global strategy on diet, physical activity and health. Western Pacific regional consultation meeting report. WHO, Geneva.

WHO (World Health Organisation) (2004) *Global Strategy on Diet, Physical Activity and Health.* WHO, Geneva.

Wofford, T.S., Greenlund, K.J., Croft, J.B. and Labarthe, D.R. (2007) Diet and physical activity of U.S. adults with heart disease following preventive advice. *Preventive Medicine*, 45(4): 295–301.

Zheng, Y. (2008) The benefit of public transport: Physical activity to reduce obesity and ecological footprint. *Preventive Medicine*, 46(1): 4–5.

12 The way forward for physical activity and health promotion: designing interventions for the future

Andy Smith with a case study from Sara Moore

Introduction

The purpose of this chapter is to challenge those with a professional and/or academic interest in promoting health-enhancing physical activity, to reach beyond their comfort zone and to think about the future. In doing this there is a danger that the author will lead the reader into speculations that are not supported by the evidence. However, it is felt that this is a risk worth taking to enable this chapter to:

1. Confront some public health dilemmas, e.g. the challenges and opportunities presented by an ageing population (see Chapter 9), yet not lose faith in the benefit of physical activity [this approach is shaped by the work of Collins (2001)].
2. Apply Schwartz's (2003) concept of 'inevitable surprises' in relation to physical activity. Schwartz's basic idea is that leaders should extrapolate from existing trends and data to identify what in the future will be surprises for others. The potential for physical activity to improve mental well-being as well as physical health (see Chapter 10) may, for example, lead to radically new ways of thinking about physical activity in the future.
3. React positively to Greenfield (2004), who has argued persuasively that what will be strange about the near future is not just the awesome technology that will have developed but also that people themselves will have changed. These insights may help us to reflect further on the work in Chapter 8 and on the type of world the children of today will live in within the coming decades.

Guided by these three approaches, this chapter will (i) comment on the content of the preceding chapters in this book, (ii) provide recommendations for the design of evidence-based interventions and (iii) discuss skills that exercise and health professionals need to develop. Nonetheless, the reader should beware that this chapter sets out to provoke and to stimulate new ways of thinking about the promotion of physical activity. Therefore, what follows should be read critically and its contents contested and challenged.

Reaching consensus?

Arguably consensus is over-rated as progress in science comes from challenging, problematising and contesting. Nonetheless, when consensus emerges from the data and as a result of mature reflection by experts in the field, it can be a powerful tool for shaping professional practice and government policy. Whilst readers are encouraged to draw their own conclusions based on what they have just read in the last 11 chapters, my observations are as follows:

1. As the content as this book demonstrates, exercise science has left the laboratory and, using a range of scholarly traditions (see Chapter 1), has developed insights into health-enhancing behaviour that can guide government policy (see Chapter 3). Health-enhancing physical activity can now be studied and applied in a range of settings including primary health care (see Chapter 5), the community (see Chapter 6) and the workplace (see Chapter 7).
2. This book illustrates that whilst the biomedical model still has relevance for some clinical contexts and disease-focused research, a health promotion model informed by scholarship from the humanities can inform interventions to help more people become more active.
3. As the preceding chapter by Jim McKenna demonstrates, this book also illustrates that the promotion of health enhancing physical activity is a global issue. Therefore, work is needed both to import best practise from around the world and export the lessons learned in the UK. This book is part of that process.

Reaching creditability

Anecdotal evidence and the experience of the author lead him to conclude that some medical doctors and scientists do not think that physical activity is a credible health intervention. Of course, this might not be your experience, and as my evidence is anecdotal, my conclusion that exercise science and health promoters lack creditability in the eyes of some decision makers and health professionals is open to challenge. Nonetheless, I am confident that some readers will agree with me that the promotion of physical activity can be seen as a Cinderella health intervention in some geographical areas and organisations.

In many ways the scepticism of some of those we encounter as we go about our work is to be applauded and used as motivation to conduct more robust research and to develop better professional practice. Indeed, one response is to point out how much sport and exercise science has done to develop its research profile (Smith, 2002).

If one accepts my position that exercise science and health promoters lack creditability in the eyes of some (and I hope that not all readers do or I will have failed in my aim to be provocative), then one has to ask why. It is only by understanding why this may be the case that we can do something about it. Perhaps it is because of the false dichotomy that appears to be held by some people that anything that is physical cannot also be important and or intellectually sound, and vice versa. Alternatively, it may be because physical activity/exercise is linked in some people's minds with education (through physical education) and sport (through training and coaching) rather than to health and well-being.

Irrespective of your position on the perceived creditability, or otherwise, of exercise and health professionals, many would agree on the importance of identifying and developing the skills required to either gain, maintain or enhance the credibility of our profession. Unfortunately, such a consensus begs the question, what skills are required and how might they be developed? Table 12.1 is an attempt to take this debate forward and should not be seen as definitive.

Reaching further

Arguably we are more successful at getting those who do most exercise to do even more, rather than getting those who do least to do a little bit more. Despite policies and frameworks [e.g. the Exercise Referral Systems: National Quality Assurance Framework (Department of Health, 2001) – see also Chapter 3] that encourage us to promote exercise to those who are socially excluded, those who are rich and empowered are still more likely to exercise than the poor and excluded. However, recently a number of interventions have been developed that reach further and out to those who are least likely to live healthy lives (many of the case studies in this book are fine examples; see Chapters 5–10). Another impressive example is HM Prisons Exercise Referral Programme, discussed by its director, Sara Moore, in the case study below.

Case study: HMPS Exercise Referral Programme

(By Sara Moore: National Programme Lead for Public Health and Physical Activity and Offender Health in the Department of Health.)

Outline of project: The Government White Paper 'Choosing Health' provided a number of opportunities to improve the health of people in prison one of which was Exercise Referral. Offender Health and the HM Prison Service jointly developed a Prison Exercise Referral programme. This started in February 2005 as a pilot involving four prisons. The programme rapidly expanded with a total of 45 prisons currently involved.

Evaluation outcomes: An evaluation of the scheme (conducted by Andy Smith) found:

1. This exercise referral scheme 'recruits' participants from a population (prisoners) that arguable are more likely to be socially excluded then one would expect from some other scheme set, e.g., in a middle-class communities. The scheme targets a population (prisoners) with significant health inequalities and is focused on this health need not exercise for its own sake.
2. Interviews with the prison officers demonstrated that they were motivated by the scheme and enthusiastic about the work.
3. 93% of the prisoners who responded to the survey ($n = 44$) enjoyed the programme.
4. 32% of the prisoners who responded to the survey instrument reported that they had their medication changed over the course of the exercise intervention.
5. 61% of the prisoners completing the survey found the advice given by the PE staff extremely helpful and 36% found it very helpful.
6. Most of the surveyed prisoners found out about the scheme from other prisoners (27%) other sources included the prison's GP (11%) and PE staff (18%). This emphasises the importance of peer education and multidisciplinary support for the programme.

Qualitative findings from the research included:

Question: 'What do you enjoy most about the programme?'

Prisoner: 'The interest and care of the Gym Instructors making sure we are doing the right exercise, also about me I enjoy every minute of the whole exercise because I'm feeling 100% better in myself'.

Application to practice: The scheme is innovative and probably the first of its kind in the world. In the examples of the types of environments in which exercise referrals might be seen listed in the National Quality Assurance Framework (NQAFD, p. 15), no mention is made of schemes based in prisons, highlighting the pioneering nature of this work. The key reasons for the success of the programme were:

■ Key stakeholder involvement including a number of governors who championed the scheme and other staff, especially health and PE, prepared to work in new and innovative ways.
■ The early involvement of a university to provide a staff training programme for prison physical training instructors.
■ Identifying barriers to success and tackling them creatively.
■ Linking the scheme into other prison health initiatives including 'Walk your way to Health'.
■ Being creative in a challenging environment where participants have significant health inequalities.

Table 12.1 Skills required to promote physical activity and how they might be developed.

Skills required to promote physical activity	Justification	How to develop the skill
'Graduate-ness'	With a government target that 50% of the population should attend University it is hard to argue against the position that every profession should be founded on a degree	Complete an honours degree which would preferably be in exercise, health or sport-related area. The subject area is not as essential as acquiring a higher education.
Understanding of exercise science	Smith (2004, p. 8) argued that exercise science 'is a theory based, research led discipline that seeks applied solutions to health problems related to physical inactivity and which seeks to understand and promote individual and public health and well being through evidence based physical activity interventions.' If those promoting physical activity want to do adopt evidence-based practice it is within this discipline that the relevant research is located.	Read, study and apply the research from exercise science published in peer-reviewed journals.
Empathy	Ross (1977) argued that people tend to have a general bias to over-emphasise dispositional explanations (e.g. their own effort and ability) for their own behaviour at the expense of situational explanations (e.g. environmental factors that effect the difficulty of the task). When applied to physical activity (Smith and Biddle, 1991), this might mean that there is a danger that those who exercise see themselves as putting a lot of effort into doing so and label those who are sedentary as 'lazy'. Clearly if you are responsible for designing and implementing interventions to promote physical activity it is important that these are informed by the evidence and address environmental factors (see e.g. Smith, 2003) and care is taken to manage any unintended attribution error.	Spend time listening to people who are sedentary so that you understand their story. It is also important to explore and understand the environment in which any intervention will be implemented. Listening, looking and understanding other people and where they live is a skill best developed by repeated practice and there is no substitute for spending time in the field.

(Continued)

Table 12.1 (Continued).

Skills required to promote physical activity	Justification	How to develop the skill
'Stickability' to life long learning and continuous professional development	As research and professional practice is developing rapidly, remaining current is both essential and challenging.	Value and reward yourself for completing continuing professional development (CPD) activities and where possible gain professional accreditation and qualifications by doing so.
Motivational skills	Most exercise scientists will need to apply motivational skills at some point in their career. If you can not help people become more active, you are unlikely to reach the top of the profession unless you are doing 'blue sky' or theoretical research.	Study as much psychology as possible and become a people watcher.
Networking skills	Somewhere someone knows something you do not about promoting physical activity. If you have good networking skills you are more likely find out what this is.	Take every opportunity to listen and talk to the widest range of people possible. Never sit next to the same person in a meeting twice and always spend more time listening to those you disagree with then talking to those who share your views.
Humility	If we knew how to get those who do the least amount of physical activity to do more we would not be faced by our current challenge and there would be no need for this book.	Find examples of self styled exercise and fitness gurus and ask yourself the question, are they role models you want to follow?

To develop other programmes that reach further (like this case study) practitioners need to:

■ Share examples of good practice globally. A challenge to overcome in this regard is the dependency of much exercise science and health promotion on the English language and perhaps a tendency to look for examples of best practice only from North America and Western Europe. Readers are directed to Chapter 11 for more thoughts on the international dimension of promoting physical activity.
■ Work with communities so far rarely touched by physical activity interventions, for example seafarers, travellers and the homeless.

Reaching to intervene with interventions

In this section, I synthesise current thinking on how to intervene, but more controversially, propose that we stop intervening in the traditional sense and embrace a bottom-up approach.

A contemporary model of interventions

Readers looking for a recent review of the evidence underpinning physical activity interventions targeting a range of populations are directed to a special edition of the *Journal of Sports Sciences* on Exercise Science and Health enhancing Physical Activity edited by the author (Volume 22, Number 8, August 2004, ISSN 0264–0414) as well as Part II of this book. Partly based on my reflections on that material and my experience as an accredited exercise scientist, I propose in Figure 12.1 a contemporary model to guide physical activity interventions.
In this I propose that:

1. In designing any intervention the starting point should be the evidence. This means ensuring that time is allocated to reading and understanding what the research tells us including those findings which we may find uncomfortable or inconvenient. Embedded within many chapters of this book, readers will find evidence that they can use and will find Chapter 4 particularly helpful.
2. Whilst most models that seek to shape health interventions prioritise evidence, they are strangely quiet about the importance of creativity. Evidence by itself will not design an intervention – that calls for a human mind. Whilst computers are good at processing and analysing lots of data, it still takes a human mind to be creative and think out of the box. It therefore surprises me that many people appear to believe that interventions can be designed in

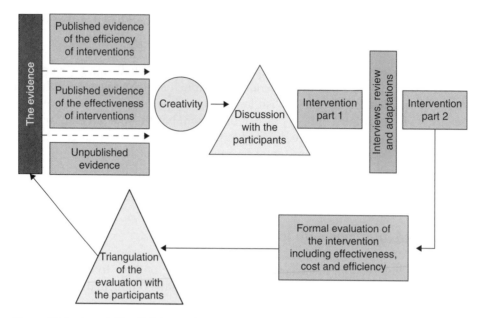

Figure 12.1   A model for PA intervention.

meetings or at a desk in an office. Are these really places that promote creativity? Perhaps we should practice what we preach and, after reading the evidence, design interventions whilst walking in the countryside or on the beach. As the neuroscientist Chris Frith (2007) observed, 'we even seem to be better at making complex decisions without conscious thought'.

3. The golden rule of interventions should be that before intervening the content of the programme must be discussed with those who will be the participants in the intervention. If the intervention is with a large population or a whole community, then a representative sample should be asked their views on the intervention before it is applied. Not to do so is at best rude and at worst unethical. The participants are the experts in what will, and what will not, help them become physically active. It surprises me that conventional wisdom highlights the importance of getting feedback from participants in the evaluation at the end of the intervention but less emphasis appears to be placed on talking to people in the design stage and pre-intervention. That is why this model proposes that you talk to the participants first.

4. The intervention can then be applied but this should be done in two stages allowing for a mid-point review and possible restructuring. Too often evaluations are conducted when it is too late to do anything with the results. If participants in the intervention think things could be improved, give them the opportunity to tell you in time to do something about it.

5. After the intervention not only should a formal evaluation be conducted that (i) asks if the programme achieved what it set out to and (ii) seeks to explore the experience of those on the intervention, but the results should be fed back to the participants to see if they recognise what has been written about and concluded regarding the intervention.

All those designing interventions should read the National Institute for Health and Clinical Excellence (NICE) guidance in this area first issued in March 2006. This considers brief interventions in primary care, exercise referral schemes, pedometers and community-based exercise programmes for walking and cycling. As others in this book have noted, these guidelines have their critics, but they should be understood to help gain a rounded perspective of physical activity interventions within the community.

To understand how complex it is to intervene to promote physical activity, and why the material in Part II of this book is so important, think about it this way. At the time of writing the UK population is about 60 million. Every one of these people have their own attitudes toward physical activity, which in turn are influenced and shaped by those around them. These attitudes are framed in a culture of societal norms toward physical activity and health. In turn these individual cognitions and community perceptions toward physical activity are facilitated or hindered by a range of factors including technologies, transport infrastructure and working hours. Given the pace of modern change, these variables may alter faster than researchers can publish the results of their studies. Participants in a health intervention to promote physical activity will spend more time away from the programme than on it or influenced by it. Away from the intervention they will be 'subjected' to the views of friends and family and the media on physical activity and struggle with the pressures to be active when confronted by a transport system dominated by machines rather then human locomotion. They will also be tempted to recreate in a seated position by exciting and often educational and socially interactive computer games and TV programmes. In my effort to understand how we might intervene in a meaningful way in such a complex situation I have become drawn to what Johnson (2001) termed 'the unknown science of self-organisation' (p. 18). In his fascinating and highly readable book Emergence he explores systems that 'solve problems by drawing on masses of relatively stupid elements, rather than a single, intelligent executive branch. They are bottom-up systems, not top down. They get their smarts from below … . They are complex adaptive systems that display emergent behaviour' (p. 18). Rather than think in terms of professionals intervening, perhaps we should be considering ways to get people active that grow upward from the grass roots. These organic methods of increasing physical activity levels will need nurturing and supporting by professionals rather than designing, implementing and evaluating. At the time of writing I am still unpacking the implications of emergence theory for the promotion of physical activity and fear this work may take a decade or more. Therefore, at this point I only feel confident enough to tentatively suggest two practical examples of what this might mean. The first is that to effectively promote physical activity, the best strategy might be to find patterns of activity that have spontaneously emerged in a community and try and reinforce and sustain them. For example, in the village I live in, the children have claimed a small piece of ground and turned it into a cycle circuit. Rather than intervene with a top-down idea perhaps it would be best to help them develop this further by including, for example, a skateboard park on the same site. The second example is promoting physical activity on the back of concerns about climate change. Rather than trying to create new attitudes about the relationship between physical activity and health, perhaps it would be more effective to promote active commuting in relation to the emerging awareness about an individual's carbon footprint. After all, the heart still gets the benefit of a brisk cycle whether the motivation be health gain or concerns about climate change. I do not claim that this second example represents an original thought on my part as it has occurred to many others and we already see this type of intervention. However, what might be new is applying emergence theory to better understand how this opportunity might be maximised.

In thinking about how we might intervene with our interventions we might also want to fundamentally reconsider what we are trying to achieve. Perhaps our definition of health is too narrow, and instead of evaluating the effectiveness of physical activity interventions in relation to, for example, reducing coronary heart disease risk factors, we should be changing our priority to focus on well-being. Instead of, or as well as, trying to prevent and treat disease, practitioners should be using physical activity to improve the quality of life of the disease free. Our focus could be on fun, enjoyment, happiness and development. Those seeking to understand and develop their thinking and professional practice in this area are encouraged to read Haworth and Hart (2007).

Reaching into the future

Thinking about the future should not be the sole preserve of Science Fiction writers although authors such as Iain M. Banks (2004; see, e.g., his book *The Algebraist*) have much to teach us about thinking beyond our preoccupation with the present. There are examples of eminent scholars (e.g. Jung, 1959) thinking in a way that gives encouragement to those who want to break the mould.

Regrettably one can create a rather pessimistic vision of the future shaped by bird flu, nuclear proliferation and terrorism (Rees, 2003). Whilst accepting that societies can collapse (Diamond, 2005), I am optimistic about our ability to muddle through and with the earth's regenerative capacities. I therefore believe that there will be a future and one worth living in, where helping people be physically activity will be an important public health issue. There will of course be major challenges and arguably the most difficult of these will be climate change. Here is not the place to review the scientific literature on climate change, but the prudent reader would be advised to do so perhaps by using Houghton (2004) as a starting point. What is worth noting is that in the future the world's climate is going to change and most places will be hotter, a few will be colder and some will be flooded. It is reasonable to assume that the physical recreation profile of a number of regions around the globe will change. In some places people will need more advice on how to exercise in hot environments and in others, traditional sports; for example skiing will no longer be available. In those areas subject to flooding it is hard to envisage those whose homes are under water will be inclined to embrace the new opportunities for water sports. However, over time things will change just as they have over millenniums of human history and people will play where their ancestors used to toil.

Whilst the author is optimistic about the future, he agrees with Greenfield (2004) that it will be a lot stranger than most people currently imagine. It is reasonable to assume that some dramatic changes may happen in the next 50 years that will be more revolutionary than the invention of powered flight, the internal combustion engine and the personal computer. If as a profession we do not attempt to predict and shape these changes, then an argument can be made that, at best, we are failing in our duty of care to prepare for future practice and, at worst, lack creativity, imagination and foresight. As a profession we should be sensitised to how technological changes can impact on human behaviour and experience. How many readers do not think that the car and the television have effected how people physically recreate or would not concede that the Industrial Revolution has shaped almost every aspect of human behaviour and experience? Yet my impression is that when we talk about these issues at conferences and in meetings it is as if technological development has ended with the silicon chip. Surely this is shortsighted and we should be asking what are going to be the future technological developments to impact on how we live our lives. In Table 12.2 I justify my statement that in the next 50 years there will be inventions more revolutionary then powered flight, the internal combustion engine and the personal computer and attempt to predict what this will mean for physical activity.

Table 12.2 Predicted scientific and technological development impacting on physical activity.

Predicted scientific and technological development in the next 50 years	Justification for prediction	Implication for the promotion of physical activity
Post and/or enhanced human evolution will begin.	Many serious scientists predict a future in which human evolution is speeded up by either genetic modification or via human-machine interfaces. Miah (2004) is perhaps the best exponent of these predictions in relation to sport.	In the future how will sports administrators be able to create a level playing field if some people are 'naturals' and others 'enhanced'? If it is possible to artificially enhance fitness, why exercise?
Nanotechnology revolutionises medical science and health care.	As Rees (2003) and others have argued, advances in nanotechnology may enable the development of miniature machines that will help both diagnose and treat illness from within the body.	If in the future medicine can fix illnesses that in the past had to be prevented by lifestyle interventions including coronary heart disease and obesity, why bother changing your behaviour? Effort, motivation and dedication may no longer be required in a world with a technological solution for almost everything.
Artificial intelligence is developed and it becomes possible to envisage non-human consciousness?	Greenfield (2004) makes a powerful case that the future is going to be a lot stranger then we think it will be. Arguably the strangest advances will the development of artificial intelligence and perhaps even self aware computers. If you think this is impossible, think how quickly computers have progressed over the last 50 years	What would it be like if your best friend was a machine? Perhaps it would mean that when you socialised you would be inactive. How wonderful would virtual reality spaces created by artificial intelligences and self-aware machines be? Would playing in these new landscapes be more exciting, interesting and developing then playing sports developed in Victorian England?

One of the reasons that I am positive about the future is that I believe that technological developments will liberate many of us from our desks and cars. Miniaturisation of hardware, increased sophistication of software and increased bandwidth will improve communication and the ability to work when and where we want to. Personally I look forward to writing and sending papers whilst riding my bike in an Alpine landscape created by virtual reality one day and through the Gobi desert the next. My fear is that whilst I may have this exciting future to look forward to that millions in the developing world will be locked into poverty, starvation, thirst and illiteracy which, to be frank, makes our work to promote health-enhancing physical activity in the West seem unimportant. That is why work such as that being conducted by Davies Banda using sport as a vehicle for HIV education in Africa is so important. In this, Banda and colleagues are using basketball and other sports as a vehicle to educate young people in the developing world about how to avoid infection by HIV.

Conclusion

Conclusions are dangerous things and none more so than short paragraphs that finish not only a chapter but also an edited book. Endings risk being written with a sense of authority that implies that nothing else can be said on the matter and that the author knows better than the reader. Clearly, there is a lot more to be said about both the determinants of physical activity and how to intervene to help people become more active. However, we hope that this book will help ensure that future dialogue is informed by evidence from a wider range of professional, theoretical and disciplinary perspectives than has sometimes been the case in the past. Finally, it is important to stress this book should make you think and draw your own conclusions. Irrespective of whether or not you agree with the positions we have adopted, we hope that this book will help you be part of the solution to the problem of physical inactivity.

References

Banks, I.M. (2004) *The Algebraist*. Orbit, London.

Collins, J. (2001) *Good to Great*. Harper Business, New York.

Department of Health (2001) *Exercise Referral Systems: A National Quality Assurance Framework*. The Stationery Office, London.

Diamond, J. (2005) *Collapse: How Societies Choose to Fail or Survive*. Penguin, London.

Frith, C. (2007) Hands up if you think you've got Free Will. *New Scientist*, 195(2616): 46–47.

Greenfield, S. (2004) *Tomorrow's People*. Penguin Books, London.

Haworth, J. and Hart, G. (Eds.) (2007) *Well-being: Individual, Community and Social Perspectives*. Palgrave McMillan, Basingstoke.

Houghton, J. (2004) *Global Warming: The Complete Briefing*. Cambridge University Press, Cambridge.

Johnson, J. (2001) *Emergence.* Penguin, London.

Jung, C. (1959) *Flying Saucers*. Routledge, London.

Miah, A. (2004) *Genetically Modified Athletes: Biomedical Ethics, Gene Doping and Sport*, Routledge, London.

Rees, M. (2003) *Our Final Century: Will Civilisation Survive the Twenty-First Century?* Arrow Books, London.

Ross, L. (1977) The intuitive psychologist and his shortcomings: Distortions in the attribution process. In: *Advances in Experimental Social Psychology* (Ed. L. Berkowitz), pp. 173–229. Academic Press, New York.

Schwartz, P. (2003) *Inevitable Surprises*. Free Press, London.

Smith, R.A. and Biddle, S.J.H. (1991) *Exercise Adherence an Attributional Perspective. VIII European Congress of Sport Psychology*. Cologne, Germany.

Smith, A. (2002) *RAE Results: Britain Is Now the Home of Sport and Exercise Science*. Bases World, Leeds.

Smith, A. (2003) Environmental determinism: How space and community can create movement. Abstract Book of the *8th Annual Congresss European Colleges of Sport Science*. Salzburg, Austria.

Smith, A. (2004) What is Exercise Science? *Journal of Hospitality, Leisure, Sport and Tourism Education*, 3(2): 5–14.

Index